Health Care Information Systems

Health Care Information Systems

A Practical Approach for Health Care Management

Fourth Edition

Karen A. Wager

Frances Wickham Lee

John P. Glaser

JB JOSSEY-BASS™

A Wiley Brand

Cover design by Wiley

Published by Jossey-Bass
A Wiley Brand
One Montgomery Street, Suite 1000, San Francisco, CA 94104-4594—www.josseybass.com

Jossey-Bass books and products are available through most bookstores. To contact Jossey-Bass directly call our Customer Care Department within the U.S. at 800-956-7739, outside the U.S. at 317-572-3986, or fax 317-572-4002.

Wiley publishes in a variety of print and electronic formats and by print-on-demand. Some material included with standard print versions of this book may not be included in e-books or in print-on-demand. If this book refers to media such as a CD or DVD that is not included in the version you purchased, you may download this material at http://booksupport.wiley.com. For more information about Wiley products, visit www.wiley.com.

Library of Congress Cataloging-in-Publication Data
Library of Congress Cataloging-in-Publication Data has been applied for and is on file with the Library of Congress.

9781119337188 (paperback)
9781119337126 (ePDF)
9781119337089 (ePub)

Printed in the United States of America

FOURTH EDITION
PB Printing   10 9 8 7 6 5 4 3 2 1

Contents

Appendixes

Tables, Figures, and Exhibits

TABLES

FIGURES

EXHIBITS

In memory of our colleague Andy Pasternack

Preface

Health care delivery is in the early stages of a profound shift in its core strategies, organization, financing, and operational and care processes.

Reactive sick care is being replaced by proactive efforts to keep people well and out of the hospital. Fragmented care delivery capabilities are being supplanted by initiatives to create and manage cross-continuum systems of care. Providers that were rewarded for volume are increasingly being rewarded for quality and efficiency.

New forms of reimbursement, such as bundles and various types of capitation, are causing this shift. To thrive in the new era of health care delivery, providers are creating health systems, such as accountable care organizations, that include venues along the care spectrum.

In addition providers are introducing new processes to support the need to manage care between encounters, keep people healthy, and ensure that utilization is appropriate. Moreover, as reimbursement shifts to incent-improved provider performance these organizations will have a common need to optimize operational efficiency, improve financial management, and effectively engage consumers in managing their health and care.

These changes in business models and processes follow on the heels of the extraordinary increase in electronic health record adoption spurred by the Meaningful Use program of the US federal government.

On top of a foundation of electronic health records, the industry will add population health management applications, systems that support extensive patient engagement, broader interoperability, and more significant use of analytics. Providers involved in patient care will need immediate access to electronic decision-support tools, the latest relevant research findings on a given topic, and patient-specific reminders and alerts. Health care executives will need to be able to devise strategic initiatives that take advantage of access to real-time, relevant administrative and clinical information.

In parallel with the changes in health care, information technology (IT) innovation continues at a remarkable pace. The Internet of Things is creating a reality of intelligent homes, cars, and equipment, such as environmental sensors and devices attached to patients. Social media use continues to grow and become more sophisticated and capable. Mobile personal devices have become the device of choice for personal and professional activities. Big data has exceptional potential to help identify new diagnostic and therapeutic algorithms, conduct most market surveillance, and assess the comparative effectiveness of treatments.

For providers to prosper in this new era they must be very effective in developing IT strategies, implementing the technology, and leveraging the technology to improve organizational performance. They must understand the nature of health care data and the challenges of privacy and security. Clinicians and managers must appreciate the breadth of health care IT and emerging health care IT trends.

The transformation of the health care industry means that IT is no longer a necessary back-office evil—it is an essential foundation if an organization is to survive. That has not been true in the past; provider organizations could do quite well in a fee-for-service world without computerized physician order entry and other advanced IT applications.

Having ready access to timely, complete, accurate, legible, and relevant information is critical to health care organizations, providers, and the patients they serve. Whether it is a nurse administering medication to a comatose patient, a physician advising a patient on the latest research findings for a specific cancer treatment, a billing clerk filing an electronic claim, a chief executive officer justifying to the board the need for building a new emergency department, or a health policy analyst reporting on the cost-effectiveness of a new prevention program to the state's Medicaid program, each individual needs access to high-quality information with which to effectively perform his or her job.

The need for quality information in health care, already strong, has never been greater, particularly as this sector of our society strives to provide quality care, contain costs, and ensure adequate access.

PURPOSE OF THIS BOOK

The purpose of this book is to prepare future health care executives with the knowledge and skills they need to manage information and information systems technology effectively in this new environment. We wrote this book with the graduate student (or upper-level undergraduate student) enrolled in a health care management program in mind.

Our definition of health care management is fairly broad and includes a range of academic programs from health administration, health information management, and public health programs to master of business administration (MBA) programs with an emphasis in health to nursing administration and physician executive educational programs. This book may also serve as an introductory text in health informatics programs.

The first (2005), second (2009), and third (2013) editions have been widely used by a variety of health care management and health information systems programs throughout the United States and abroad. Although we have maintained the majority of the chapters from the third edition, this edition has gone through significant changes in composition and structure reflecting feedback from educators and students and the need to discuss topics such as population health and recent changes in payment reform initiatives. We have removed the section on the international perspective on health care information technology and updated the case studies of organizations experiencing management-related information system challenges. We also added a new chapter on the role of information systems in managing population health.

ORGANIZATION OF THIS BOOK

The chapters in this book are organized into four major parts:

- Part One: "Major Environmental Forces That Shape the National Health Information System Landscape" (Chapters One through Four)
- Part Two: "Selection, Implementation, Evaluation, and Management of Health Care Information Systems" (Chapters Five through Eight)
- Part Three: "Laws, Regulations, and Standards That Affect Health Care Information Systems" (Chapters Nine through Eleven)
- Part Four: "Senior-Level Management Issues Related to Health Care Information Systems Management" (Chapters Twelve through Fourteen)

In addition Appendix A provides an overview of the health care IT industry. Appendix B provides a compendium of a sample project charter, sample job descriptions, and a sample user satisfaction survey.

The purpose of Part One ("Major Environmental Forces That Shape the National Health Information System Landscape") is to provide the reader with the foundation needed for the rest of the book. This foundation includes an overview of the major environmental forces that are shaping the national health IT landscape, such as Medicare's alternative payment programs. The reader will gain insight into the different types of clinical, administrative, and external data used by health care provider organizations. Additionally, the reader will gain an understanding of the adoption, use, and functionality of health care information systems with focus on electronic health records (EHRs), personal health records (PHRs), and systems need to support population health management (e.g., data analytics, telehealth).

Specifically Part One has four chapters:

- *Chapter One: National Health Information Technology Landscape.* This chapter discusses the various forces and activities that are shaping health information systems nationally. The chapter reviews the HITECH Act, the Affordable Care Act, HIPAA, and national efforts to advance interoperability.

- *Chapter Two: Health Care Data.* This chapter examines the range of health care data and issues with data quality and capture. This examination is conducted from a cross-continuum, health system perspective.

- *Chapter Three: Health Care Information Systems.* This chapter provides an overview of clinical and administrative information systems. The chapter focuses on the electronic health record and personal health record and describes in greater detail the major initiatives that have led to current adoption and use of EHRs by hospitals and physician practices (e.g., Meaningful Use and health information exchanges). The chapter also includes discussion on the state of EHRs in settings across the care continuum (e.g., behavioral health, community care, long-term care). It concludes with a discussion on important health care information system issues including interoperability, usability, and health IT safety.

- *Chapter Four: Information Systems to Support Population Health Management.* This is a new chapter. Its purpose is to focus on the key data and information needs of health systems to effectively manage population health. Key topics include population health, telehealth, patient engagement (including social media), data analytics, and health information exchange (HIE).

The purpose of Part Two ("Selection, Implementation, Evaluation, and Management of Health Care Information Systems") is to provide the reader with an overview of what is needed to effectively select, implement, evaluate, and manage health care information systems. This section discusses issues mid- and senior-level managers are likely to encounter related to managing change and managing projects. The reader will also gain insight into the role and functions of the IT organization or department.

Specifically Part Two has four chapters:

- *Chapter Five: System Acquisition.* This chapter discusses the processes that organizations use to select information systems. We have included a discussion on the importance of system architecture.

- *Chapter Six: System Implementation and Support.* This chapter reviews the processes and activities need to implement and support health care information systems. We have included an examination of change management and project management.

- *Chapter Seven: Assessing and Achieving Value in Health Care Information Systems.* This chapter discusses the nature of the value that can be obtained from health care information systems and the approaches to achieving that value.

- *Chapter Eight: Organizing Information Technology Services.* This chapter reviews the structure and responsibilities of the IT organization. This chapter discusses IT senior management roles such as the chief information officer and the chief medical information officer.

The purpose of Part Three ("Laws, Regulations, and Standards That Affect Health Care Information Systems") is to provide the reader with an overview of the laws, regulations, and standards that affect health care information systems. Emphasis is given to system security.

Specifically Part Three has three chapters:

- *Chapter Nine: Privacy and Security.* This chapter examines privacy and security regulations and practices.

- *Chapter Ten: Performance Standards and Measures.* This chapter discusses the wide range of regulations that affect health care information systems, with an emphasis on new regulations related to the focus on the continuum of care.

- *Chapter Eleven: Health Care Information Systems Standards.* This chapter reviews the new and emerging standards that govern health care data, transactions, and quality measures.

The purpose of Part Four ("Senior-Level Management Issues Related to Health Care Information Systems Management") is to provide the reader with an understanding of senior-level management responsibilities and activities related to IT management.

Specifically Part Four has three chapters:

- *Chapter Twelve: IT Alignment and Strategic Planning.* This chapter discusses the processes used by organizations to develop an IT strategic plan. The chapter reviews the challenges faced in developing these plans.
- *Chapter Thirteen: IT Governance and Management.* This chapter discusses several topics that must be addressed by senior leadership if IT is to be leveraged effectively: establishing IT governance, developing the IT budget, and ensuring that projects are successful.
- *Chapter Fourteen: Health IT Leadership Case Studies.* This chapter comprises case studies that provide real-world situations that touch on the content of this textbook.

Each chapter in the book (except Chapter Fourteen) begins with a set of chapter learning objectives and an overview and concludes with a summary of the material presented and a set of learning activities. These activities are designed to give students an opportunity to explore more fully the concepts introduced in the chapter and to gain hands-on experience by visiting and talking with IT and management professionals in a variety of health care settings.

Two appendixes offer supplemental information. Appendix A presents an overview of the health care IT industry: the companies that provide IT hardware, software, and a wide range of services to health care organizations. Appendix B contains a sample project charter, sample job descriptions, and a sample user satisfaction survey: documents referenced throughout the book.

Depending on the nature and interests of the students, various chapters are worth emphasizing. Students and courses that are targeted for current or aspiring senior executive positions may want to emphasize Chapter One (National Health Care IT Landscape), Chapter Four (Population Health), Chapter Seven (IT Value), Chapter Twelve (IT Strategy), and Chapter Thirteen (IT Governance and Management). For classes focused on mid-level management, Chapter One (National Health Care IT Landscape), Chapter Five (System Selection), Chapter Six (System Implementation), and Chapter Seven (IT Value) will merit attention.

Regardless of role, Chapter Two (Health Care Data), Chapter Three (Health Care Information Systems), Chapter Eight (IT Organization), and Part Three (Laws, Regulations, and Standards) provide important foundational knowledge.

One final comment. Two terms, *health information technology (HIT)* and *health care information systems (HCIS),* are frequently used throughout the text. Although it may seem that these terms are interchangeable, they are, in fact, related but different. As used in this text, HIT encompasses the technologies (hardware, software, networks, etc.) used in the management of health information. HCIS describes a broader concept that not only encompasses HIT but also the processes and people that the HIT must support. HCIS delivers value to individual health care organizations, patients, and providers, as well as across the continuum of care and for entire communities of individuals. HIT delivers little value on its own. Both HCIS and HIT must be managed, but the management of HCIS is significantly more difficult and diverse.

Health care and health care information technology are in the early stages of a profound transformation. We hope you find this textbook helpful as we prepare our students for the challenges that lie ahead.

Acknowledgments

We wish to extend a special thanks to Juli Wilt for her dedication and assistance in preparing the final manuscript for this book. We also wish to thank the following MUSC students in the doctoral program in health administration, who contributed information systems management stories and experiences to us for use as case studies: Penney Burlingame, Barbara Chelton, Stuart Fine, David Freed, David Gehant, Patricia Givens, Shirley Harkey, Victoria Harkins, Randall Jones, Michael Moran, Catrin Jones-Nazar, Ronald Kintz, Lauren Lent, George Mikatarian, Lorie Shoemaker, and Gary Wilde.

To all of our students whom we have learned from over the years, we thank you.

Finally, we wish to extend a very special thanks to Molly Shane Grasso for her many contributions to Chapter Four, "Information Systems to Support Population Health Management."

The Authors

Karen A. Wager is professor and associate dean for student affairs in the College of Health Professions at the Medical University of South Carolina (MUSC), where she teaches management and health information systems courses to graduate students. She has more than thirty years of professional and academic experience in the health information management profession and has published numerous articles, case studies, and book chapters. Recognized for her excellence in interprofessional education and in bringing practical research to the classroom, Wager received the 2016 College Teacher of the Year award and the 2008 MUSC outstanding teaching award in the educator-lecturer category and the 2008 Governor's Distinguished Professor Award. She currently serves as the chair of the Accreditation Council for the Commission on Accreditation of Healthcare Management Education (CAHME), is a member of the CAHME board of directors, and is a past fellow of CAHME. Wager previously served as a member of the HIMSS-AUPHA-CAHME Task Force responsible for the development of a model curriculum in health information systems appropriate for educating graduate students in health administration programs. She is past president of the South Carolina chapter of the Healthcare Information and Management Systems Society (HIMSS) and past president of the South Carolina Health Information Management Association. Wager holds a doctor of business administration (DBA) degree with an emphasis in information systems from the University of Sarasota.

Frances Wickham Lee is professor and director of instructional operations for Healthcare Simulation South Carolina at the Medical University of South Carolina (MUSC). She recently joined the faculty at Walden University to teach in the Master of Healthcare Administration program. Lee has more than thirty years of professional and academic experience in the health information management, including publication of numerous articles and book chapters related to the field. She is past president of the North Carolina Health Information Management Association and South Carolina chapter of the Healthcare Information and Management Systems Society (HIMSS). Since 2007, Lee has broadened her expertise as a health care educator through her membership in a pioneering team charged with bringing health care simulation to students and practicing professionals across the state of South Carolina. She holds a DBA degree with an emphasis in information systems from the University of Sarasota.

John P. Glaser currently serves as the senior vice president of population health for Cerner. He joined Cerner in 2015 as part of the Siemens Health Services acquisition, where he was CEO. Prior to Siemens, Glaser was vice president and CIO at Partners HealthCare. He also previously served as vice president of information systems at Brigham and Women's Hospital.

Glaser was the founding chair of the College of Healthcare Information Management Executives (CHIME) and the past president of the Healthcare Information and Management Systems Society (HIMSS). He has served on numerous boards including eHealth Initiative, the American Telemedicine Association (ATA), and the American Medical Informatics Association (AMIA). He is a fellow of CHIME, HIMSS, and the American College of Health Informatics. He is a former senior advisor to the Office of the National Coordinator for Health Information Technology (ONC).

Glaser has published more than two hundred articles, three books on the strategic application of information technology in health care. Glaser holds a PhD in health care information systems from the University of Minnesota.

Health Care Information Systems

PART ONE

Major Environmental Forces That Shape the National Health Information System Landscape

CHAPTER 1

The National Health Information Technology Landscape

LEARNING OBJECTIVES

- To be able to discuss some of the most significant influences shaping the current and future health information technology landscapes in the United States.
- To understand the roles national private sector and government initiatives have played in the advancement of health information technology in the United States.
- To be able to describe major events since the 1990s that have influenced the adoption of health information technologies and systems.

Since the early 1990s, the use of **health information technology (HIT)** across all aspects of the US health care delivery system has been increasing. **Electronic health records (EHRs),** telehealth, social media, mobile applications, and so on are becoming the norm—even commonplace—today. Today's health care providers and organizations across the continuum of care have come to depend on reliable HIT to aid in managing population health effectively while reducing costs and improving quality patient care. Chapter One will explore some of the most significant influences shaping the current and future HIT landscapes in the United States. Certainly, advances in information technology affect HIT development, but national private sector and government initiatives have played key roles in the adoption and application of the technologies in health care. This chapter will provide a chronological overview of the significant government and private sector actions that have directly or indirectly affected the adoption of HIT since the Institute of Medicine landmark report, *The Computer-Based Patient Record: An Essential Technology for Health Care,* authored by Dick and Steen and published in 1991. Knowledge of these initiatives and mandates shaping the current HIT national landscape provides the background for understanding the importance of the health information systems that are used to promote excellent, cost-effective patient care.

1990s: THE CALL FOR HIT

Institute of Medicine CPR Report

The Institute of Medicine (IOM) report *The Computer-Based Patient Record: An Essential Technology for Health Care* (Dick & Steen, 1991) brought international attention to the numerous problems inherent in paper-based medical records and called for the adoption of the **computer-based patient record (CPR)** as the standard by the year 2001. The IOM defined the CPR as "an electronic patient record that resides in a system specifically designed to support users by providing accessibility to complete and accurate data, alerts, reminders, clinical decision support systems, links to medical knowledge, and other aids" (Dick & Steen, 1991, p. 11). This vision of a patient's record offered far more than an electronic version of existing paper records—the IOM report viewed the CPR as a tool to assist the clinician in caring for the patient by providing him or her with reminders, alerts, clinical decision–support capabilities, and access to the latest research findings on a particular diagnosis or treatment modality. CPR systems and related applications, such as EHRs, will be further discussed in Chapter Three. At this point, it is important to understand the IOM report's impact on the vendor community and health care organizations. Leading vendors and health care organizations saw this report as an impetus toward radically changing the ways in which patient information would be managed and patient care delivered. During the 1990s, a number of vendors developed CPR systems. However, despite the fact that these systems were, for the most part, reliable and technically mature by the end of the decade, only 10 percent of hospitals and less than 15 percent of physician practices had implemented them (Goldsmith, 2003). Needless to say, the IOM goal of widespread CPR adoption by 2001 was not met. The report alone was not enough to entice organizations and individual providers to commit to the required investment of resources to make the switch from predominantly paper records.

Health Insurance Portability and Accountability Act (HIPAA)

Five years after the IOM report advocating CPRs was published, President Clinton signed into law the **Health Insurance Portability and Accountability Act (HIPAA)** of 1996 (which is discussed in detail in Chapter Nine). HIPAA was designed primarily to make health insurance more affordable and accessible, but it included important provisions to simplify administrative processes and to protect the security and confidentiality of personal health information. HIPAA was part of a larger health care reform effort and a federal interest in HIT for purposes beyond reimbursement. HIPAA also brought national attention to the issues surrounding the use of personal health information in electronic form. The Internet had revolutionized the way that consumers, providers, and health care organizations accessed health information, communicated with each other, and conducted business, creating new risks to patient privacy and security.

2000–2010: THE ARRIVAL OF HIT
IOM Patient Safety Reports

A second IOM report, *To Err Is Human: Building a Safer Health Care System* (Kohn, Corrigan, & Donaldson, 2000), brought national attention to research estimating that 44,000 to 98,000 patients die each year because of medical errors. A subsequent related report by the IOM Committee on Data Standards for Patient Safety, *Patient Safety: Achieving a New Standard for Care* (Aspden, 2004), called for health care organizations to adopt information technology capable of collecting and sharing essential health information on patients and their care. This IOM committee examined the status of standards, including standards for health data interchange, terminologies, and medical knowledge representation. Here is an example of the committee's conclusions:

- As concerns about **patient safety** have grown, the health care sector has looked to other industries that have confronted similar challenges, in particular, the airline industry. This industry learned long ago that information and clear communications are critical to the safe navigation of an airplane. To perform their jobs well and guide their plane safely to its destination, pilots must communicate with the airport controller concerning their destination and current circumstances (e.g., mechanical or other problems), their flight plan, and environmental factors (e.g., weather conditions) that could necessitate a change in course. Information must also pass seamlessly from one controller to another to ensure a safe and smooth journey for planes flying long distances, provide notification of airport delays or closures because of weather conditions, and enable rapid alert and response to extenuating circumstance, such as a terrorist attack.

- Information is as critical to the provision of safe health care—which is free of errors of commission and omission—as it is to the safe operation of aircraft. To develop a treatment plan, a doctor must have access to complete patient information (e.g., diagnoses, medications, current test results, and available social supports) and to the most current science base (Aspden, 2004).

Whereas *To Err Is Human* focused primarily on errors that occur in hospitals, the 2004 report examined the incidence of serious safety issues in other settings as well, including ambulatory care facilities and nursing homes. Its authors point out that earlier research on patient safety focused on errors of commission, such as prescribing a medication that has a potentially fatal interaction with another medication the patient is taking, and they argue that errors of omission are equally important. An example of an error of omission is failing to prescribe a medication from which the patient would likely have benefited (Institute of Medicine, Committee on Data Standards for Patient Safety, 2003). A significant contributing factor to the unacceptably high rate of medical errors reported in these two reports and many others is poor information management practices. Illegible prescriptions, unconfirmed verbal orders, unanswered telephone calls, and lost medical records could all place patients at risk.

Transparency and Patient Safety

The federal government also responded to quality of care concerns by promoting health care transparency (for example, making quality and price information available to consumers) and furthering the adoption of HIT. In 2003, the **Medicare Modernization Act** was passed, which expanded the program to include prescription drugs and mandated the use of electronic prescribing (**e-prescribing**) among health plans providing prescription drug coverage to Medicare beneficiaries. A year later (2004), President Bush called for the widespread adoption of EHR systems within the decade to improve efficiency, reduce medical errors, and improve quality of care. By 2006, he had issued an executive order directing federal agencies that administer or sponsor health insurance programs to make information about prices paid to health care providers for procedures and information on the quality of services provided by physicians, hospitals, and other health care providers publicly available. This executive order also encouraged adoption of HIT standards to facilitate the rapid exchange of health information (The White House, 2006).

During this period significant changes in reimbursement practices also materialized in an effort to address patient safety, health care quality, and cost concerns. Historically, health care providers and organizations had been paid for services rendered regardless of patient quality or outcome. Nearing the end of the decade, payment reform became a hot item. For example, **pay for performance (P4P)** or value-based purchasing pilot programs became more widespread. P4P reimburses providers based on meeting predefined quality measures and thus is intended to promote and reward quality. The **Centers for Medicare and Medicaid Services (CMS)** notified hospitals and physicians that future increases in payment would be linked to improvements in clinical performance. Medicare also announced it would no longer pay hospitals for the costs of treating certain conditions that could reasonably have been prevented—such as bedsores, injuries caused by falls, and infections resulting from the prolonged use of catheters in blood vessels or the bladder—or for treating "serious preventable" events—such as leaving a sponge or other object in a patient during surgery or providing the patient with incompatible blood or blood products. Private health plans also followed Medicare's lead and began denying payment for such mishaps. Providers began to recognize the importance of adopting improved HIT to collect and transmit the data needed under these payment reforms.

Office of the National Coordinator for Health Information Technology

In April 2004, President Bush signed Executive Order No. 13335, 3 C.F.R., establishing the **Office of the National Coordinator for Health Information Technology (ONC)** and charged the office with providing "leadership for the development and nationwide implementation of an interoperable health information technology infrastructure to improve the quality and efficiency of health care." In 2009, the role of the ONC (organizationally located within the US Department of Health and Human Services) was strengthened when the **Health Information Technology for Economic and Clinical Health (HITECH) Act** legislatively mandated it to provide leadership and oversight of the national efforts to support the adoption of EHRs and **health information exchange (HIE)** (ONC, 2015).

In spite of the various national initiatives and changes to reimbursement during the first decade of the twenty-first century, by the end of the decade only 25 percent of physician practices (Hsiao, Hing, Socey, & Cai, 2011) and 12 percent of hospitals (Jha, 2010) had implemented "basic" EHR systems. The far majority of solo and small physician practices continued to use paper-based medical record systems. Studies show that the relatively low adoption rates among solo and small physician practices were because of the cost of HIT and the misalignment of incentives (Jha et al., 2009). Patients, payers, and purchasers had the most to gain from physician use of EHR systems, yet it was the physician who was expected to bear the total cost. To address this misalignment of incentives issue, to provide health care organizations and providers with some funding for the adoption and **Meaningful Use of EHRs,** and to promote a national agenda for HIE, the HITECH Act was passed as a part of the **American Recovery and Reinvestment Act** in 2009.

2010–PRESENT: HEALTH CARE REFORM AND THE GROWTH OF HIT

HITECH and Meaningful Use

An important component of HITECH was the establishment of the Medicare and Medicaid EHR Incentive Programs. Eligible professionals and hospitals that adopt, implement, or upgrade to a certified EHR received incentive payments. After the first year of adoption, the providers had to prove successfully that they were "demonstrating Meaningful Use" of certified EHRs to receive additional incentive payments. The criteria, objectives, and measures for demonstrating Meaningful Use evolved over a five-year period from 2011 to 2016. The first stage of Meaningful Use criteria was implemented in 2011–2012 and focused on data capturing and sharing. Stage 2 (2014) criteria are intended to advance clinical processes, and Stage 3 (2016) criteria aim to show improved outcomes. Table 1.1 provides a broad overview of the Meaningful Use criteria by stage.

Through the Medicare EHR Incentive Program, each eligible professional who adopted and achieved meaningful EHR use in 2011 or 2012 was able to earn up to $44,000 over a five-year period. The amount decreased over the period, creating incentives to providers to start sooner rather than later.

Table 1.1 Stages of Meaningful Use

Stage 1: Meaningful Use criteria focus	Stage 2: Meaningful Use criteria focus	Stage 3: Meaningful Use criteria focus
Electronically capturing health information in a standardized format	More rigorous HIE	Improving quality, safety, and efficiency leading to improved health outcomes
Using that information to track key clinical conditions	Increased requirements for e-prescribing and incorporating lab results	Decision support for national high-priority conditions
Communicating that information for care coordination processes	Electronic transmission of patient summaries across multiple settings	Patient access to self-management tools
Initiating the reporting of clinical quality measures and public health information	More patient-controlled data	Access to comprehensive patient data through patient-centered HIE
Using information to engage patients and their families in their care		Improving population health

Source: ONC (n.d.a.).

Eligible hospitals could earn over $2 million through the Medicare EHR Incentive Program, and the Medicaid program made available up to $63,500 for each eligible professional (through 2021) and over $2 million to each eligible hospital. As of December 2015, more than 482,000 health care providers received a total of over $31 billion in payments for participating in the Medicare and Medicaid EHR Incentive Programs (CMS, n.d.). See Table 1.2 for primary differences between the two incentive programs.

Within the ONC, the Office of Interoperability and Standards oversees certification programs for HIT. The purpose of certification is to provide assurance to EHR purchasers and other users that their EHR system has the technological capability, functionality, and security needed to assist them in meeting Meaningful Use criteria. Eligible providers who apply for the EHR Medicare and Medicaid Incentive Programs are required to use certified EHR technology. The ONC has authorized certain organizations to perform the actual testing and certification of EHR systems.

Other HITECH Programs

Many small physician practices and rural hospitals do not have the in-house expertise to select, implement, and support EHR systems that meet certification standards. To address these needs, HITECH funded sixty-two **regional extension centers (RECs)** throughout the nation to support providers in adopting and becoming meaningful users of EHRs. The RECs are primarily intended to provide advice and technical assistance to primary care providers, especially those in small practices, and to small rural hospitals, which often do not have information technology (IT) expertise. Furthermore, HITECH provided funding for various workforce training programs to support the education of HIT professionals. The education-based programs included curriculum development, community college consortia, competency examination, and university-based training programs, with the overarching goal of training an additional forty-five thousand HIT professionals. Funding was also made available to seventeen **Beacon communities** and **Strategic Health IT Advanced Research Projects (SHARP)** across the nation. The Beacon programs are leading organizations that are demonstrating how HIT can be used in innovative ways to target specific health problems within communities (HealthIT.gov, 2012). These programs are illustrating HIT's role in improving individual and population health outcomes and in overcoming barriers such as **coordination of care,** which plagues our nation's health care system (McKethan et al., 2011).

Achieving Meaningful Use requires that health care providers are able to share health information electronically with others using a secure network for HIE. To this end, HITECH provided state grants to help build the HIE

Table 1.2 Differences between Medicare and Medicaid EHR incentive programs

Medicare EHR Incentive Program	Medicaid EHR Incentive Program
Federally implemented and available nationally	Implemented voluntarily by states
Medicare Advantage professionals have special eligibility accommodations.	Medicaid managed care professionals must meet regular eligibility requirements.
Open to physicians, subsection (d) hospitals, and critical access hospitals	Open to five types of professionals and three types of hospitals
Same definition of Meaningful Use applied to all participants nationally	States can adopt a more rigorous definition of Meaningful Use.
Must demonstrate Meaningful Use in first year	Adopt, implement, or upgrade option in first year
Maximum incentive for eligible professionals is $44,000; 10 percent for HPSA (health professional shortage area).	Maximum incentive for eligible professionals is $63,750.
2014 is the last year in which a professional can initiate participation.	2016 is the last year in which a professional can initiate participation.
Payments over five years	Payments over six years
In 2015 fee reductions (penalties) begin for those who do not demonstrate Meaningful Use of a certified HER.	No fee reductions (penalties)
2016 is the last incentive payment year.	2021 is the last incentive payment year.
No Medicare patient population minimum is required.	Eligible professionals must have a 30 percent Medicaid population (20 percent for pediatricians) to participate; this must be demonstrated annually.

Source: Carson, Garr, Goforth, and Forkner (2010).

infrastructure for exchange of electronic health information among providers and between providers and consumers. Nearly all states have approved strategic and operational plans for moving forward with implementation of their HIE cooperative agreement programs.

Affordable Care Act

In addition to the increased efforts to promote HIT through legislated programs, the early 2010s brought dramatic change to the health care sector as a whole with the passage of significant health care reform legislation. Americans have grappled for decades with some type of "health care reform" in an attempt to achieve the simultaneous "triple aims" for the US health care delivery system:

- Improve the patient experience of care
- Improve the health of populations
- Reduce per capita cost of health care (IHI, n.d.)

Full achievement of these aims has been challenging within a health care delivery system managed by different stakeholders—payers, providers, and patients—whose goals are frequently not well aligned. The latest attempt at reform occurred in 2010, when President Obama signed into law the Patient Protection and Affordable Care Act (PPACA), now known as the **Affordable Care Act (ACA).**

Along with mandating that individuals have health insurance and expanding Medicaid programs, the ACA created the structure for health insurance exchanges, including a greater role for states, and imposed changes to private insurance, such as prohibiting health plans from placing lifetime limits on the dollar value of coverage and prohibiting preexisting condition exclusions. Numerous changes were to be made to the Medicare program, including continued reductions in Medicare payments to certain hospitals for hospital-acquired conditions and excessive preventable hospital readmissions. Additionally, the CMS established an innovation center to test, evaluate, and expand different payment structures and methodologies to reduce program expenditures while maintaining or improving quality of care. Through the innovation center and other means, CMS has been aggressively pursuing implementation of **value-based payment** methods and exploring the viability of alternative models of care and payment.

The final assessment of the success of ACA is still unknown; however, what is certain is that its various programs will rely heavily on quality HIT to achieve their goals. A greater emphasis than ever is placed on facilitating patient engagement in their own care through the use of technology. On the other end of the spectrum, new models of care and payment include improved health for populations as an explicit goal, requiring HIT to manage the sheer volume and complexity of data needed.

Value-Based Payment Programs

Shortly after the ACA was passed, CMS implemented several value-based payment programs in an effort to reward health care providers with incentive payments for the quality of care they provide to Medicare patients. In 2015, the **Medicare Access and CHIP Reauthorization Act (MACRA)** was signed into law. Among other things, MACRA outlines a timetable for the 2019 implementation of a **merit-based incentive payment system (MIPS)** that will replace other value-based payment programs, including the EHR Incentive Programs. MIPS will use a set of performance measures, divided into categories, to calculate a score (between 0 and 100) for eligible professionals. Each category of performance will be weighted as shown in Table 1.3.

Health care providers meeting the established threshold score will receive no adjustment to payment; those scoring below will receive a negative adjustment, and those above, a positive adjustment. Exceptional performers may receive bonus payments (CMS, n.d.).

Alternate Payment Methods

Providers who meet the criteria to provide an **alternate payment method (APM)** will receive bonus payments and will be exempt from the MIPS. Although there are likely to be other APMs identified over time, three types are receiving a great deal of attention currently: **accountable care organizations (ACOs), bundled payments,** and **patient-centered medical homes (PCMHs).** ACOs are "networks of . . . health care providers that share responsibility for coordinating care and meeting health care quality and cost metrics for a defined patient population" (Breakaway Policy Strategies for FasterCures, 2015, p. 2). Bundled payments aim to incentivize providers to improve care coordination, promote teamwork, and lower costs. Payers will compensate

Table 1.3 MIPS performance categories

Category	Weight (%)
Quality	50
Advancing care information	25
Clinical practice improvement activities	15
Resource use	10

providers with a single payment for an episode of care. PCMHs are APMs that are rooted in the private sector. In 2007, four physician societies published a joint statement of principles emphasizing a personal physician–led coordination of care. All of the APMs rely heavily on HIT. ACOs and PCMHs, in particular, require that HIT support the organization and its providers in the carrying out the following functions:

- Manage and coordinate integrated care.
- Identify, manage, and reduce or contain costs.
- Adhere to evidence-based practice guidelines and standards of care; ensure quality and safety.
- Manage population health.
- Engage patients and their families and caregivers in their own care.
- Report on quality outcomes.

HIT Interoperability Efforts

Despite efforts dating back to the first reports on the need for adoption of computerized patient records, complete interoperability among HIT systems, which is key to supporting an integrated health care delivery system that provides improved care to individuals and populations while managing costs, remains elusive. The federal government, along with other provider, vendor, and professional organizations, however, recognize this need for interoperability. The ONC defines interoperability as "the ability of a system to exchange electronic health information with and use electronic health information from other systems without special effort on the part of the user" (ONC, n.d.a). Interoperability among HIT encompasses far more than just connected EHRs across systems. Home health monitoring systems are becoming commonplace, telehealth is on the rise, and large public health databases exist at state and national levels. True interoperability will encompass any electronic sources with information needed to provide the best possible health care.

Some of the more notable efforts toward **HIT interoperability** include the efforts by the government under the direction of the ONC and several other national public and private organizations. In 2015, the ONC published "Connecting Health and Care for the Nation: A Shared **Nationwide Interoperability Roadmap**," a ten-year plan for achieving HIT interoperability in the United States. Figure 1.1 summarizes the key milestones identified in the ONC road map. The ultimate goal for 2024 is "a learning health system enabled by nationwide interoperability." The goal of the learning health system is to

Figure 1.1 Milestones for a supportive payment and regulatory environment

2015–2017	2018–2020	2021–2024
Send, receive, find, and use priority data domains to improve health and health care quality	Expand interoperable health IT and users to improve health and lower cost	A learning health system enabled by nationwide interoperability
A1.1 CMS will aim to administer 30% of all medicare payments to providers through alternative payment models that reward quality and value, and encourage interoperability, by the end of 2016.	A1.2 CMS will administer 50% of all Medicare payments to providers through alternative payment models that reward quality and value by the end of 2018.	A1.3 The federal government will use value-based payment models as the dominant mode of payment for providers.

Source: ONC (2015).

improve the health of individuals and populations by "generating information and knowledge from data captured and updated over time... and sharing and disseminating what is learned in timely and actionable forms that directly enable individuals, clinicians, and public health entities to... make informed decisions" (ONC, 2015, p. 18).

Health Level Seven International (HL7), a not-for-profit, **ANSI (American National Standards Institute)**–accredited, standards-developing organization, is focused on technical standards for HIE. The HL7 **Fast Healthcare Interoperability Resources (FHIR) standards** were introduced in 2012 and are under development to improve the exchange of EHR data. About this same time Healtheway, now **the Sequoia Project,** was chartered as a nonprofit organization to "advance the implementation of secure, interoperable nationwide health information exchange" (Sequoia Project, n.d.a). The Sequoia Project supports several initiatives, including the **eHealth Exchange,** a group of government and nongovernment organizations devoted to improving patient care through "interoperable health information exchange" (Sequoia Project, n.d.a). Unlike HL7, which focuses on technical standards, eHealth Exchange's primary focus is on the legal and policy barriers associated with nationwide interoperability. Another Sequoia initiative, Carequality, strives to connect private HIE networks. Another private endeavor, **Commonwell Health Alliance,** is a consortium of HIT vendors and other organizations that are committed to achieving interoperability. Commonwell began in 2013 with six EHR vendors. In 2015, their membership represented 70 percent of hospitals. Provider members of Commonwell register their patients in order to exchange easily information with other member providers (Jacob, 2015).

Although HIT has become commonplace across the continuum of care, seamless interoperability among the nation's HIT systems has not yet been realized. One author describes the movement toward HIT interoperability in the United States not as a straight path but rather as a jigsaw puzzle with multiple public and private organizations "working on different pieces"

(Jacob, 2015). Interoperability requires not only technical standards but also a national health information infrastructure, along with an effective governing system. Concerns about the misalignment of incentives for achieving interoperability remain. Most experts agree that technology is not the barrier to interoperability. Governance and alignment of agendas among disparate organizations are cited as the most daunting barriers. Because of its potential to affect seriously the progress of interoperability, in 2015, the ONC reported to Congress on the phenomenon of **health information blocking,** which is defined as occurring "when persons or entities knowingly and unreasonably interfere with the exchange or use of electronic health information" (ONC, 2015). The report charged that current economic incentives were not supportive of information exchange and that some of the current market practices actually discouraged sharing health information (DeSalvo & Daniel, 2015).

SUMMARY

Chapter One provides a brief chronological overview of the some of the most significant national drivers in the development, growth, and use of HIT in the United States. Since the 1990s and the publication of *The Computer-Based Patient Record: An Essential Technology for Health Care,* the national HIT landscape has certainly evolved, and it will continue to do so. Challenges to realizing an integrated national HIT infrastructure are numerous, but the need for one has never been greater. Recognizing that the technology is not the major barrier to the national infrastructure, the government, through legislation, CMS incentive programs, the ONC, and other programs, will continue to play a significant role in the Meaningful Use of HIT, pushing for the alignment of incentives within the health care delivery system.

In a 2016 speech, CMS acting chief Andy Slavitt summed up the government's role in achieving its HIT vision with the following statements:

> The focus will move away from rewarding providers for the use of technology and towards the outcome they achieve with their patients.
>
> Second, providers will be able to customize their goals so tech companies can build around the individual practice needs, not the needs of the government. Technology must be user-centered and support physicians, not distract them.
>
> Third, one way to aid this is by leveling the technology playing field for start-ups and new entrants. We are requiring open APIs... that allow apps, analytic tools, and connected technologies to get data in and out of an EHR securely.

We are deadly serious about interoperability. We will begin initiatives... pointing technology to fill critical use cases like closing referral loops and engaging a patient in their care.

Technology companies that look for ways to practice "data blocking" in opposition to new regulations will find that it won't be tolerated. (Nerney, 2016)

Many of the initiatives discussed in Chapter One will be explored more fully in subsequent chapters of this book. The purpose of Chapter One is to provide the reader with a snapshot of the national HIT landscape and enough historical background to set the stage for why health care managers and leaders must understand and actively engage in the implementation of effective health information systems to achieve better health for individuals and populations while managing costs.

KEY TERMS

Accountable Care Organizations (ACOs)

Affordable Care Act (ACA)

Alternate payment methods (APM)

American Recovery and Reinvestment Act

ANSI (American National Standards Institute)

Beacon communities

Bundled payments

Centers for Medicare and Medicaid Services (CMS)

Commonwell Health Alliance

Computer-based patient record (CPR)

Coordination of care

eHealth Exchange

Electronic health records (EHRs)

e-prescribing

Fast Healthcare Interoperability Resources (FHIR) standards

Health information blocking

Health information exchange (HIE)

Health information technology (HIT)

Health Information Technology for Economic and Clinical Health (HITECH) Act

Health Insurance Portability and Accountability Act (HIPAA)

Health Level Seven International (HL7)

HIT interoperability

Meaningful Use of EHR

Medicare Access and CHIP Reauthorization Act (MACRA)

Medicare Modernization Act

Merit-based incentive payment system (MIPS)

Nationwide Interoperability Roadmap

Office of the National Coordinator for Health Information Technology (ONC)

Patient-centered medical homes (PCMHs)

Patient safety

Pay for performance (P4P)

Regional extension centers (RECs)

Strategic Health IT Advanced Research Projects (SHARP)

The Sequoia Project

Value-based payment

LEARNING ACTIVITIES

1. Investigate the latest Meaningful Use criteria for eligible professionals or eligible hospitals. Visit either a physician practice or hospital in your community. Have they participated in the Medicare or Medicaid EHR Incentive Program? Why or why not? If the organization or provider has participated in the program, what has the experience been like? What lessons have they learned? Find out the degree to which the facility uses EHRs and what issues or challenges they have had in achieving Meaningful Use.

2. Evaluate different models of care within your local community or state. Did you find any examples of accountable care organizations or patient-centered medical homes? Explain. Working as a team, visit or interview a leader from a site that uses an innovative model of care. Describe the model, its use, challenges, and degree of patient coordination and integration. How is HIT used to support the delivery of care and reporting of outcomes?

3. Investigate one of the Beacon communities to find out how they are using HIT to improve quality of care and access to care within their region. Be prepared to share with the class a summary of your findings. Do you think the work that this Beacon community has done could be replicated in your community? Why or why not?

4. Explore the extent to which health information exchange is occurring within your community, region, or state. Who are the key players? What types of models of health information exchange exist? To what extent is information being exchanged across organizations for patient care purposes?

5. Investigate the CMS website to determine their current and proposed value-based or pay-for-performance programs. Compare one or more of the programs to the traditional fee-for-service payment method. What are the advantages and disadvantages of each to a physician provider in a small practice?

REFERENCES

Aspden, P. (2004). *Patient safety: Achieving a new standard for care.* Washington, DC: National Academies Press.

Breakaway Policy Strategies for FasterCures. (2015). *A closer look at alternative payment models.* FasterCures value and coverage issue brief. Retrieved August 4, 2016, from http://www.fastercures.org/assets/Uploads/PDF/VC-Brief-Alternative PaymentModels.pdf

Carson, D. D., Garr, D. R., Goforth, G. A., & Forkner, E. (2010). *The time to hesitate has passed: The age of electronic health records is her*e (pp. 2–11). Columbia, SC: South Carolina Medical Association.

Centers for Medicare & Medicaid Services (CMS). (n.d.). *The merit-based incentive payment system: MIPS scoring methodology overview.* Retrieved August 4, 2016, from https://www.cms.gov/Medicare/Quality-Initiatives-Patient-Assessment-Instruments/Value-Based-Programs/MACRA-MIPS-and-APMs/MIPS-Scoring-Methodology-slide-deck.pdf

DeSalvo, K., & Daniel, J. (2015, April 10). Blocking of health information undermines health system interoperability and delivery reform. *HealthIT Buzz.* Retrieved August 4, 2016, from https://www.healthit.gov/buzz-blog/from-the-onc-desk/health-information-blocking-undermines-interoperability-delivery-reform/

Dick, R. S., & Steen, E. B. (1991). *The computer-based patient record: An essential technology for health care.* Washington, DC: National Academy Press.

Goldsmith, J. C. (2003). *Digital medicine: Implications for healthcare leaders.* Chicago, IL: Health Administration Press.

HealthIT.gov. (2012). *The Beacon community program improving health through health information technology* [Brochure]. Retrieved August 3, 2016, from https://www.healthit.gov/sites/default/files/beacon-communities-lessons-learned.pdf

Hsiao, C., Hing, E., Socey, T., & Cai, B. (2011, Nov.). Electronic medical record/electronic health record systems of office-based physicians: United States, 2009 and preliminary 2010 state estimates. *NCHS Data Brief* (79). Washington, DC: US Department of Health and Human Services, National Center for Health Statistics, Division of Health Care Statistics.

Institute for Healthcare Improvement (IHI). (n.d.). *The IHI triple aim.* Retrieved September 22, 2016, from http://www.ihi.org/Engage/Initiatives/TripleAim/Pages/default.aspx

Institute of Medicine, Committee on Data Standards for Patient Safety. (2003). *Reducing medical errors requires national computerized information systems: Data standards are crucial to improving patient safety.* Retrieved from http://www8.nationalacademies.org/onpinews/newsitem.aspx?RecordID=10863

Jacob, J. A. (2015). On the road to interoperability, public and private organizations work to connect health care data. *JAMA, 314*(12), 1213.

Jha, A. K. (2010). Meaningful use of electronic health records. *JAMA, 304*(15), 1709. doi:10.1001/jama.2010.1497

Jha, A. K., Desroches, C. M., Campbell, E. G., Donelan, K., Rao, S. R., Ferris, T. G. . . . Blumenthal, D. (2009). Use of electronic health records in US hospitals. *New England Journal of Medicine, 360*(16), 1628–1638. doi:10.1056/nejmsa0900592

Kohn, L. T., Corrigan, J., & Donaldson, M. S. (2000). *To err is human: Building a safer health system.* Washington, DC: National Academy Press.

McKethan, A., Brammer, C., Fatemi, P., Kim, M., Kirtane, J., Kunzman, J. . . . Jain, S. H. (2011). An early status report on the Beacon Communities' plans for transformation via health information technology. *Health Affairs, 30*(4), 782–788. doi:10.1377/hlthaff.2011.0166

Nerney, C. (2016, January). *CMS acting chief Slavitt on interoperability.* Retrieved August 3, 2016, from http://www.hiewatch.com/news/cms-acting-chief-slavitt-interoperability

Office of the National Coordinator for Health Information Technology (ONC). (2015). *Connecting health and care for the nation: A shared nationwide interoperability roadmap.* Retrieved August 3, 2016, from https://www.healthit.gov/sites/default/files/nationwide-interoperability-roadmap-draft-version-1.0.pdf

Office of the National Coordinator for Health Information Technology (ONC). (n.d.a). *EHR incentives & certification.* Retrieved September 21, 2016, from https://www.healthit.gov/providers-professionals/how-attain-meaningful-use

Office of the National Coordinator for Health Information Technology (ONC). (n.d.b). *Interoperability.* Retrieved September 21, 2016, from https://www.healthit.gov/policy-researchers-implementers/interoperability

The Sequoia Project. (n.d.a). *About the Sequoia Project.* Retrieved August 4, 2016, from http://sequoiaproject.org/about-us/

The Sequoia Project. (n.d.b). *What is eHealth exchange.* Retrieved from http://sequoiaproject.org/ehealth-exchange/

The White House. (2006, August). *Fact sheet: Health care transparency: Empowering consumers to save on quality care.* Retrieved September 22, 2016, from https://georgewbush-whitehouse.archives.gov/news/releases/2006/08/20060822.html

CHAPTER 2

Health Care Data

LEARNING OBJECTIVES

- To be able to define health care data and information.
- To be able to understand the major purposes for maintaining patient records.
- To be able to discuss basic patient health record and claims content.
- To be able to discuss basic uses of health care data, including big and small data and analytics.
- To be able to identify common issues related to health care data quality.

Central to health care information systems is the actual health care data that is collected and subsequently transformed into useful **health care information**. In this chapter we will examine key aspects of health care data. In particular, this chapter is divided into four main sections:

- Health care data and information defined (What are health data and health information?)
- Health care data and information sources (Where does health data originate and why? When does health care data become health care information?)
- Health care data uses (How do health care organizations use data? What is the impact of the trend toward analytics and big data on health care data?)
- Health care data quality (How does the quality of health data affect its use?)

HEALTH CARE DATA AND INFORMATION DEFINED

Often the terms *health care data* and *health care information* are used interchangeably. However, there is a distinction, if somewhat blurred in current use. What, then, is the difference between health data and health information? The simple answer is that *health information* is *processed health data*. (We interpret *processing* broadly to cover everything from formal analysis to explanations supplied by the individual decision maker's brain.) Health care data are raw health care facts, generally stored as characters, words, symbols, measurements, or statistics. One thing apparent about health care data is that they are generally not very useful for decision making. Health care data may describe a particular event, but alone and unprocessed they are not particularly helpful. Take, for example, this figure: 79 percent. By itself, what does it mean? If we process this datum further by indicating that it represents the average bed occupancy for a hospital for the month of January, it takes on more meaning. With the additional facts attached, is this figure now information? That depends. If all a health care executive wants or needs to know is the bed occupancy rate for January, this could be considered information. However, for the hospital executive who is interested in knowing the trend of the bed occupancy rate over time or how the facility's bed occupancy rate compares to that of other, similar facilities, this is not yet the information he needs. A clinical example of raw data would be the lab value, hematocrit (HCT) = 32 or a diagnosis, such as diabetes. These are single facts, data at the most granular level. They take on meaning when assigned to particular patients in the context of their health care status or analyzed as components of population studies.

Knowledge is seen by some as the highest level in a hierarchy with data at the bottom and information in the middle (Figure 2.1). *Knowledge* is defined by Johns (1997, p. 53) as "a combination of rules, relationships, ideas, and experience." Another way of thinking about knowledge is that it is information applied to rules, experiences, and relationships with the result that it can be used for decision making. Data analytics applied to health care information and research

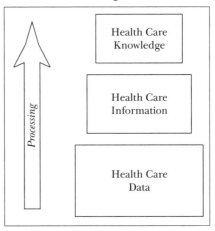

Figure 2.1 Health care data to health care knowledge

studies based on health care information are examples of transforming health care information into new knowledge. To carry out our example from previous paragraphs, the 79 percent occupancy rate could be related to additional information to lead to knowledge that the health care facility's referral strategy is working.

Where do health care data end and where does health care information begin? Information is an *extremely* valuable asset at *all* levels of the health care community. Health care executives, clinical staff members, and others rely on information to get their jobs accomplished. The goal of this discussion is not to pinpoint where data end and information begins but rather to further an understanding of the relationship between health care data and information— health care data are the beginnings of health care information. You cannot create information without data. Through the rest of this chapter the terms *health care data* and *health care information* will be used to describe either the most granular components of health care information or data that have been processed, respectively (Lee, 2002).

The first several sections of this chapter focus primarily on the health care data and information levels, but the content of the section on **health care data quality** takes on new importance when applied to processes for seeking knowledge from health care data. We will begin the chapter exploring where some of the most common health care data originate and describe some of the most common organizational and provider uses of health care information, including patient care, billing and reimbursement, and basic **health care statistics.** Please note there are many other uses for health information that go beyond these basics that will be explored throughout this text.

HEALTH CARE DATA AND INFORMATION SOURCES

The majority of health care information created and used in health care information systems within and across organizations can be found as an entry in a patient's health record or claim, and this information is readily matched to a specific, identifiable patient.

The **Health Insurance Portability and Accountability Act (HIPAA),** the federal legislation that includes provisions to protect patients' health information from unauthorized disclosure, defines *health information* as any information, whether oral or recorded in any form or medium, that does the following:

- Is created or received by a health care provider, health plan, public health authority, employer, life insurer, school or university, or health care clearinghouse
- Relates to the past, present, or future physical or mental health or condition of an individual, the provision of health care to an individual, or the past, present, or future payment for the provision of health care to an individual

HIPAA refers to this type of identifiable information as **protected health information (PHI).**

The Joint Commission, the major accrediting agency for many types of health care organizations in the United States, has adopted the HIPAA definition of protected health information as the definition of "health information" listed in their accreditation manuals' glossary of terms (The Joint Commission, 2016). Creating, maintaining, and managing quality health information is a significant factor in health care organizations, such as hospitals, nursing homes, rehabilitation centers, and others, who want to achieve Joint Commission accreditation. The accreditation manuals for each type of facility contain dozens of standards that are devoted to the creation and management of health information. For example, the hospital accreditation manual contains two specific chapters, Record of Care, Treatment, and Services (RC) and Information Management (IM). The RC chapter outlines specific standards governing the components of a complete medical record, and the IM chapter outlines standards for managing information as an important organizational resource.

Medical Record versus Health Record

The terms *medical record* and *health record* are often used interchangeably to describe a patient's clinical record. However, with the advent and subsequent evolution of electronic versions of patient records these terms actually describe different entities. The Office of the National Coordinator for Health

Information Technology (ONC) distinguishes the electronic medical record and the electronic health record as follows.

Electronic medical records (EMRs) are a digital version of the paper charts. An EMR contains the medical and treatment history of the patients in one practice (or organization). EMRs have advantages over paper records. For example, EMRs enable clinicians (and others) to do the following:

- Track data over time
- Easily identify which patients are due for preventive screenings or checkups
- Check how their patients are doing on certain parameters—such as blood pressure readings or vaccinations
- Monitor and improve overall quality of care within the practice

But the information in EMRs doesn't travel easily *out* of the practice (or organization). In fact, the patient's record might even have to be printed out and delivered by mail to specialists and other members of the care team. In that regard, EMRs are not much better than a paper record.

Electronic health records (EHRs) do all those things—and more. EHRs focus on the total health of the patient—going beyond standard clinical data collected in the provider's office (or during episodes of care)—and is inclusive of a broader view on a patient's care. EHRs are designed to reach out beyond the health organization that originally collects and compiles the information. They are built to share information with other health care providers (and organizations), such as laboratories and specialists, so they contain information from all the clinicians involved in the patient's care (Garrett & Seidman, 2011). Another distinguishing feature of the EHR (discussed in more detail in Chapter Three) is the inclusion of decision-support capabilities beyond those of the EMR.

Patient Record Purposes

Health care organizations maintain patient clinical records for several key purposes. As we move into the discussion on clinical information systems in subsequent chapters, it will be important to remember these purposes, which remain constant regardless of the format or infrastructure supporting the records. In considering the purposes listed, the scope of care is also important. Records support not only managing a single episode of care but also a patient's continuum of care and population health. **Episode of care** generally refers to the services provided to a patient with a specific condition for a specific period of time. **Continuum of care,** as defined by HIMSS (2014), is a concept involving a system that guides and tracks patients over time through a comprehensive array of health services spanning all levels and intensity of care. **Population health** is a relatively new term and definitions vary. However, the concept behind managing population health is to improve health outcomes within defined communities (Stoto, 2013). The following list comprises the most commonly recognized purposes for creating and maintaining patient records.

1. **Patient care.** Patient records provide the documented basis for planning patient care and treatment, for a single episode of care and across the care continuum. This purpose is considered the number-one reason for maintaining patient records. As our health care delivery system moves toward true population health management and patient-focused care, the patient record becomes a critical tool for documenting each provider's contribution to that care.

2. **Communication.** Patient records are an important means by which physicians, nurses, and others, whether within a single organization or across organizations, can communicate with one another about patient needs. The members of the health care team generally interact with patients at different times during the day, week, or even month or year. Information from the patient's record plays an important role in facilitating communication among providers across the continuum of care. The patient record may be the only means of communication among various providers. It is important to note that patients also have a right to access their records, and their engagement in their own care is often reflected in today's records.

3. **Legal documentation.** Patient records, because they describe and document care and treatment, are also legal records. In the event of a lawsuit or other legal action involving patient care, the record becomes the primary evidence for what actually took place during the care. An old but absolutely true adage about the legal importance of patient records says, "If it was not documented, it was not done."

4. **Billing and reimbursement.** Patient records provide the documentation patients and payers use to verify billed services. Insurance companies and other third-party payers insist on clear documentation to support any claims submitted. The federal programs Medicare and Medicaid have oversight and review processes in place that use patient records to confirm the accuracy of claims filed. Filing a claim for a service that is not clearly documented in the patient record may be construed as fraud.

5. **Research and quality management.** Patient records are used in many facilities for research purposes and for monitoring the quality of care provided. Patient records can serve as source documents from which information about certain diseases or procedures can be taken, for example. Although research is most prevalent in large academic medical centers, studies are conducted in other types of health care organizations as well.

6. **Population health.** Information from patient records is used to monitor population health, assess health status, measure utilization of services, track quality outcomes, and evaluate adherence to evidence-based practice guidelines. Health care payers and consumers are increasingly demanding to know the cost-effectiveness and efficacy of different treatment options and modalities. Population health focuses on prevention as a means of achieving cost-effective care.

7. **Public health.** Federal and state public health agencies use information from patient records to inform policies and procedures to ensure that they protect citizens from unhealthy conditions.

Patient Records as Legal Documents

The importance of maintaining complete and accurate patient records cannot be underestimated. They serve not only as a basis for planning patient care but also as the legal record documenting the care that was provided to patients. The data captured in a patient record become a permanent record of that patient's diagnoses, treatments, response to treatments, and case management. Patient records provide much of the source data for health care information that is created, maintained, and managed within and across health care organizations.

When the patient record was a file folder full of paper housed in the health information management department of the hospital, identifying the **legal health record (LHR)** was fairly straightforward. Records kept in the usual course of business (in this case, providing care to patients) represent an exception to the hearsay rule, are generally admissible in a court, and therefore can be subpoenaed—they are legal documentation of the care provided to the patients. With the implementation of comprehensive EHR systems the definition of an LHR remains the same, but the identification of the boundaries for it may be harder to determine. In 2013, the ONC's National Learning Consortium published the *Legal Health Record Policy Template* to guide health care organizations and providers in defining which records and record sets constitute their legal health record for administrative, business, or evidentiary purposes. The media on which the records are maintained does not determine the legal status; rather, it is the purpose for which the record was created and is maintained. The complete template can be found at www .healthit.gov/sites/default/files/legal_health_policy_template.docx.

Because of the legal nature of patient records, the majority of states have specific retention requirements for information contained within them. These state requirements should be the basis for the health care organization's formal retention policy. (The Joint Commission and other accrediting agencies also address retention but generally refer organizations back to their own state regulations for specifics.) When no specific retention requirement is made by the state, all patient information that is a part of the LHR should be maintained for at least as long as the state's statute of limitations or other regulation requires. In the case of minor children the LHR should be retained until the child reaches the age of majority as defined by state law, usually eighteen or twenty-one. Health care executives should be aware that statutes of limitations may allow a patient to bring a case as long as ten years after the patient learns that his or her care caused an injury (Lee, 2002). Although some specific retention requirements and general guidelines exist, it is becoming increasingly popular for health care organizations to keep all LHR information indefinitely, particularly if the information is stored in an electronic format. If an organization does decide to destroy LHR information, this destruction must be carried out in accordance with all applicable laws and regulations.

Another important aspect related to the legal nature of patient records is the need for them to be authenticated. State and federal laws and accreditation standards require that medical record entries be authenticated to ensure that the legal document shows the person or persons responsible for the care provided. Generally, authentication of an LHR entry is accomplished when the physician or other health care professional signs it, either with a handwritten signature or an electronic signature.

Personal Health Records

An increasingly common type of patient record is maintained by the individual to track personal health care information: the personal health record (PHR). According to the American Health Information Management Association (AHIMA, 2016), a PHR "is a tool . . . to collect, track and share past and current information about your health or the health of someone in your care." A PHR is not the same as a health record managed by a health care organization or provider, and it does not constitute a legal document of care, but it should contain all pertinent health care information contained in an individual's health records. PHRs are an effective tool enabling patients to be active members of their own health care teams (AHIMA, 2016).

Patient Record Content

The following components are common to most patient records, regardless of facility type or record system (AHIMA, 2016). Specific patient record content is determined to a large extent by external requirements, standards, and regulations (discussed in Chapter Nine). Keep in mind, a patient record may contain some or all of the documentation listed. Depending on the patient's illness or injury and the type of treatment facility, he or she may need additional specialized health care services. These services may require specific documentation. For example, long-term care facilities and behavioral health facilities have special documentation requirements. Our list is intended to introduce the common components of patient records, not to provide a comprehensive list of all possible components. The following provides a general overview of record content and the person or persons responsible for capturing the content during a single episode of care. It reveals that the patient record is a repository for a variety of health care data and information that is captured by many different individuals involved in the care of the patient.

- **Identification screen.** Information found on the identification screen of a health or medical record originates at the time of registration or admission. The identification data generally includes at least the patient name, address, telephone number, insurance carrier, and policy number, as well as the patient's diagnoses and disposition at discharge. These diagnoses are recorded by the physicians and coded by administrative personnel. (Diagnosis coding is discussed following in this chapter.) The identification component of the data is used as a clinical and an administrative document. It provides a quick view of the diagnoses that required care during the encounter. The codes and other demographic information are used for reimbursement and planning purposes.

- **Problem list.** Patient records frequently contain a comprehensive problem list, which identifies significant illnesses and operations the patient has experienced. This list is generally maintained over time. It is not specific to a single episode of care and may be maintained by the attending or primary care physician or collectively by all the health care providers involved in the patient's care.

- **Medication record.** Sometimes called a *medication administration record (MAR),* this record lists medicines prescribed for and subsequently administered to the patient. It often also lists any medication allergies the patient may have. Nursing personnel are generally responsible for documenting and maintaining medication information in acute care settings, because they are responsible for administering medications according to physicians' written or verbal orders.

• **History and physical.** The history component of the report describes any major illnesses and surgeries the patient has had, any significant family history of disease, patient health habits, and current medications. The information for the history is provided by the patient (or someone acting on his or her behalf) and is documented by the attending physician or other care provider at the beginning of or immediately prior to an encounter or treatment episode. The physical component of this report states what the physician found when he or she performed a hands-on examination of the patient. The history and physical together document the initial assessment of the patient for the particular care episode and provide the basis for diagnosis and subsequent treatment. They also provide a framework within which physicians and other care providers can document significant findings. Although obtaining the initial history and physical is a one-time activity during an episode of care, continued reassessment and documentation of that reassessment during the patient's course of treatment is critical. Results of reassessments are generally recorded in progress notes.

• **Progress notes.** Progress notes are made by the physicians, nurses, therapists, social workers, and other staff members caring for the patient. Each provider is responsible for the content of his or her notes. Progress notes should reflect the patient's response to treatment along with the provider's observations and plans for continued treatment. There are many formats for progress notes. In some organizations all care providers use the same note format; in others each provider type uses a customized format. A commonly used format for a progress note is the SOAP format. Providers are expected to enter notes divided into four components:

  o Subjective findings

  o Objective findings

  o Assessment

  o Plan

• **Consultation.** A consultation note or report records opinions about the patient's condition made by another health care provider at the request of the attending physician or primary care provider.

Consultation reports may come from physicians and others inside or outside a particular health care organization, but this information is maintained as part of the patient record.

- **Physician's orders.** Physician's orders are a physician's directions, instructions, or prescriptions given to other members of the health care team regarding the patient's medications, tests, diets, treatments, and so forth. In the current US health care system, procedures and treatments must be ordered by the appropriate licensed practitioner; in most cases this will be a physician.

- **Imaging and X-ray reports.** The radiologist is responsible for interpreting images produced through X-rays, mammograms, ultrasounds, scans, and the like and for documenting his or her interpretations or findings in the patient's record. These findings should be documented in a timely manner so they are available to the appropriate provider to facilitate the appropriate treatment. The actual digital images are generally maintained in the radiology or imaging departments in specialized computer systems. These images are typically not considered part of the legal patient record, per se, but in modern EHRs they are available through the same interface.

- **Laboratory reports.** Laboratory reports contain the results of tests conducted on body fluids, cells, and tissues. For example, a medical lab might perform a throat culture, urinalysis, cholesterol level, or complete blood count. There are hundreds of specific lab tests that can be run by health care organizations or specialized labs. Lab personnel are responsible for documenting the lab results into the patient record. Results of the lab work become part of the permanent patient record. However, lab results must also be available during treatment. Health care providers rely on accurate lab results in making clinical decisions, so there is a need for timely reporting of lab results and a system for ensuring that physicians and other appropriate care providers receive the results. Physicians or other primary care providers are responsible for documenting any findings and treatment plans based on the lab results.

- **Consent and authorization forms.** Copies of consents to admission, treatment, surgery, and release of information are an important component of the patient record related to its use as a legal document. The practitioner who actually provides the treatment must obtain informed consent for the treatment. Patients must sign informed consent documents before treatment takes place. Forms authorizing release of information must also be signed by patients before any patient-specific health care information is released to parties not directly involved in the care of the patient.

- **Operative report.** Operative reports describe any surgery performed and list the names of surgeons and assistants. The surgeon is responsible for documenting the information found in the operative report.

- **Pathology report.** Pathology reports describe tissue removed during any surgical procedure and the diagnosis based on examination of that tissue. The pathologist is responsible for documenting the information contained within the pathology report.

- **Discharge summary.** Each acute care patient record contains a discharge summary. The discharge summary summarizes the hospital stay, including the reason for admission, significant findings from tests, procedures performed, therapies provided, responses to treatments, condition at discharge, and instructions for medications, activity, diet, and follow-up care. The attending physician is responsible for documenting the discharge summary at the conclusion of the patient's stay in the hospital.

With the passage of the **Accountable Care Act (ACA)** and other health care payment reform measures, organizations and communities have begun to shift focus from episodic care to population health. By definition, population health focuses on maintaining health and managing health care utilization for a defined population of patients or community with the goal of decreasing costs. Along with other key components, successful population health will require extensive care coordination across care providers and community organizations. Care managers are needed to interact with patients on a regular basis during and in between clinical encounters (Institute for Health Technology Transformation, 2012). Needless to say, this will have a significant impact on the form and structure of the future EHRs. These care managers will document all plan findings, clinical and social, within the patient's record and rely on other providers' notes and findings to effectively coordinate care. Baker, Cronin, Conway, DeSalvo, Rajkumar, and Press (2016), for example, describes a new tool to support "person-centered care by a multidisciplinary team," the **comprehensive shared care plan (CSCP),** which will rely on HIT to enable collaboration across settings. A stakeholder group organized by the US Department of Health and Human Services developed key goals for the CSCP as they envision it:

- It should enable a clinician to electronically view information that is directly relevant to his or her role in the care of the person, to easily identify which clinician is doing what, and to update other members of an interdisciplinary team on new developments.

- It should put the person's goals (captured in his or her own words) at the center of decision making and give that individual direct access to his or her information in the CSCP.

- It should be holistic and describe clinical and nonclinical (including home- and community-based) needs and services.

- It should follow the person through high-need episodes (e.g., acute illness) as well as periods of health improvement and maintenance (Baker et al., 2016).

Figures 2.2 through 2.5 display screens from one organization's EHR.

Claims Content

As we have seen in the previous section, health care information is captured and stored as a part of the patient record. However, there is more to the story: health care organizations and providers must be paid for the care they provide. Generally, the health care organization's accounting or billing

Figure 2.2 Sample EHR information screen

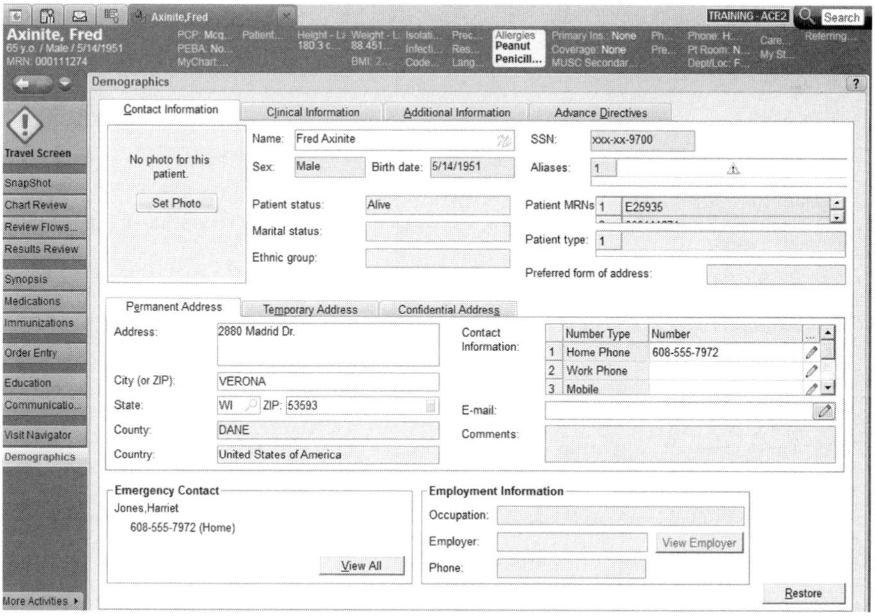

Source: Medical University of South Carolina; Epic.

Figure 2.3 Sample EHR problem list

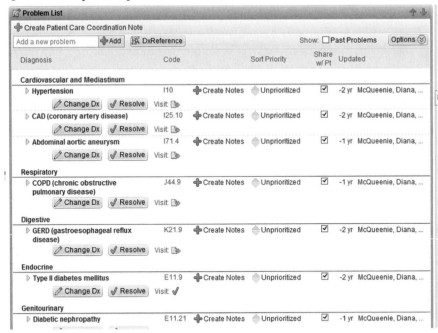

Source: Medical University of South Carolina; Epic.

Figure 2.4 Sample EHR progress notes

Progress Notes			Fred Axinite (MR# 000111274)
Progress Notes by Diana McQueenie, MD signed at 9/30/2016 3:51 AM			

Author: Diana McQueenie, MD   Service: (none)   Author Type: Physician
Date of Service: 9/30/2016   Filed: 9/30/2016 3:51 AM   Status: Signed
Editor: Diana McQueenie, MD (Physician)
Subjective:
Patient presents for follow-up of Type 2 diabetes mellitus, severe headaches, and a request for a referral to bariatrics to help with his severe obesity.

Known diabetic complications: none
Cardiovascular risk factors: advanced age (older than 55 for men, 65 for women), hypertension, male gender, current smoker, and sedentary lifestyle
Current diabetic medications include intensive insulin injection program.
Eye exam current (within one year): yes
Weight trend: fluctuating a bit
Prior visit with dietician: no
Current diet: in general, an ""unhealthy"" diet, diabetic, high salt
Current exercise: walking and yard work

Current monitoring regimen: home blood tests - 4 times daily and office lab tests - 4 times yearly
Home blood sugar records: fasting range: 120-150 and trend: increasing steadily
Any episodes of hypoglycemia? yes

Patient's medications, allergies, past medical, surgical, social and family histories were reviewed and updated as appropriate.

Source: Medical University of South Carolina; Epic.

Figure 2.5 Sample EHR lab report

CBC AND DIFFERENTIAL						Normal
Status: Final result Visible to patient: Not Released			Next appt: None	Dx: Diabetes		
	Ref Range	6:24 AM (11/10/16)	1mo ago (9/30/16)	1mo ago (9/30/16)	1yr ago (5/18/15)	
RED BLOOD CELL COUNT	<null>	4.86 MCL			4.60 R	
HEMATOCRIT		39.0%	46		36 (A)	
HEMOGLOBIN		13.7 GRMS/DL		15.3	13.5	
WHITE BLOOD CELL COUNT	10^3/mL	5.5 B/L			8.4 R	
Resulting Agency		MUSCLAB				

Last Resulted: 11/10/16 6:24 AM

R=Reference range differs from displayed range

Result Base Name Information

Use the names listed under the Component Base Name column to pull lab results into a note with SmartPhrases.

Result Component	Component Base Name	Component Common Name
RED BLOOD CELL COUNT [1577212]	RBC	RBC
HEMATOCRIT [655]	HEMATOCRIT	HEMATOCRIT
HEMOGLOBIN [656]	HEMOGLOBIN	HEMOGLOBIN
WHITE BLOOD CELL COUNT [1577876]	WBC	WBC

Source: Medical University of South Carolina; Epic.

department is responsible for processing claims, an activity that includes verifying insurance coverage; billing third-party payers (private insurance companies, Medicare, or Medicaid); and processing the payments as they are received. Centers for Medicare and Medicaid Services (CMS) currently requires health care providers to submit claims electronically using a set of standard elements. As early as the 1970s the health care community strived to develop standard insurance claim forms to facilitate payment collection. With the nearly universal adoption of electronic billing and government-mandated transaction standards, standard claims content has become essential.

Depending on the type of service provided to the patient, one of two standard data sets will be submitted to the third-party payer. The UB-04, or CMS-1450, is submitted for inpatient, hospital-based outpatient, home health care, and long-term care services. The CMS-1500 is submitted for health care provider services, such as those provided by a physician's office. It is also used for billing by some Medicaid state agencies. The standard requirements for the parallel electronic counterparts to the CMS-1450 and CMS-1500 are defined by ANSI ASC X12N 837I (Institutional) and ANSI ASC X12N 837P (Professional), respectively. Therefore, the claims standards are frequently referred to as 837I and 837P.

UB-04/CMS-1450/837I

In 1975, the **American Hospital Association (AHA)** formed the **National Uniform Billing Committee (NUBC),** bringing the major national provider and payer organizations together for the purpose of developing a single billing form and standard data set that could be used for processing health care claims by institutions nationwide. The first uniform bill was the UB-82. It has since been modified and improved on, resulting, first, in the UB-92 data set and now in the currently used UB-04, also known as CMS-1450. UB-04 is the de facto institutional provider claim standard. Its content is required by CMS and has been widely adopted by other government and private insurers. In addition to hospitals, UB-04 or 837I is used by skilled nursing facilities, end stage renal disease providers, home health agencies, hospices, rehabilitation clinics and facilities, community mental health centers, critical access hospitals, federally qualified health centers, and others to bill their third-party payers. The NUBC is responsible for maintaining and updating the specifications for the data elements and codes that are used for the **UB-04/CMS-1450 and 837I.** A full description of the elements required and the specifications manual can be found on the NUBC website, www.nubc.org (CMS 2016a; NUBC, 2016).

CMS-1500/837P

The **National Uniform Claim Committee (NUCC)** was created by the American Medical Association (AMA) to develop a standardized data set for the noninstitutional or "professional" health care community to use in the submission of claims (much as the NUBC has done for institutional providers). Members of this committee represent key provider and payer organizations, with the AMA appointing the committee chair. The standardized claim form developed and overseen by NUCC is the **CMS-1500** and its electronic counterpart is the **837P.** This standard has been adopted by CMS to bill Medicare fee-for-service, and similar to UB-04 and 837I for institutional care, it has become the de facto standard for all types of noninstitutional provider claims, such as those for private physician services. NUCC maintains a crosswalk between the 837P and CMS-1500 explaining the specific data elements, which can be found on their website at www.nucc.org (CMS, 2013; NUCC, 2016).

It is important to recognize that the UB-04 and the CMS-1500 and their electronic counterparts incorporate standardized data sets. Regardless of a health care organization's location or a patient's insurance coverage, the same data elements are collected. In many states UB-04 data and CMS-1500 data must be reported to a central state agency responsible for aggregating and analyzing the state's health data. At the federal level the CMS aggregates the data from these claims forms for analyzing national health care reimbursement and clinical and population trends. Having uniform data sets means that data can be compared not only within organizations but also within states and across the country.

Diagnostic and Procedural Codes

Diagnostic and procedural codes are captured during the patient encounter, not only to track clinical progress but also for billing, reimbursement, and other administrative purposes. This diagnostic and procedural information is initially captured in narrative form through physicians' and other health care providers' documentation in the patient record. This documentation is subsequently translated into numerical codes. Coding facilitates the classification of diagnoses and procedures for reimbursement purposes, clinical research, and comparative studies.

Two major coding systems are employed by health care providers today:

- **ICD-10 (International Classification of Diseases)**
- **CPT (Current Procedural Terminology),** published by the American Medical Association

Use of these systems is required by the federal government for reimbursement, and they are recognized by health care agencies nationally and internationally. The UB-04 and CMS-1500 have very specific coding requirements for claim submission, which include use of these coding sets.

ICD-10-CM

The ICD-10 classification system used to code diseases and other health statuses in the United States is derived from the *International Classification of Diseases, Tenth Revision,* which was developed by the World Health Organization (WHO) (CDC, 2016) to capture disease data. The precursors to the current ICD system were developed to enable comparison of morbidity (illness) and mortality (death) statistics across nations. Over the years this basic purpose has evolved and today **ICD-10-CM (Clinical Modification)** coding plays major role in reimbursement to hospitals and other health care institutions. ICD-10-CM codes used for determining the **diagnosis related group (DRG)** into which a patient is assigned. DRGs are in turn the basis for determining appropriate inpatient reimbursements for Medicare, Medicaid, and many other health care insurance beneficiaries. Accurate ICD coding has, as a consequence, become vital to accurate institutional reimbursement.

The National Center of Health Statistics (NVHS) is the federal agency responsible for publishing ICD-10-CM (Clinical Modification) in the United States. Procedure information is similarly coded using the **ICD-10-PCS (Procedural Coding System).** ICD-10-PCS was developed by CMS for US inpatient

Exhibit 2.1 Excerpt from ICD-10-CM 2016

Malignant neoplasms (C00-C96)

Malignant neoplasms, stated or presumed to be primary (of specified sites), and certain specified histologies, except neuroendocrine, and of lymphoid, hematopoietic, and related tissue (C00-C75)

Malignant neoplasms of lip, oral cavity, and pharynx (C00-C14)

C00   Malignant neoplasm of lip

   Use additional code to identify:

   alcohol abuse and dependence (F10.-)

   history of tobacco use (Z87.891)

   tobacco dependence (F17.-)

   tobacco use (Z72.0)

   Excludes 1: malignant melanoma of lip (C43.0)

      Merkel cell carcinoma of lip (C4A.0)

      other and unspecified malignant neoplasm of skin of lip (C44.0-)

C00.0   **Malignant neoplasm of external upper lip**

   Malignant neoplasm of lipstick area of upper lip

   Malignant neoplasm of upper lip NOS

   Malignant neoplasm of vermilion border of upper lip

C00.1   **Malignant neoplasm of external lower lip**

   Malignant neoplasm of lower lip NOS

   Malignant neoplasm of lipstick area of lower lip

   Malignant neoplasm of vermilion border of lower lip

hospital settings only. The ICD-10-CM and ICD-10-PCS publications are considered federal government documents whose contents may be used freely by others. However, multiple companies republish this government document in easier-to-use, annotated, formally copyrighted versions. In general, the ICD-10-CM and ICD-10-PCS are updated on an annual basis (CMS, 2015, 2016b).

Exhibits 2.1 and 2.2 are excerpts from the ICD-10-CM and ICD-10-PCS classification systems. They show the system in its text form, but large health care organizations generally use encoders, computer applications that facilitate accurate coding. Whether a book or text file or encoder is used, the classification system follows the same structure.

C00.2   **Malignant neoplasm of external lip, unspecified**

Malignant neoplasm of vermilion border of lip NOS

C00.3   **Malignant neoplasm of upper lip, inner aspect**

Malignant neoplasm of buccal aspect of upper lip

Malignant neoplasm of frenulum of upper lip

Malignant neoplasm of mucosa of upper lip

Malignant neoplasm of oral aspect of upper lip

C00.4   **Malignant neoplasm of lower lip, inner aspect**

Malignant neoplasm of buccal aspect of lower lip

Malignant neoplasm of frenulum of lower lip

Malignant neoplasm of mucosa of lower lip

Malignant neoplasm of oral aspect of lower lip

C00.5   **Malignant neoplasm of lip, unspecified, inner aspect**

Malignant neoplasm of buccal aspect of lip, unspecified

Malignant neoplasm of frenulum of lip, unspecified

Malignant neoplasm of mucosa of lip, unspecified

Malignant neoplasm of oral aspect of lip, unspecified

C00.6   **Malignant neoplasm of commissure of lip, unspecified**

C00.7   **Malignant neoplasm of overlapping sites of lip**

C00.8   **Malignant neoplasm of lip, unspecified**

Source: CMS (2016b).

CPT and HCPCS

The American Medical Association (AMA) publishes an updated CPT each year. Unlike ICD-9-CM, CPT is copyrighted, with all rights to publication and distribution held by the AMA. CPT was first developed and published in 1966. The stated purpose for developing CPT was to provide a uniform language for describing medical and surgical services. In 1983, however, the government adopted CPT, in its entirety, as the major component (known as Level 1) of the **Healthcare Common Procedure Coding System (HCPCS).** Since then CPT has become the standard for physician's office, outpatient, and ambulatory care coding for reimbursement purposes. Exhibit 2.3 is a simplified example of a patient encounter form with HCPCS/CPT codes.

Exhibit 2.2 Excerpt from ICD-10 PCS 2017 OCW

Section **0** Medical and Surgical

Body System **C** Mouth and Throat

Operation **W** Revision: Correcting, to the extent possible, a portion of a malfunctioning device or the position of a displaced device

Body Part	Approach	Device	Qualifier
A Salivary Gland	**0** Open	**0** Drainage Device	**Z** No Qualifier
	3 Percutaneous	**C** Extraluminal Device	
	X External		
S Larynx	**0** Open	**0** Drainage Device	**Z** No Qualifier
	3 Percutaneous	**7** Autologous Tissue Substitute	
	7 Via Natural or Artificial Opening	**D** Intraluminal Device	
	8 Via Natural or Artificial Opening Endoscopic	**J** Synthetic Substitute	
	X External	**K** Nonautologous Tissue Substitute	
Y Mouth and Throat	**0** Open	**0** Drainage Device	**Z** No Qualifier
	3 Percutaneous	**1** Radioactive Element	
	7 Via Natural or Artificial Opening	**7** Autologous Tissue Substitute	
	8 Via Natural or Artificial Opening Endoscopic	**D** Intraluminal Device	
	X External	**J** Synthetic Substitute	
		K Nonautologous Tissue Substitute	

Source: CMS (2016c).

Exhibit 2.3 Patient encounter form coding standards

Pediatric Associates P.A. 123 Children's Avenue, Anytown, USA

Office Visits

99211 Estab Pt—minimal
99212 Estab Pt—focused
99213 Estab Pt—expanded
99214 Estab Pt—detailed
99215 Estab Pt—high complexity

99201 New Pt—problem focused
99202 New Pt—expanded
99203 New Pt—detailed
99204 New Pt—moderate complexity

99205 New Pt—high complexity

99050 After Hours
99052 After Hours—after 10 pm
99054 After Hours—Sundays and Holidays

Outpatient Consult
99241 99242 99243 99244 99245

Preventive Medicine—New
99381 Prev Med 0-1 years
99382 Prev Med 1-4 years
99383 Prev Med 5-11 years
99384 Prev Med 12-17 years
99385 Prev Med 18-39 years

Preventive Medicine—Established
99391 Prev Med 0-1 years
99392 Prev Med 1-4 years
99393 Prev Med 5-11 years
99394 Prev Med 12-17 years
99395 Prev Med 18-39 years

99070 10 Arm Sling
99070 11 Sterile Dressing
99070 45 Cervical Cap

Immunizations, Injections, and Office Laboratory Services

90471 Adm of Vaccine 1
90472 Adm of Vaccine > 1
90648 HIB
90658 Influenza
90669 Prevnar
90701 DTP
90702 DT
90707 MMR
90713 Polio Injection
90720 DTP/HIB
90700 DTaP
90730 Hepatitis A
90733 Meningococcal
90744 Hepatitis B 0-11
90746 Hepatitis B 18+ years

81000 Urinalysis w/ micro
81002 Urinalysis w/o micro
82270 Hemoccult Stool
82948 Dextrostix
83655 Lead Level
84030 PKU
85018 Hemoglobin
87086 Urine Culture
87081 Throat Culture
87205 Gram Stain
87208 Ova Smear (pin worm)
87210 Wet Prep
87880 Rapid Strep

Diagnosis

Patient Name
No.
Date
Time
Address
DOB
Name of Insured   ID
Insurance Company
Return Appointment _____

As coding has become intimately linked to reimbursement, directly determining the amount of money a health care organization can receive for a claim from insurers, the government has increased its scrutiny of coding practices. There are official guidelines for accurate coding, and health care facilities that do not adhere to these guidelines are liable to charges of fraudulent coding practices. In addition, the **Office of Inspector General of the Department of Health and Human Services (HHS OIG)** publishes compliance guidelines to facilitate health care organizations' adherence to ethical and legal coding practices. The OIG is responsible for (among other duties) investigating fraud involving government health insurance programs. More specific information about compliance guidelines can be found on the OIG website (www.oig.hhs.gov) and will be more thoroughly discussed in Chapter Nine.

HEALTH CARE DATA USES

The previous sections of this chapter examine how health care data is captured in patient records and billing claims. Even with this brief overview you can begin to see what a rich source of health care data these records could be. However, before health care data can be used, it must be stored and retrieved. How do we retrieve that data so that the information can be aggregated, manipulated, or analyzed for health care organizations to improve patient care and business operations? How do we combine this patient care data created and stored internally with other pertinent data from external sources?

As we discussed previously in the chapter, data need to be processed to become information. We also noted that data and information may be considered along a continuum, one person's data may be another person's information depending on the level of processing required. In this section of the chapter we will focus on the use of data analysis to transform data into information. There is a lot of discussion about the current and future impact of so-called **big data** on the health care community. We will start the discussion of data analysis by looking at the basic elements required to perform effective health care data analysis, followed by a comparison of "small" data analysis examples to the emerging big data.

Regardless of the scope of the data or the tools used, health care data analysis requires basic elements. First, there must be a source of data, for example, the EHR, claims data, laboratory data, and so on. Second, these data must be stored in a retrievable manner, for example, in a database or data warehouse. Next, an analytical tool, such as mathematical statistics, probability models, predictive models, and so on, must be applied to the stored data. Finally, to be meaningful, the analyzed data must be reported in a usable manner.

Databases and Data Warehouses

A **database** generally refers to any structured, accessible set of data stored electronically; it can be large or small. The back end of EHR and claims systems are examples of large databases. A **data warehouse** differs from a database in its structure and function. In health care, data warehouses that are derived from health care information systems may be referred to as clinical data repositories. The data in a data warehouse come from a variety of sources, such as the EHR, claims data, and ancillary health care information systems (laboratory, radiology, etc.). The data from the sources are extracted, "cleaned," and stored in a structure that enables the data to be accessed along multiple dimensions, such as time (e.g., day, month, year); location; or diagnosis. Data warehouses help organizations transform large quantities of data from separate transactional files or other applications into a single decision-support database. The important concept to understand is that the database or data warehouse provides organized storage for data so that they can be retrieved and analyzed. Before useful information can be obtained, the data must be analyzed. In the most straightforward uses, the data from the data stores are aggregated and reported using simple reporting or statistical methods.

Small versus Big Data

Data stores and data analytics are not new to health care. However, the scope and speed with which we are now capable of analyzing data and discovering new information has increased tremendously. Big data is not a data store (warehouse or database), nor is it a specific analytical tool, but rather it refers to a combination of the two. Experts describe big data as characterized by three Vs (the fourth V—veracity, or accuracy—is sometimes added). These characteristics are present in big but not small data:

- Very large **volume** of data
- A **variety** (e.g., images, text, discrete) of types and sources (EHR, wearable fitness technology, social media, etc.) of data
- The **velocity** at which the data is accumulated and processed (Glaser, 2014; Macadamian, n.d.)

Harris and Schneider (2015) describe a useful metaphor for explaining the difference between big data and traditional data storage and analysis systems. They tell us to consider "even enormous databases, such as the Medicare claims database as 'filing cabinets,' while big data is more like a 'conveyor belt.' The filing cabinet no matter how large, is static, while the conveyor belt is constantly moving and presenting new data points and even data sources" (p. 53). They further provide the following examples of questions answered by big versus **small data** in health care:

- o What are the effects of our immunization programs? versus Is my child growing as expected?
- o What are some the healthiest regions? versus Is this medication improving my (or my patients') blood pressure?

Small Data Examples

Disease and Procedure Indexes

Health care management often wants to know summary information about a particular disease or treatment. Examples of questions that might be asked are What is the most common diagnosis among patients treated in the facility? What percentage of patients with diabetes is African American? What is the most common procedure performed on patients admitted with gastritis (or heart attack or any other diagnosis)? Traditionally, such questions have been answered by looking in **disease and procedure indexes.** Prior to EHRs and their resulting databases, disease and procedure indexes were large card catalogues or books that kept track of the numbers of diseases treated and procedures occurring in a facility by disease and procedure codes. Now that repositories of health care data are common, the disease and procedure index function is generally handled as a component of the EHR. The retrieval of information related to diseases and procedures is still based on ICD and CPT codes, but the queries are limitless. Users can search the disease and procedure database for general frequency statistics for any number of combinations of data. Figure 2.6 is an example of a screen resulting from a query for a specific patient, Iris Hale, who has been identified as a member of both the Heart Failure and Hypertension registries.

Many other types of aggregate clinical reports are used by health care providers and executives. Ad hoc reporting capability applied to clinical databases gives providers and executives access to any number of summary reports based on the data elements from patient health and claims records.

Health Care Statistics

Utilization and performance statistics are routinely gathered for health care executives. This information is needed for facility and health care provision planning and improvement. Statistical reports can provide managers and executives a snapshot of their organization's performance.

Two categories of statistics directly related to inpatient stays are routinely captured and reported. Many variations of these reports and others that drill down to more granular level of data also exist.

- *Census statistics.* These data reveal the number of patients present at any one time in a facility. Several commonly computed rates are based on these census data, including the *average daily census* and *bed occupancy rates.*

- *Discharge statistics.* This group of statistics is calculated from data accumulated when patients are discharged. Some commonly computed rates based on discharge statistics are average *length of stay, death rates, autopsy rates, infection rates, and consultation rates.*

Outpatient facilities and group practices, specialty providers, and so on also routinely collect utilization statistics. Some of the more common statistics are average patient visits per month (or year) and percentage of patients achieving a health status goal, such as immunizations or smoking cessation. The number of descriptive health care statistics that can be produced is limitless. Health care organizations also track a wide variety of financial

Figure 2.6 Sample heart failure and hypertension query screen

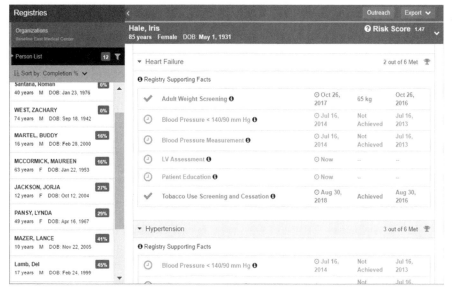

Source: Cerner Corporation (2016). Used with permission.

performance, patient satisfaction, and employee satisfaction data. Patient and employee data generally come from surveys that are routinely administered. The body of data collected and analyzed is driven by the mission of the organization, along with reporting requirements from state, federal, and accrediting organizations.

Health care organizations also look to data to guide improved performance and patient satisfaction. Performance data are essential to health care leaders; however, because they are generally managed within a quality or performance improvement department and are not derived from health care data, per se, they will not be discussed in depth in this chapter. A few significant external agencies that report performance data, however, will be discussed in Chapter Nine.

Although each organization will determine which daily, monthly, and yearly statistics they need to track based on their individual service missions, Rachel Fields (2010) in an article published by *Becker's Hospital Review* provides a list of ten common measures identified by a panel of five hospital leaders, as shown in Table 2.1.

Big Data Examples

Health care organizations today contend with data from EHRs, internal databases, data warehouses, as well as the availability of data from the growing volume of other health-related sources, such as diagnostic imaging equipment, aggregated pharmaceutical research, social media, and personal devices such as Fitbits and other wearable technologies. No longer is the data needed to support health care decisions located within the organization or any single data source. As we begin to manage populations and care continuums we have to bring together data from hospitals, physician practices, long-term care facilities, the patient, and so on. These data needs are bigger than the data needs we had (and still have) when we focused primarily on inpatient care.

Big data is a practice that is applied to a wide range of uses across a wide range of industries and efforts, including health care. There is no single big data product, application, or technology, but big data is broadening the range of data that may be important in caring for patients. For instance, in the case of Alzheimer's and other chronic diseases such as diabetes and cancer, online social sites not only provide a support community for like-minded patients but also contain knowledge that can be mined for public health research, medication use monitoring, and other health-related activities. Moreover, popular social networks can be used to engage the public and monitor public perception and response during flu epidemics and other public health threats (Glaser, 2014).

Table 2.1 Ten common hospital statistical measures

Daily	Monthly	Yearly
1. Quality measures, such as	4. Point-of-service cash collections	9. Colleague satisfaction scores
Infection rates	5. Percentage of charity care	10. Market share and service line development
Patient falls	6. Percentage of budget spent for each department	
Overall mortality		
2. Patient census statistics	7. Door-to-discharge time	
	8. Patient satisfaction scores	
By physician		
By service line		
3. Discharged but not final billed		

Source: Fields (2010).

As important and perhaps more important than the data themselves are the novel analytics that are being developed to analyze these data. In health care we see an impressive range of analytics:

- Post-market surveillance of medication and device safety
- Comparative effectiveness research (CER)
- Assignment of risk, for example, readmissions
- Novel diagnostic and therapeutic algorithms in areas such as oncology
- Real-time status and process surveillance to determine, for example, abnormal test follow-up performance and patient compliance with treatment regimes
- Determination of structure including intent, for example, identifying treatment patterns using a range of structured and unstructured and EHR and non-EHR data
- Machine correction of data-quality problems

The potential impact of applying data analytics to big data is huge. McKinsey & Company (Kayyil, Knott, & Van Kuiken, 2013) estimates that big data initiatives could account for $300 to $450 billion in reduced health care spending, or 12 to 17 percent of the $2.6 trillion baseline in US health care costs. There are several early examples of possibly profound impact. For example, an analysis of the cumulative sum of monthly hospitalizations because of myocardial infarction, among other clinical and cost data, led to the discovery of arthritis drug Vioxx's adverse effects and its subsequent withdrawal from the market in 2004.

A Deloitte (2011) analysis identified five areas of analysis that will be crucial in the emerging era of providers being held more accountable for the care delivered to a patient and a population:

- **Population management analytics.** Producing a variety of clinical indicator and quality measure dashboards and reports to help improve the health of a whole community, as well as help identify and manage at-risk populations
- **Provider profiling/physician performance analytics.** Normalizing (severity and case mix–adjusted profiling), evaluating, and reporting the performance of individual providers (PCPs and specialists) compared to established measures and goals
- **Point of care (POC) health gap analytics.** Identifying patient-specific health care gaps and issuing a specific set of actionable recommendations and notifications either to physicians at the point of care or to patients via a patient portal or PHR
- **Disease management.** Defining best practice care protocols over multiple care settings, enhancing the coordination of care, and monitoring and improving adherence to best practice care protocols
- **Cost modeling/performance risk management/comparative effectiveness.** Managing aggregated costs and performance risk and integrating clinical information and clinical quality measures

HEALTH CARE DATA QUALITY

Up to this point, this chapter has examined health care data and information with a focus on the origins and uses of such. Changes to the health care delivery system and payment reform are amending the ways in which we use health care information. Traditionally, patient clinical and claims records were used primarily to document episodic care or, at best, the care received by an individual across the continuum, as long as that care was provided through a single organization. In today's environment, care providers, care coordinators, analysts, and researchers are all looking to EHRs and electronic claims records as a source of data beyond the episodic scope. Any discussion of health care data analytics and big data include the EHR as a key data source. This expanded use of electronic records and the push for bigger and better data analytics has raised the bar for ensuring the quality of the health care data. Quality health care data has always been important, but the criteria for what constitute high-quality data have shifted.

There are many operational definitions for quality. Two of the best known were developed by the well-known quality "gurus," Philip B. Crosby and Joseph M. Juran. Crosby (1979) defines quality as "conformance to requirements" or conformance to standards. Juran (Juran & Gryna, 1988) defines quality as "fitness for use," products or services must be free of deficiencies. What these definitions have in common is that the criteria against which quality is measured will change depending on the product, service, or use. Herein lies the problem with adopting a single standard for health care data quality—it depends on the use of the data.

EHRs evolved from patient medical records, whose central purpose was to document and communicate episodes of patient care. Today EHRs are being evaluated as source data for complex data analytics and clinical research. Before an organization can measure the quality of the information it produces and uses, it must establish data standards. And before it can establish data standards it must identify all endorsed uses of the EHR.

Consider this scenario. EHRs contain two basic types of data: structured data that is quantifiable or predefined and unstructured data that is narrative. Within a health care organization, the clinicians using the EHR for patient care prefer unstructured data, because it is easier to dictate a note than to follow a lengthy point and click pathway to create a structured note. The clinicians feel that the validation screens cost time that is too valuable for them to waste. The researchers within the organization, however, want as much of the data in the record as possible to be structured to avoid missing data and data entry errors. What should the organization adopt as its standard? Structured or unstructured data? Who will decide and based on what criteria? This discussion between the primary use of EHR data and secondary, or reuse, of data is likely to continue. However, to effectively use EHR data to create new knowledge, either through analytics or research, will require HIT leaders to adopt the more stringent data quality criteria posed by these uses. Wells, Nowacki, Chagin, and Kattan (2013) identify missing data as particularly problematic when using the EHR for research purposes. They further identify two main sources of missing EHR data:

1. Data were not collected. A patient was never asked about a condition. This is most likely directly related to the clinician's lack of interest in what would be considered irrelevant to the current episode of

care. Few clinicians will take a full history, for example, at every encounter.

2. Documentation was not complete. The patient was asked, but it was not noted in the record. This is common in the EHR when clinicians only note positive values and leave negative values blank. For example, if a patient states that he or she does not have a history of cancer, no note will be made, either positive or negative. For a researcher this creates issues. Is this missing data or a negative value?

Although there is no single common standard against which health care data quality can be measured, there are useful frameworks for organizations to use to evaluate health care quality (once the purpose for the data is clearly determined).

The following section will examine two different frameworks for evaluating health care data quality. The first was developed by the American Health Information Management Association (AHIMA) (Davoudi et al., 2015), the second by Weiskopf and Weng (2013). The AHIMA framework is set in the context of managing health care data quality across the enterprise. The Weiskopf and Weng framework was delineated after in-depth research into the quality of data specifically found within an EHR, as currently used. Common health data quality issues will be examined using each framework.

AHIMA Data Quality Characteristics

AHIMA developed and published a set of health care **data quality characteristics** as a component of a comprehensive data quality management model. They define data quality management as "the business processes that ensure the integrity of an organization's data during collection, application (including aggregation), warehousing, and analysis" (Davoudi et al., 2015). These characteristics are to be measured for conformance during the entire data management process.

- **Data accuracy.** Data that reflect correct, valid values are accurate. Typographical errors in discharge summaries and misspelled names are examples of inaccurate data.

- **Data accessibility.** Data that are not available to the decision makers needing them are of no value to those decision makers.

- **Data comprehensiveness.** *All* of the data required for a particular use must be present and available to the user. Even relevant data may not be useful when they are incomplete.

- **Data consistency.** Quality data are consistent. Use of an abbreviation that has two different meanings is a good example of how lack of consistency can lead to problems. For example, a nurse may use the abbreviation *CPR* to mean *cardiopulmonary resuscitation* at one time and *computer-based patient record* at another time, leading to confusion.

- **Data currency.** Many types of health care data become obsolete after a period of time. A patient's admitting diagnosis is often not the same as the diagnosis recorded on discharge. If a health care executive needs a report on the diagnoses treated during a particular time frame, which of these two diagnoses should be included?

- **Data definition.** Clear definitions of data elements must be provided so that current and future data users will understand what the data mean. This issue is exacerbated in today's health care environment of collaboration across organizations.

- **Data granularity.** Data granularity is sometimes referred to as *data atomicity.* That is, individual data elements are "atomic" in the sense that they cannot be further subdivided. For example, a typical patient's name should generally be stored as three data elements (last name, first name, middle name—"Smith" and "John" and "Allen"), not as a single data element ("John Allen Smith"). Again, granularity is related to the purpose for which the data are collected. Although it is possible to subdivide a person's birth date into separate fields for the month, the date, and the year, this is usually not desirable. The birth date is at its lowest practical level of granularity when used as a patient identifier. Values for data should be defined at the correct level for their use.

- **Data precision.** Precision often relates to numerical data. Precision denotes how close to an actual size, weight, or other standard a particular measurement is. Some health care data must be very precise. For example, in figuring a drug dosage it is not all right to round up to the nearest gram when the drug is to be dosed in milligrams.

- **Data relevancy.** Data must be relevant to the purpose for which they are collected. We could collect very accurate, timely data about a patient's color preferences or choice of hairdresser, but are these matters relevant to the care of the patient?

Table 2.2 Terms used in the literature to describe the five common dimensions of data quality

Completeness	Correctness	Concordance	Plausibility	Currency
Accessibility	Accuracy	Agreement	Accuracy	Recency
Accuracy	Corrections made	Consistency	Believability	Timeliness
Availability	Errors	Reliability	Trustworthiness	
Missingness	Misleading	Variation	Validity	
Omission	Positive predictive value			
Presence	Quality			
Quality	Validity			
Rate of recording				
Sensitivity				
Validity				

Source: Weiskopf and Weng (2013). Reproduced with permission of Oxford University Press.

- **Data timeliness.** Timeliness is a critical dimension in the quality of many types of health care data. For example, critical lab values must be available to the health care provider in a timely manner. Producing accurate results after the patient has been discharged may be of little or no value to the patient's care.

Weiskopf and Weng Data Quality Dimensions

Weiskopf and Weng (2013) published a review article in the *Journal of the American Medical Informatics Association* that identified five dimensions of EHR data quality. They based their findings on a pool of ninety-five articles that examined EHR data quality. Their context was using the EHR for research, that is, "reusing" the EHR data. Although different terms were used in the articles, the authors were able to map the terms to one of the five dimensions (see Table 2.2):

- **Completeness:** Is the truth about a patient present?
- **Correctness:** Is an element that is in the EHR true?
- **Concordance:** Is there agreement between elements in the EHR or between the EHR and another data source?
- **Plausibility:** Does an element in the EHR make sense in light of other knowledge about what that element is measuring?

PERSPECTIVE
Problems with Reusing EHR Data: Examples from the Literature

Botsis, T., Hartvigsen, G., Chen, F., & Weng, C. (2010). Secondary use of EHR: Data quality issues and informatics opportunities. *Summit on Translational Bioinformatics, 2010*, 1–5.

The authors report on data quality issues they encountered when attempting to use data that originated in an EHR to conduct survival analysis of pancreatic cancer patients treated at a large medical center in New York City. They found that of 3,068 patients within the clinical data warehouse, only 1,589 had appropriate disease documentation within a pathology report. The sample size was further reduced to 522 when the researchers discovered incompleteness of key study variables. Other instances of incompleteness and inaccuracies were found within the remaining 522 subjects' documentation, causing the researchers to make inferences regarding some of the non-key study variables.

Bayley, K. B., Belnap, T., Savitz, L., Masica, A. L., Shah, N., & Fleming, N. S. (2013). Challenges in using electronic health record data for CER. *Medical Care, 51*(8 Suppl 3), S80–S86. doi:10.1097/mlr.0b013e31829b1d48

The authors conducted research to determine the "strengths and challenges" of using EHRs for CER across four major health care systems with mature EHR systems. They looked at comparing the effectiveness of antihypertensive medications on blood pressure control for a population of patients with hypertension who were being followed by primary care providers within the health systems. Data quality problems that were identified included the following:

- Missing data
- Erroneous data
- Uninterpretable data
- Inconsistent data
- Text notes and noncoded data

The authors concluded that the potential for EHRs as a source of longitudinal data for comparative effectiveness studies in populations is high, but they note that "improving data quality within the EHR in order to facilitate research will remain a challenge as long as research is seen as a separate activity from clinical care."

- **Currency:** Is an element in the EHR a relevant representation of the patient state at a given point in time?

The authors further identify completeness, correctness, and currency as "fundamental," stating that concordance and plausibility "appear to be proxies for the fundamental dimensions when it is not possible to assess them directly."

Strategies for Minimizing Data Quality Issues

As a beginning point, health care data standardization requires clear, consistent definitions. One essential tool for identifying and ensuring the use of standard data definitions is to use a data dictionary. AHIMA defines a data dictionary as "a descriptive list of names (also called 'representations' or 'displays'), definitions, and attributes of data elements to be collected in an information system or database" (Dooling, Goyal, Hyde, Kadles, & White, 2014, p. 7) (see Table 2.3).

Regardless of how well data are defined, however, errors in entry will occur. These errors can be discussed in terms of two types of underlying cause—systematic errors and random errors. *Systematic errors* are errors that can be attributed to a flaw or discrepancy in the system or in adherence to standard operating procedures or systems. *Random errors,* however, are caused by carelessness, human error, or simply making a mistake.

Consider these scenarios:

- A nurse is required to document vital signs into each patient's EHR at the beginning of each visit. However, the data entry screen is cumbersome and often the nurse must wait until the end of day and go back to update the vital signs. On occasion the EHR locks up and does not allow the nurse to update the information. This is an example of a *systematic error.*
- A physician uses the structured history and physical module of the EHR within her practice. However, to save time she cuts and pastes information from one visit to another. During cutting and pasting, she fails to reread her note and leaves in the wrong encounter date. Although there are some elements of systematic error in this situation (not following protocol), the error is primarily a *random error.*

Effective systems are needed to ensure preventable errors are minimized and errors that are not preventable are easily detected and corrected. Clearly, there are multiple points during data collection and processing when the system design can reduce data errors.

The Markle Foundation (2006, p. 4) argues that comprehensive data quality programs are needed by health care organizations to prevent "dirty data" and subsequently improve the quality of patient care. They propose that a data quality program include "automated and human strategies":

- Standardizing data entry fields and processes for entering data
- Instituting real-time quality checking, including the use of validation and feedback loops
- Designing data elements to avoid errors (e.g., using check digits, algorithms, and well-designed user interfaces)
- Developing and adhering to guidelines for documenting the care that was provided
- Building human capacity, including training, awareness-building, and organizational change

Health care data quality problems are exacerbated by inter-facility collaborations and health information exchange. Imagine standardizing processes and definitions across multiple organizations.

Certainly, information technology has tremendous potential as a tool for improving health care data quality. Through the use of electronic data entry, users can be required to complete certain fields, prompted to add information, or warned when a value is out of prescribed range. When health care providers respond to a series of prompts, rather than dictating a free-form narrative, they are reminded to include all necessary elements of a health record entry. Data quality is improved when these systems also incorporate error checking. Structured data entry, drop-down lists, and templates can be incorporated to promote accuracy, consistency, and completeness (Wells et al., 2013). To date some of this potential for technology-enhanced improvements has been realized, but many opportunities remain. As noted in the Perspective many of the data in existing EHR systems are recorded in an unstructured format, rather than in data fields designated to contain specific pieces of information, which can lead to poor health care data quality. Natural language processing (NLP) is a promising, evolving technology that will enable efficient data extraction from the unstructured components of the EHR, but it is not yet commonplace with health care systems.

A clear example of data quality improvement achieved through information technology is the result seen from incorporating medication administration systems designed to prevent medication error. With structured data input and sophisticated error prevention, these systems can significantly

Table 2.3 Excerpt from data dictionary used by AHRQ surgical site infection risk stratification/outcome detection

Table	Field	Datatype	Description
PATIENT			Include patients who had surgery that meet inclusion CPT, SNOMED, or ICD-9 criteria between 1/1/2007 and 1/30/2009.
PATIENT	DOB	Date	The birthdate for the patient
PATIENT	PATIENT_ID	Integer	A unique ID for the patient
PATIENT	DATA_SOURCE_ID	Varchar(10)	An identifier for the source of the patient record data (UU, IHC, DH for example)
DIAGNOSIS			Include ICD-9 CM discharge codes within one month of surgery. A list of included codes is in table 2 of Stevenson et al. AJIC vol 36 (3) 155–164.
DIAGNOSIS	DIAGNOSIS_ID	Integer	A unique ID for the diagnosis
DIAGNOSIS	DIAGNOSIS_CODE	Varchar(64)	The code for the patient's diagnosis
DIAGNOSIS	DIAGNOSIS_CODE_SOURCE	Varchar(64)	The nomenclature that the diagnosis code is taken from (ICD9, etc.)
DIAGNOSIS	CLINICAL_DTM	Date	The date and time of the diagnosis's onset or exacerbation

MICROBIOLOGY			Include all Microbiology specimens taken within one month before or after a surgery. (For risk, this might be expanded to one year or more.)
MICROBIOLOGY	MICRO_ID	Integer	A unique ID for the procedure
MICROBIOLOGY	SPECIMEN_CODE	Varchar(64)	The site that the specimen was collected from
MICROBIOLOGY	SPECIMEN_CODE_SOURCE	Varchar(64)	The nomenclature that the specimen code is taken from (SNOMED, LOINC, etc.)
MICROBIOLOGY	PATHOGEN_CODE	Varchar(64)	The code of the pathogen cultured from the collected specimen
MICROBIOLOGY	PATHOGEN_CODE_SOURCE	Varchar(64)	The nomenclature that the pathogen code is taken from (SNOMEN, LOINC, etc.)
MICROBIOLOGY	COLLECT_DTM	Date	The date and time the specimen was collected
ENCOUNTER			Include all Encounters within one month before or after surgery.
ENCOUNTER	ENCOUNTER_ID	Integer	A unique ID for the visit. This will serve to tie all of the different data tables together via foreign key relationship.
ENCOUNTER	ADMIT_DTM	Date	The admission date and time for a patient's visit
ENCOUNTER	DISCH_DTM	Date	The discharge date and time for a patient's visit
ENCOUNTER	ENCOUNTER_TYPE	Varchar(64)	The type of patient encounter such as inpatient, outpatient, observation, etc.

Source: Agency for Healthcare Research and Quality (2012).

reduce medication errors. The challenge for the foreseeable future is to balance the need for structured data with the associated costs (time and money). Further in the future, new challenges will appear as the breadth of data contained in patient records is likely to increase. Genomic and proteomic data, along with enhanced behavioral and social data, are likely to be captured (IOM, 2014). These added data will introduce new quality issues to be resolved.

SUMMARY

Without health care data and information, there would be no need for health care information systems. Health care data and information are valuable assets in health care organizations, and they must be managed similar to other assets. To that end, health care executives need an understanding of the sources of health care data and information and recognize the importance of ensuring the quality of health data and information. In this chapter, after defining health care data and information, we examined patient record and claims content as sources for health care data. We looked at disease and procedure indexes and health care statistics as examples of basic uses of the health care data. The emerging use of data analytics and big data were introduced and the chapter concluded with a discussion of two frameworks for examining health care data quality and a discussion of how information technology, in general, and the EHR, in particular, can be leveraged to improve the quality of health care data.

KEY TERMS

Accountable Care Act (ACA)
American Hospital Association (AHA)
Big data
CMS-1500/837P
Completeness
Comprehensive shared care plan
   (CSCP)
Concordance
Consent and authorization forms
Consultation
Continuum of care
Correctness

CPT (Current Procedural Terminology)
Currency
Data accessibility
Data accuracy
Data comprehensiveness
Data consistency
Data currency
Data definition
Data granularity
Data precision
Data quality characteristics
Data relevancy

Data timeliness

Databases

Data warehouses

Diagnosis related group (DRG)

Diagnostic and procedural codes

Discharge summary

Disease and procedure indexes

Electronic health records (EHRs)

Electronic medical records
(EMRs)

Episode of care

Healthcare Common Procedure
Coding System (HCPCS)

Health care data

Health care data quality

Health care information

Health care statistics

Health Insurance Portability and
Accountability Act (HIPAA)

Health record

History and physical

ICD-10 (International Classification of
Diseases)

ICD-10-CM (Clinical Modification)

ICD-10-PCS (Procedural Coding
System)

Identification screen

Imaging and X-ray reports

Knowledge

Laboratory reports

Legal health record (LHR)

Medical record

Medication record

The National Center of Health
Statistics (NVHS)

National Uniform Billing Committee
(NUBC)

National Uniform Claim Committee
(NUCC)

Office of Inspector General of the
Department of Health and Human
Services (HHS OIG)

Operative report

Pathology report

Physician's orders

Plausibility

Population health

Problem list

Progress notes

Protected health information (PHI)

Small data

UB-04/CMS-1450/837I

LEARNING ACTIVITIES

1. Contact a health care facility (hospital, nursing home, physician's office, or other organization) to ask permission to view a sample of the health records they maintain. Answer the following questions for each record:

   a. What is the primary reason (or condition) for which the patient was seen?

   b. How long has the patient had this condition?

   c. Did the patient have a procedure performed? If so, what procedure(s) was (were) done?

    d. Did the patient experience any complications? If so, what were they?

    e. How does the physician's initial assessment of the patient compare with the nurse's initial assessment? Where in the record would you find this information?

    f. To where was the patient discharged?

    g. What were the patient's discharge orders or instructions? Where in the record should you find this information?

2. Make an appointment to meet with the business manager at a physician's office or health care clinic. Discuss the importance of ICD-10 coding or CPT coding (or both) for that office. Ask to view the system that the office uses to assign diagnostic and procedure codes. After the visit, write a brief summary of your findings and impressions.

3. Visit www.oig.hhs.gov. What are the major responsibilities of the Office of Inspector General as they relate to coded health care data? What other responsibilities related to health care fraud and abuse does this office have?

4. Consider a patient (real or imagined) with a chronic health condition. Identify at least three actual health care providers that this patient has seen in the past twelve months. Draw a diagram to illustrate the timeline of the patient's encounters. Considering these encounters, how easy is it for each provider to share health care information regarding this patient with the others? What are the barriers to the communication and sharing of health care information? How will this affect the patient's overall care?

5. Contact a health care facility (hospital, nursing home, physicians' office, or other facility) to ask permission to view a sample of the health records it maintains. These records may be in paper or electronic form. For each record, answer the following questions about data quality:

    a. How would you assess the quality of the data in the patient's record?

    b. What proportion of the data in the patient's medical record is captured electronically? What information is recorded manually? Do you think the method of capture affects the quality of the information?

    c. How does the data quality compare with what you expected?

REFERENCES

Agency for Healthcare Research and Quality. (2012). *Improving the measurement of surgical site infection risk stratification/outcome detection. Appendix C: Data dictionary.* Retrieved from http://www.ahrq.gov/research/findings/final-reports/ssi/ssiapc.html

AHIMA. (2016). *What is a personal health record (PHR)?* Retrieved May 29, 2016, from http://myphr.com/StartaPHR/what_is_a_phr.aspx

Baker, A., Cronin, K., Conway, P., DeSalvo, K., Rajkumar, R., & Press, M. (2016, May 18). *Making the comprehensive shared care plan a reality.* Retrieved June 1, 2016, from http://catalyst.nejm.org/making-the-comprehensive-shared-care-plan-a-reality/

Bayley, K. B., Belnap, T., Savitz, L., Masica, A. L., Shah, N., & Fleming, N. S. (2013). Challenges in using electronic health record data for CER. *Medical Care, 51*(8 Suppl 3), S80–S86. doi:10.1097/mlr.0b013e31829b1d48

Botsis, T., Hartvigsen, G., Chen, F., & Weng, C. (2010). Secondary use of EHR: Data quality issues and informatics opportunities. *Summit on Translational Bioinformatics, 2010,* 1–5.

CDC. (2016). *International classification of diseases, tenth revision.* Clinical Modification (ICD-10-CM). Retrieved May 30, 2016, from http://www.cdc.gov/nchs/icd/icd10cm.htm

Centers for Medicare and Medicaid Services (CMS). (2013). *Medicare billing: 837P and form CMS-1500* [Brochure]. Retrieved March 2013 from https://www.cms.gov/Outreach-and-Education/Medicare-Learning-Network-MLN/MLNProducts/downloads/form_cms-1500_fact_sheet.pdf

Centers for Medicare and Medicaid Services (CMS). (2015). *ICD-10-CM/PCS: The next generation of coding* [Brochure]. Retrieved May 30, 2016, from https://www.cms.gov/Medicare/Coding/ICD10/downloads/ICD-10Overview.pdf

Centers for Medicare and Medicaid Services (CMS). (2016a). *Medicare billing: 837I and form CMS-1450* [Brochure]. Retrieved May 30, 2016, from https://www.cms.gov/Outreach-and-Education/Medicare-Learning-Network-MLN/MLNProducts/Downloads/837I-FormCMS-1450-ICN006926.pdf

Centers for Medicare and Medicaid Services (CMS). (2016b). *2016 ICD-10-CM and GEMS.* Retrieved August 2016 from https://www.cms.gov/Medicare/Coding/ICD10/2016-ICD-10-CM-and-GEMs.html

Centers for Medicare and Medicaid Services (CMS). (2016c). *2017 ICD-10 PCS and GEMS.* Retrieved August 2016 from https://www.cms.gov/Medicare/Coding/ICD10/2017-ICD-10-PCS-and-GEMs.html

Crosby, P. B. (1979). *Quality is free: The art of making quality certain.* New York, NY: McGraw-Hill.

Davoudi, S., Dooling, J., Glondys, B., Jones, T., Kadlec, L., Overgaard, S., . . .

& Wendicke, A. (2015, Oct.). Data quality management model (2015 update). *Journal of AHIMA, 86*(10). Retrieved from http://bok.ahima.org/doc?oid=107773#.V6ILzfkrIuU

Deloitte Consulting. (2011) *Integrated care organizations' information technology requirements.* New York, NY: Author.

Dooling, J., Goyal, P., Hyde, L., Kadles, L., & White, S. (2014). *Health data analysis toolkit.* Chicago, IL: AHIMA. Retrieved September 22, 2016, from http://library.ahima.org/PdfView?oid=107504

Fields, R. (2010, Sept. 2). 10 statistics your hospital should track. *Becker's Hospital Review.* Retrieved May 30, 2016, from http://www.beckershospitalreview.com/hospital-management-administration/10-statistics-your-hospital-should-track.html

Garrett, P., & Seidman, J. (2011, Jan. 4). EMR vs. EHR—what is the difference? *Health IT Buzz.* Retrieved May 30, 2016, from http://www.healthit.gov/buzz-blog/electronic-health-and-medical-records/emr-vs-ehr-difference/

Glaser, J. (2014, Dec. 9). *Solving big problems with big data.* Retrieved October 11, 2016, from http://www.hhnmag.com/articles/3809-solving-big-problems-with-big-data

Harris, Y., & Schneider, C. D. (2015). *Health information technology in the United States, 2015: Transition to a post-HITECH world* (Ch. 4). Published jointly by the Robert Wood Johnson Foundation, Mathematica Policy Research, Harvard School of Public Health, and University of Michigan, School of Information. Available online.

Health Information Management and Systems Society (HIMSS). (2014). *Definition of continuum of care* [Brochure]. Retrieved June 1, 2016, from http://s3.amazonaws.com/rdcms-himss/files/production/public/2014-05-14-DefinitionContinuumofCare.pdf

Institute for Health Technology Transformation. (2012). *Population health management: A roadmap for provider-based automation in a new era of healthcare.* Retrieved May 29, 2016, from http://ihealthtran.com/pdf/PHMReport.pdf

Institute of Medicine (IOM). (2014) *Capturing social and behavioral domains and measures in electronic health records.* Washington, DC: National Academies.

Johns, M. (1997). *Information management for health professionals.* Albany, NY: Delmar.

The Joint Commission. (2016). *Comprehensive accreditation manual for hospitals.* Oakbrook Terrace, IL: Author.

Juran, J. M., & Gryna, F. M. (1988). *Juran's quality control handbook.* New York, NY: McGraw-Hill.

Kayyil, B., Knott, D., & Van Kuiken, S. (2013). *The "big data" revolution in healthcare.* New York, NY: McKinsey and Co. Retrieved July 8, 2016, from http://healthcare.mckinsey.com/sites/default/files/The_big-data_revolution_in_US_health_care_Accelerating_value_and_innovation%5B1%5D.pdf

Lee, F. W. (2002). Data and information management. In K. LaTour & S. Eichenwald (Eds.), *Health information management concepts, principles, and practice* (pp.83–100). Chicago, IL: American Health Information Management Association.

Macadamian. (n.d.). *Big data vs. small data: Turning big data into actionable insights.* Retrieved August 3, 2016, from http://www.macadamian.com/guide-to-healthcare-software-development/big-data-vs-small-data/

Markle Foundation. (2006). *Connecting for health common framework: Background issues on data quality.* Retrieved September 22, 2016, from http://www.markle.org/sites/default/files/T5_Background_Issues_Data.pdf

National Learning Consortium. (2013). *Legal health record policy template.* Office of the National Coordinator for Health Information Technology. Retrieved August 18, 2016, from www.healthit.gov/sites/default/files/legal_health_policy_template.docx

National Uniform Billing Committee (NUBC). (2016). *About us.* Retrieved August 2016 from http://www.nubc.org/aboutus/index.dhtml

National Uniform Claim Committee (NUCC). (2016). *Who are we?* Retrieved August 2016 from http://www.nucc.org/index.php/22-active-home-page/23-who-are-we

Stoto, M. A. (2013, Feb. 21). *Population health in the Affordable Care Act era.* Academy Health. Retrieved June 1, 2016, from https://www.academyhealth.org/files/AH2013pophealth.pdf

Wells, B. J., Nowacki, A. S., Chagin, K., & Kattan, M. W. (2013). Strategies for handling missing data in electronic health record derived data. EGEMs *(Generating Evidence & Methods to Improve Patient Outcomes),* 1(3). doi:10.13063/2327-9214.1035

Weiskopf, N. G., & Weng, C. (2013). Methods and dimensions of electronic health record data quality assessment: Enabling reuse for clinical research. *Journal of the American Medical Informatics Association, 20*(1), 144–151. doi:10.1136/amiajnl-2011-000681

CHAPTER 3

Health Care Information Systems

LEARNING OBJECTIVES

- To be able to identify the major types of administrative and clinical information systems used in health care.
- To be able to give a brief explanation of the history and evolution of health care information systems.
- To be able to discuss the key functions and capabilities of electronic health record systems and current adoption rates in hospitals, physician practices, and other settings.
- To be able to describe the use and adoption of personal health records and patient portals.
- To be able to discuss current issues pertaining to the use of HCIS systems including interoperability, usability, and health IT safety.

After reading Chapters One and Two, you should have a general understanding of the national health IT landscape and the types and uses of clinical and administrative data captured in provider organizations. In this chapter we build on these fundamental concepts and introduce *health care information systems,* a broad category that includes clinical and administrative applications. We begin by providing a brief history and overview of information systems used in health care provider organizations. The chapter focuses on the **electronic health record (EHR)** and **personal health record (PHR),** including patient portals and the major initiatives that have led to the adoption and use of EHRs in hospitals and physician practices. Included is a discussion on the state of EHR adoption and use in other health care settings, including behavioral health, community health, and long-term care. Applications such as computerized provider order entry and decision support are described in the context of the EHR. (*Note:* Other health IT systems and applications needed to support population health and value-based payment—such as patient engagement tools, telemedicine, and telehealth—are described in Chapter Four.) Finally, the chapter concludes with a discussion on important key issues in the use of HCIS including usability, interoperability, and health IT safety.

We begin first with a brief review of key terms.

REVIEW OF KEY TERMS

An *information system (IS)* is an arrangement of data (information), processes, people, and information technology that interact to collect, process, store, and provide as output the information needed to support the organization (Whitten & Bentley, 2007). Note that information technology is a component of every information system. *Information technology (IT)* is a contemporary term that describes the combination of computer technology (hardware and software) with data and telecommunications technology (data, image, and voice networks). Often in current management literature the terms *information system (IS)* and *information technology (IT)* are used interchangeably.

Within the health care sector, health care IS and IT include a broad range of applications and products and are used by a wide range of constituent groups such as payers, government, life sciences, and patients, as well as providers and provider organizations. For our purpose, however, we have chosen to focus on health care information systems from the provider organization's perspective. The *provider organization* is the hospital, health system, physician practice, integrated delivery system, nursing home, or rural health clinic. That is, it is any setting where health-related services are delivered. The organization (namely, the capacity, decisions about how health IT is applied, and incentives) and the external environment (regulations and public opinion) are important elements in how systems are used by clinicians and other users (IOM, 2011). We also examine the use of patient engagement tools such as PHRs and secure patient portals. Yet our focus is from an organization or provider perspective.

MAJOR HEALTH CARE INFORMATION SYSTEMS

There are two primary categories of health care information systems: *administrative* and *clinical*. A simple way to distinguish them is by purpose and the type of data they contain. An **administrative information system** (or an *administrative application*) contains primarily administrative or financial data and is generally used to support the management functions and general operations of the health care organization. For example, an administrative information system might contain information used to manage personnel, finances, materials, supplies, or equipment. It might be a system for human resource management, materials management, patient accounting or billing, or staff scheduling. Revenue cycle management is increasingly important to health care organizations and generally includes the following:

- Charge capture
- Coding and documentation review
- Managed care contracting
- Denial management of claims
- Payment posting
- Accounts receivable follow-up
- Patient collections
- Reporting and benchmarking

By contrast, a *clinical information system* (or *clinical application*) contains clinical or health-related information used by providers in diagnosing and treating a patient and monitoring that patient's care. **Clinical information systems** may be departmental systems—such as radiology, pharmacy, or laboratory systems—or clinical decision support, medication administration, computerized provider order entry, or EHR systems, to name a few. They may be limited in their scope to a single area of clinical information (for example, radiology, pharmacy, or laboratory), or they may be comprehensive and cover virtually all aspects of patient care (as an EHR system does, for example). Table 3.1 lists common types of clinical and administrative health care information systems.

Health care organizations, particularly those that have implemented EHR systems, generally provide patients with access to their information electronically through a patient portal. A *patient portal* is a secure website through which patients may communicate with their provider, request refill on prescriptions, schedule appointments, review test results, or pay bills (Emont, 2011). Another term that is frequently used is *personal health record (PHR)*. Different from an EHR or patient portal, which is managed by the provider or health care organization, the PHR is managed by the consumer. It may

Table 3.1. Common types of administrative and clinical information systems

Administrative Applications	Clinical Applications
Patient administration systems	Ancillary information systems
Admission, discharge, transfer (ADT) tracks the patient's movement of care in an inpatient setting	Laboratory information supports collection, verification, and reporting of laboratory tests
Registration may be coupled with ADT system; includes patient demographic and insurance information as well as date of visit(s), provider information	Radiology information supports digital image generation (picture archiving and communication systems [PACS]), image analysis, image management
Scheduling aids in the scheduling of patient visits; includes information on patients, providers, date and time of visit, rooms, equipment, other resources	Pharmacy information supports medication ordering, dispensing, and inventory control; drug compatibility checks; allergy screening; medication administration
Patient billing or accounts receivable includes all information needed to submit claims and monitor submission and reimbursement status	Other clinical information systems
Utilization management tracks use and appropriateness of care	Nursing documentation facilitates nursing documentation from assessment to evaluation, patient care decision support (care planning, assessment, flow-sheet charting, patient acuity, patient education)
Other administrative and financial systems	
Accounts payable monitors money owed to other organizations for purchased products and services	Electronic health record (EHR) facilitates electronic capture and reporting of patient's health history, problem lists, treatment and outcomes; allows clinicians to document clinical findings, progress notes, and other patient information; provides decision-support tools and reminders and alerts
General ledger monitors general financial management and reporting	

Administrative Applications	Clinical Applications
Personnel management manages human resource information for staff, including salaries, benefits, education, and training	**Computerized provider order entry** (CPOE) enables clinicians to directly enter orders electronically and access decision-support tools and clinical care guidelines and protocols
Materials management monitors ordering and inventory of supplies, equipment needs, and maintenance	**Telemedicine and telehealth** supports remote delivery of care; common features include image capture and transmission, voice and video conferencing, text messaging
Payroll manages information about staff salaries, payroll deductions, tax withholding, and pay status	
Staff scheduling assists in scheduling and monitoring staffing needs	**Rehabilitation service documentation** supports the capturing and reporting of occupational therapy, physical therapy, and speech pathology services
Staff time and attendance tracks employee work schedules and attendance	
Revenue cycle management monitors the entire flow of revenue generation from charge capture to patient collection; generally relies on integration of a host of administrative and financial applications	**Medication administration** is typically used by nurses to document medication given, dose, and time

include health information and wellness information, such as an individual's exercise and diet. The consumer decides who has access to the information and controls the content of the record. The adoption and use of patient portals and PHRs are discussed further on in this chapter. For now, we begin with a brief historical overview of how these various clinical and administrative systems evolved in health care.

HISTORY AND EVOLUTION

Since the 1960s, the development and use of health care information systems has changed dramatically with advances in technology and the impact of environmental influences and payment reform (see Figure 3.1). In the 1960s to 1970s, health care executives invested primarily in administrative and financial information systems that could automate the patient billing process and facilitate accurate Medicare cost reporting. The administrative applications that were used were generally found in large hospitals, such as those affiliated with academic medical centers. These larger health care organizations were often the only ones with the resources and staff available to develop,

Figure 3.1 History and evolution of health care information systems (1960s to today)

1960–70s	1980s	1990s	2000s	2010–present
• Administrative and financial • Mainframe computing • Designed primarily in house in large hospitals	• Need for clinical and administrative data • Advent of microcomputer	• Internet and WWW and e-mail • IOM Calls for widespread adoption of CPR • Continued growth of clinical applications	• IOM reports on patient safety • Leapfrog recommends CPOE • E-prescribing expands • PHRs available	• ACA and HITECH • CMS EHR incentive programs and Meaningful Use • Payment reform • Population health management • Big data and data analytics • Cloud computing • Mobile applications

implement, and support such systems. It was common for these facilities to develop their own administrative and financial applications in-house in what were then known as "data processing" departments. The systems themselves ran on large **mainframe computers**, which had to be housed in large, environmentally controlled settings. Recognizing that small, community-based hospitals could not bear the cost of an in-house, mainframe system, leading vendors began to offer shared systems, so called because they enabled hospitals to share the use of a mainframe with other hospitals. Vendors typically charged participating hospitals for computer time and storage, for the number of terminal connects, and for reports.

By the 1970s, departmental systems such as clinical laboratory or pharmacy systems began to be developed, coinciding with the advent of minicomputers. **Minicomputers** were smaller and more powerful than some of the mainframe computers and available at a cost that could be justified by revenue-generating departments. Clinical applications including departmental systems such as laboratory, pharmacy, and radiology systems became more commonplace. Most systems were stand-alone and did not interface well with other clinical and administrative systems in the organization.

The 1980s brought a significant turning point in the use of health care information systems primarily because of the development of the **microcomputer,** also known as the *personal computer (PC)*. Sweeping changes in reimbursement practices designed to rein in high costs of health care also had a significant impact. In 1982, Medicare shifted from a cost-based reimbursement system to a prospective payment system based on diagnosis related groups (DRGs). This new payment system had a profound effect on hospital billing practices. Reimbursement amounts were now dependent on the accuracy of the patient's diagnosis and procedures(s) and other information contained in the patient's record. With hospital reimbursement changes occurring, the advent of the microcomputer could not have been more timely. The microcomputer was smaller, often as or more powerful, and far more affordable than a mainframe computer. Additionally, the microcomputer was not confined to large hospitals. It brought computing capabilities to a host of smaller organizations including small community hospitals, physician practices, and other care delivery settings. Sharing information among micro-computers also became possible with the development of *local area networks.* The notion of **best of breed** systems was also common; individual clinical departments would select the best application or system for meeting their unique unit's needs and attempt to get the "systems to talk to each other" using interface engines.

Rapid technological advances continued into the 1990s, with the most profound being the evolution and widespread use of the *Internet* and *electronic mail* (e-mail). The Internet provided health care consumers, patients, providers, and industries with access to the World Wide Web and new and innovative opportunities to access care, promote services, and share information. Concurrently, the Institute of Medicine (IOM, 1991) published its first landmark report *The Computer-Based Patient Record: An Essential Technology for Health Care,* which called for the widespread adoption of computerized patient records (CPRs) as the standard by the year 2001. CPRs were the precursor to what we refer to today as EHR systems. Numerous studies had revealed the problems with paper-based medical records (Burnum, 1989; Hershey, McAloon, & Bertram, 1989; IOM, 1991). Records are often illegible, incomplete, or unavailable when and where they are needed. They lack any type of *active* decision-support capability and make data collection and analysis very cumbersome. This passive role for the medical record was no longer sufficient. Health care providers needed access to active tools that afforded them clinical decision-support capabilities and access to the latest relevant research findings, reminders, alerts, and other knowledge aids. Along with patients, they needed access to systems that would support the integration of care across the continuum.

By the start of the new millennium, health care quality and patient safety emerged as top priorities. In 2000, the IOM published the report *To Err Is Human: Building a Safer Health Care System,* which brought national attention to research estimating that 44,000 to 98,000 patients die each year to medical errors. Since then, additional reports have indicated that these figures are grossly underestimated and the incidents of medical errors are much higher

(Classen et al., 2011; James, 2013; Makary & Daniel, 2016;). A subsequent report, *Patient Safety: Achieving a New Standard of Care* (2004), called for health care providers to adopt information technology to help prevent and reduce errors because of illegible prescriptions, drug-to-drug interactions, and lost medical records, for example.

By 2009, the US government launched an "unprecedented effort to reengineer" the way we capture, store, and use health information (Blumenthal, 2011, p. 2323). This effort was realized in the Health Information Technology for Economic and Clinical Health (HITECH) Act. Nearly $30 billion was set aside over a ten-year period to support the adoption and Meaningful Use of EHRs and other types of health information technology with the goal of improving health and health care. Rarely, if ever, have we seen public investments in the advancement of health information technology of this magnitude (Blumenthal, 2011). Interest also grew in engaging patients more fully in providing access to their EHR through patient portals or the concept of a PHR. We have also seen significant advances in telemedicine and telehealth, cloud computing, and mobile applications that monitor and track a wide range of health data.

ELECTRONIC HEALTH RECORDS

Features and Functions

Let's first examine the features and functions of an EHR because it is core to patient care. An EHR can electronically collect and store patient data, supply that information to providers on request, permit clinicians to enter orders directly into a **computerized provider order entry (CPOE)** system, and advise health care practitioners by providing decision-support tools such as reminders, alerts, and access to the latest research findings or appropriate evidence-based guidelines. CPOE at its most basic level is a computer application that accepts provider orders electronically, replacing handwritten or verbal orders and prescriptions. Most CPOE systems provide physicians and other providers with decision-support capabilities at the point of ordering. For example, an order for a laboratory test might trigger an alert to the provider that the test has already been ordered and the results are pending. An order for a drug to which the patient is allergic might trigger an alert warning to the provider of an alternative drug. These decision-support capabilities make the EHR far more robust than a digital version of the paper medical record.

Figure 3.2 illustrates an EHR alert reminding the clinician that the patient is allergic to certain medication or that two medications should not be taken

Figure 3.2 Sample drug alert screen

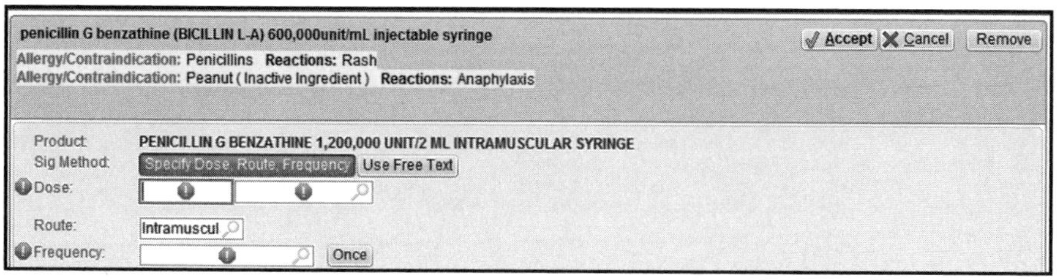

Source: Medical University of South Carolina, Epic. Used with permission.

in combination with each other. Reminders might also show that the patient is due for a health maintenance test such as a mammography or a cholesterol test or for an influenza vaccine (Figure 3.2).

Up until the passage of the HITECH Act of 2009, EHR adoption and use was fairly low. HITECH made available incentive money through the Medicare and Medicaid EHR Incentive Programs for eligible professionals and hospitals to adopt and become "meaningful users" of EHR. As mentioned in Chapter One, the Meaningful Use criteria were established and rolled out in three phases. Each phase built on the previous phase in an effort to further the advancement and use of EHR technology as a strategy to improve the nation's health outcome policy priorities:

- Improve health care quality, safety, and efficiency and reduce health disparities.
- Engage patients and families in their health care.
- Improve care coordination.
- Improve population and public health.
- Ensure adequate privacy and security of personal health information.

To accomplish these goals and facilitate patient engagement in managing their health and care, health care organizations provide patients with access to their records typically through a ***patient portal***. A patient portal is a secure website through which patients can electronically access their medical records. Portals often also enable users to complete forms online, schedule appointments, communicate with providers, request refills on prescriptions, review test results, or pay bills (Emont, 2011) (see Figure 3.3). Some providers offer patients the opportunity to schedule e-visits for a limited number of nonurgent medical conditions such as allergic skin reactions, colds, and nosebleeds.

Figure 3.3 Sample patient portal

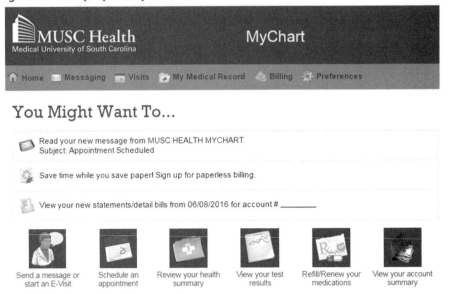

Source: Medical University of South Carolina.

EHR Adoption Rates in US Hospitals

As of 2015, nearly 84 percent of US nonfederal acute care hospitals had adopted basic EHR systems representing a nine-fold increase from 2008 (Henry, Pylypchuck, Searcy, & Patel, 2016) (see Figure 3.4). Table 3.2 lists the difference functionality between a basic system and a fully functional system (DesRoches et al., 2008). A key distinguishing characteristic is fully functional EHRs provide order entry capabilities (beyond ordering medications) and decision-support capabilities.

The Veterans Administration (VA) has used an EHR system for years, enabling any veteran treated at any VA hospital to have electronic access to his or her EHR. Likewise, the US Department of Defense is under contract with Cerner to replace its EHR system. EHR adoption among specialty hospitals such as children's (55 percent) and psychiatric hospitals (15 percent) is significantly lower than general medicine hospitals because these types of hospitals were not eligible for HITECH incentive payments. Small, rural, and critical access hospitals that have historically lagged behind in EHR adoption are now closing the gap with general acute care hospitals (Henry et al., 2016).

Figure 3.4 Percent of non-federal acute care hospitals with adoption of at least a basic EHR with notes system and position of a certified EHR: 2008–2015

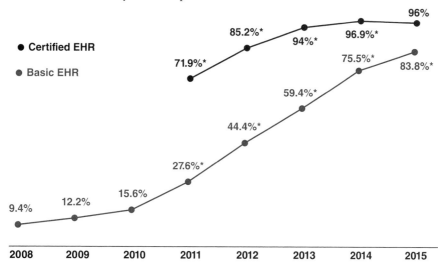

Note: Basic EHR adoption requires the EHR system to have a set of EHR functions defined in Table 3.2. A certified EHR is EHR technology that meets the technological capability, functionality, and security requirements adopted by the Department of Health and Human Services. Possession means that the hospital has a legal agreement with the EHR vendor but is not equivalent to adoption. *Significantly different from previous year ($p<0.05$).
Source: ONC (2015a).

EHR Adoption in Office-Based Physician Practices

In addition to EHR use in hospitals, we have also seen significant increases in the adoption and use of EHR systems among office-based physician practices. By 2014, 79 percent of primary care physicians had adopted a certified EHR system and 70 percent of medical and surgical specialties had as well (Heisey-Grove & Patel, 2015) (see Figure 3.5).

Ninety-eight percent of physicians in community health centers had adopted an EHR, three-quarters of them using a certified EHR. Not surprisingly, physicians in solo and small group practices were less likely to have adopted EHR systems (Heisey-Grove & Patel, 2015).

EHR Adoption in Other Settings

Less is known nationally about EHR adoption rates in settings other than hospitals and physician practices. Among home health and hospice agencies,

Table 3.2 Functions defining the use of EHRs

	Basic System	Fully Functional System
Health Information Data		
Patient demographics	X	X
Patient problem lists	X	X
Electronic lists of medications taken by patients	X	X
Clinical notes	X	X
Notes including medical history and follow-up		X
Order Entry Management		
Orders for prescriptions	X	X
Orders for laboratory tests		X
Orders for radiology tests		X
Prescriptions sent electronically		X
Orders sent electronically		X
Results Management		
Viewing laboratory results	X	X
Viewing imaging results	X	X
Electronic images returned		X
Clinical Decision Support		
Warnings of drug interactions or contraindications provided		X
Out-of-range test levels highlighted		X
Reminders regarding guidelines-based interventions or screening		X

the latest national estimates based on data from the 2007 National Home and Hospice Care survey indicate that 44 percent of home health and hospice agencies have adopted EHR systems (16 percent EHRs only and 28 percent EHRs and mobile technologies such as tablets or hand-held devices

Figure 3.5. Office-based physician practice EHR adoption since 2004

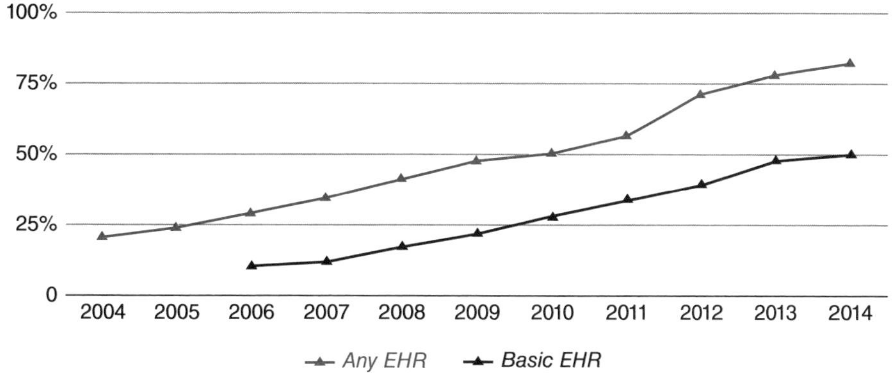

Source: ONC (2015a).

used to gather information at the point of care) (Bercovitz, Park-Lee, & Jamoom, 2013).

Some states, such as New York, have attempted to assess EHR adoption in long-term care facilities such as nursing homes. One study found that among 473 nursing homes in New York, 56.3 percent had implemented an EHR system (Abramson, Edwards, Silver, & Kaushal, 2014). Among the nursing homes that did not have EHRs, the majority had plans to implement one within two years. One-fifth had plans to implement one in more than two years, and 11.7 percent had no EHR implementation plans (Abramson et al., 2014). The majority of nursing homes indicated the biggest barriers to health IT investment were the initial cost, a lack of IT staff members, and the lack of fiscal incentives. National estimates on EHR adoption in long-term care are nearly nonexistent. Most are qualitative studies examining the experiences of early adopters (Cherry, Ford, & Peterson, 2011).

Impact of EHR Systems

Numerous studies over the years have demonstrated the value of using EHR systems and other types of clinical applications within health care organizations. The majority of benefits fall into three broad categories: (1) quality, outcomes, and safety; (2) efficiency, improved revenues, and cost reduction; and (3) provider and patient satisfaction. Following is a brief discussion of these major categories, along with several recent examples and reports illustrating the value of EHRs to the health care process. It is important to note, however, that despite the benefits, some studies have found mixed results or negative consequences.

- **Quality, outcomes, and safety**. EHR systems can have a significant impact on patient quality, outcomes, and safety. Three major effects on quality are increased adherence to evidence-based care, enhanced surveillance and monitoring, and decreased medication errors. Banger and Graber (2015) recently conducted a review of the literature on the impact of health IT (including EHR systems) on patient quality and safety and found four major systematic reviews had been conducted from 2006 through 2014 each using a consistent methodology (Buntin, Burke, Hoaglin, & Blumenthal, 2011; Chaudhry et al., 2006; Goldzweig, Towfigh, Maglione, & Shekelle, 2009; Jones, Rudin, Perry, & Shekelle, 2014). Two of the reviews were published before the HITECH Act and two afterward. Collectively, 59 percent of the studies examined demonstrated positive effects on quality and safety, 25 percent had mixed-positive outcomes, 9 percent were neutral, and 8 percent were negative (Banger & Graber, 2015). Limitations of most of the earlier studies were based on the fact that they did not include many commercially available EHR systems. Since then, more than half of EHR evaluation studies involved commercially available EHR systems (Jones et al., 2014). Findings from the most recent systematic review conclude that CPOE effectively decreases medication errors. Hydari, Telang, and Marella (2014) studied the incidence of adverse patient safety events reported from 231 Pennsylvania hospitals from 2005 to 2012 in relation to their level of health IT use. After controlling for several possibly confounding factors, the authors found that hospitals adopting advanced EHRs (as defined by HIMSS) experienced a 27 percent overall reduction in reported patient safety events. Using advanced EHRs was associated with a 30 percent decline in medication errors and a 25 percent decline in procedure-related errors (Hydari et al., 2014).

- **Efficiency, improved revenue, and cost reduction**. In addition to improving quality and safety, some studies have shown that the EHR can improve efficiency, increase revenues, and lead to cost reductions (Barlow, Johnson, & Steck, 2004; Grieger, Cohen, & Krusch, 2007). A fairly recent study by Howley, Chou, Hansen, and Dalrymple (2014) examined the financial impact of EHRs on ambulatory practices by tracking the productivity (e.g., the number of patient visits) and reimbursement of thirty practices for two years after EHR implementation. They found that practice revenues increased during EHR implementation despite seeing fewer patients. Another study looked at seventeen primary care clinics that used EHR systems and found that the clinics recovered their EHR investments within an average period of ten months (95 percent CI 6.2–17.4 months), seeing more patients with an average increase of 27 percent in the active-patients-to-clinicians full-time equivalent ratio, and an increase in the clinic net revenue ($p<.001$) (Jang, Lortie, & Sanche, 2014).

• **Provider and patient satisfaction.** Provider and patient satisfaction are common factors to assess when implementing EHR systems. Results from satisfaction surveys are often mixed. In a 2008 national survey of physicians, 90 percent of providers using EHRs reported they were satisfied or very satisfied with them and a large majority could point to specific quality benefits (DesRoches et al., 2008). Those who had systems in place for two or more years were more likely to be satisfied (Menachemi, Powers, Au, & Brooks, 2010). A study that examined EHR satisfaction among obstetrics/gynecology (OB/GYN) physicians found that 63 percent reported being satisfied with their EHR system, and nearly 31 percent were not satisfied (Raglan, Margolis, Paulus, & Schulkin, 2014). Among study participants, younger OB/GYN physicians were more satisfied with their EHR than older physicians. A study by Rand (in collaboration with the AMA) found that although many physicians approved of EHRs in concept (for example, they appreciated the fact that they could remotely access patient information and provide improved patient care), they expressed frustrations with usability and work flow (Friedberg et al., 2013). The time-consuming nature of data entry, interference with face-to-face patient care, inefficiency, and the inability to exchange health information between EHR products led to dissatisfaction. Physicians across the full range of specialties and practice models also described other concerns regarding the degradation of clinical documentation.

Among US hospitals, a 2011 national study found that those with EHRs had significantly higher patient satisfaction scores on items such as "staff always giving patients information about what to do for the recovery at home," "patients rating the hospital as a 9 or 10 overall," and "patients would definitely recommend the hospital to others" than hospitals that did not (Kazley, Diana, Ford, & Menachemi, 2011, p. 26). Yet the same study found that the EHR use was not statistically associated with other patient satisfaction measures (such as having clean rooms) that one would not expect to be affected by EHR use. A more recent study by Jarvis and colleagues (2013) assessed the impact of using advanced EHRs (as defined as Stages 6 or 7 on the **HIMSS Analytics EMR Adoption Model [EMRAM]** level of health IT adoption) on hospital quality patient satisfaction using a composite score for measuring patient experience. (See the following Perspective.) They found that hospitals with the most advanced EHRs had the greatest gains in improving clinical process of care scores, without negatively affecting the patient experience (Jarvis et al., 2013). Another study found that physicians using EHRS that met Meaningful Use criteria and had two or more years EHR experience were more likely to report clinical benefits (King, Patel, Jamoon, & Furukawa, 2014).

Limitations and Need for Further Research

Not all studies have demonstrated positive outcomes from using EHR systems. For example, the same EHR or clinical information system can be implemented in different organizations and have different results. As example of variability, two children's hospitals implemented the same EHR (including CPOE) in their pediatric intensive care units. One hospital experienced a significant increase in mortality (Han et al., 2005), and the other did not (Del Beccaro, Jeffries, Eisenberg, & Harry, 2006). The hospital that experienced an increase in mortality noted that several implementation factors contributed to the deterioration in quality; specific order sets for critical care were not created, changes in workflow were not well executed, and orders for patients arriving via critical care transportation could not be written before the patient arrived at the hospital, delaying life-saving treatments. Many factors can influence the successful use and adoption of EHR systems. These are discussed more fully in Chapter Six.

PERSONAL HEALTH RECORDS

In addition to EHRs and patient portals, the broader concept of a personal health record has emerged in recent years. Initially, the PHR was envisioned as a tool to enable individuals to keep their own health records, and they could share information electronically with their physicians or other health care professionals and receive advice, reminders, test results, and alerts from them. Unlike the EHR and patient portal, which is managed by health care provider organizations, the PHR is managed by the consumer. It may include health and wellness information, such as an individual's exercise and diet. The consumer decides who has access to the information and controls the content of the record. Personal data the consumer gathers through use of health apps such as My Fitness Pal or Fitbits may be included.

What is the value of the PHR, and how does it relate to the EHR? Tang and Lansky (2005) believe the PHR enables individuals to serve as copilots in their own care. Patients can receive customized content based on their needs, values, and preferences. PHRs should be lifelong and comprehensive and should support information exchange and portability. Patients are often seen by multiple health care providers in different settings and locations over

PERSPECTIVE

HIMSS Analytics EHR Adoption Levels among US Hospitals

Stage	Cumulative Capabilities	2016—Q1
Stage 7	Complete EHR is used; data warehousing and data analytics is used to improve care; clinical information can be shared via standardized electronic transactions across continuum of care.	4.3%
Stage 6	Physician documentation with structured templates and discrete data is implemented for at least one inpatient area. Full CCSS. The closed loop medication administration with bar coding is used. The five rights of medication administration are verified.	29.1%
Stage 5	A full complement of radiology PACS system provides medical images to physicians via an intranet.	34.4%
Stage 4	Computerized provider order entry (CPOE) used to create orders; CDSS is used with clinical protocols.	10.0%
Stage 3	Nursing/clinical documentation has been implemented including electronic medication administration record (MAR); clinical decision support (CDS) capabilities allow for error checking with order entry. Medical image access from picture archive and communication systems (PACS) is available within organization.	15.3%
Stage 2	Major clinical systems feed into clinical data repository (CDR) that enables viewing of orders and results. CDR contains a controlled medical vocabulary, and clinical decision support system (CDSS) capabilities. Hospital may have health information exchange (HIE) capabilities and can share CDR information with patient care stakeholders.	2.5%
Stage 1	All three major ancillary clinical systems (laboratory, pharmacy, radiology) are installed.	1.8%
Stage 0	All three key ancillary department systems (laboratory, pharmacy, radiology) are not installed.	2.6%
		N=5,456

Source: Adapted from HIMSS Analytics EMR Adoption Model (EMRAM). © HIMSS Analytics 2016. Retrieved from http://www.himssanalytics.org/provider-solutions. Used with permission.

the course of a lifetime. In our fragmented health care system, this means patients are often left to consolidate information from the various participants in their care. A PHR that brings together important health information across an individual's lifetime and that is safe, secure, portable, and easily accessible can reduce costs by avoiding unnecessary duplicate tests and improving health care communications. The concept of patient portals and PHRs are also inherent in the CMS Meaningful Use program. Stage 3 Meaningful Use recommendations (originally scheduled for implementation in 2017 but now under policy reconsideration) state that patients should be able to (1) communicate electronically using secure messaging, (2) access patient education materials on the Internet, (3) generate health data into their providers' EHRs, and (4) view, download, and transmit their provider-managed EHRs. Taken together, Ford, Hesse, and Huerta (2016) argue that these requirements outline the basic functionalities of a consumer-managed PHR.

Ford and his colleagues (2016) examined US consumers PHR use over time, the factors that influence use, and projected the diffusion of PHR under three scenarios. Not surprisingly, they found that consumers were increasingly using electronic means for storing health data and communicating with their clinical providers. An estimated 5 percent of consumers used PHRs in 2008, and by 2013, this number had reached 17 percent (Ford et al., 2016), still relatively low. Using various prediction models, they estimate that PHR use will increase significantly within the next decade.

PHRs and personal health applications have the potential to positively affect medication adherence and quality of life for patients with chronic diseases. For example, a recent controlled study examined the impact of a text-based message reminder system on medication adherence among adolescents with asthma (Johnson et al., 2016). Compared to adolescents in the control group, they found improvements in self-reported medication adherence (p = .011), quality of life (p = .037), and self-efficacy (p = .016). System use varied considerably, however, with lower use among African American adolescents (Johnson et al., 2016).

Consumers are also increasingly capturing health, wellness, and clinical data about themselves using a wide range of mobile technologies and applications—everything from wrist-worn devices that track steps and sleep patterns to web-based food diaries, networked weight scales, and blood pressure machines (Rosenbloom, 2016). They also use social media networks to connect with others who share a similar health condition. Such approaches are referred to as *person-generated health data (PGHD)* technologies given that consumers may use these technologies independent of situations in which they are patients per se. According to Rosenbloom (2016) the field of PGHD and related technologies is in its infancy, particularly in studying the real value these technologies add to health care delivery. Shaw and his colleagues (2016) found, for example, that individuals with chronic illnesses (who may have the most to benefit from using mobile health devices) may be less likely to adopt and use these devices compared to healthy individuals. As health care organizations and providers move to managing population health and cohorts of patients under value-based payment models, the use of such technologies with certain populations of patients may be incredibly useful. Chapter Four discusses further the health IT tools needed to support population health management.

KEY ISSUES AND CHALLENGES

Despite the proliferation in the adoption and use of EHR systems, health care providers and organizations still face critical issues and challenges related to **interoperability, usability,** and **health IT safety.** Following is a brief discussion of each.

Interoperability

In simple terms, *interoperability* is "the ability of a system to exchange electronic health information with and use electronic health information from other systems without special effort on the part of the [user]" (Institute for Electrical and Electronics Engineering [IEEE], n.d.). The ONC's report *Connecting Health and Care for the Nation: A Shared Nationwide Interoperability Roadmap* (ONC, 2015a) describes the importance of interoperability in a creating a "learning health system" in which "health information flows seamlessly and is available to the right people, at the right place, at the right time." The overarching vision of a learning health system is to put patients at the center of their care—"where providers can easily access and use secure health information from different sources; where an individual's health information is not limited to what is stored in EHRs, but includes information from other sources (including technologies that individuals use) and portrays a longitudinal picture of their health, not just episodes of care; where diagnostic tests are only repeated when necessary, because the information is readily available; and where public health agencies and researchers can rapidly learn, develop and deliver cutting edge treatments" (ONC, 2015a, p. vi) (see Figure 3.6).

Today, providers are challenged to knit together multiple EHRs, financial systems, and analytic solutions in an effort to effectively manage population health and facilitate care coordination. As health care providers

Figure 3.6 The ONC's roadmap to interoperability

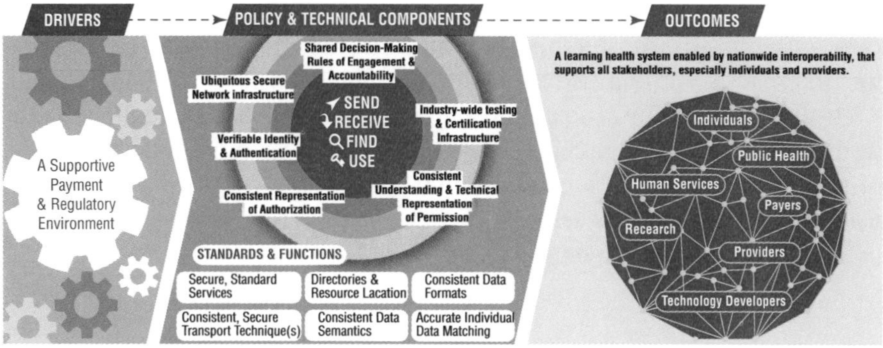

Source: ONC (2015a).

and organizations coalesce to manage performance and utilization risk in their communities, they need high degrees of interoperability among these systems (Glaser, 2015). The systems must also fit well into the clinical workflow and patient care process while ensuring patient safety and quality. Additionally, interoperability will enable data generated by personal fitness and wearable devices to be included in the patient's EHR (Glaser, 2015).

True interoperability has yet to be realized. Several factors make interoperability among health care information systems complicated. EHR systems are often developed using different platforms with inconsistent use of standards, no universal patient identifier exists, and pulling together from a wide range of sources is complicated (Glaser, 2015). Moreover, historically there has not been a great deal of incentive for providers to share information, nor for health IT vendors to bridge together a number of different systems, giving rise to the concept of information blocking. According to the ONC, **information blocking** occurs "when persons or entities knowingly and unreasonably interfere with exchange or use of electronic health information" (ONC, 2015b). The concept of information blocking implies that the entity intentionally and knowingly interferes with sharing the data and is objectively unreasonable in light of public policy. The ONC has developed comprehensive strategies for identifying, deterring, and remedying information blocking and coordinating with other federal agencies that can investigate and take action against certain types of information blocking.

The ONC *Roadmap to Interoperability* postulates that work is needed in three critical areas: (1) requiring standards, (2) motivating the use of those standards through appropriate incentives, and (3) creating a trusted environment for collecting, sharing, and using electronic health information. Broad stakeholder involvement is critical to achieving interoperability. Stakeholders include those who receive or support care, those who deliver care, those who pay for care, and people and organizations that support health IT capabilities, oversight of health care organizations, and those who develop and maintain standards (ONC, 2015b). (See the following Perspective.) In addition to the ONC, which resides in the Department of Health and Human Services, CMS and state governments also play key roles in advancing interoperability. Statewide health information exchanges can be found in Massachusetts, New York, and Delaware (Glaser, 2015). Interoperability efforts and standards development are discussed more fully in Chapter Ten.

Partnerships are also occurring within the private sector to advance interoperability among systems by creating standards and promoting the sharing of data. CommonWell Health Alliance has created and implemented patient identification and record-locating service capabilities, Carequality is developing an interoperability and governance framework, and the Argonaut Project is testing the next generation of interoperability standards. Glaser (2015) argues that we must focus on several important goals in making interoperability in health care a reality by doing the following:

- Advancing standards development and pursuing new technical approaches to effecting standards-based interoperability
- Strengthening sanctions, perhaps through the certification process, to minimize business practices that thwart interoperability
- Increasing transparency of vendor and provider progress in achieving interoperability
- Developing a trust framework that balances the need for efficient exchange with the privacy rights of patients
- Promoting collaborative multi-stakeholder efforts, such as CommonWell Health Alliance, Carequality, and eHealth Initiative
- Encouraging provider-led activities within communities to broaden the range of interconnections and include stakeholders such as safety net providers
- Creating a governance mechanism that ensures an effective interchange across a wide range of health information exchanges
- Making reimbursement changes that emphasize care coordination and population health management, all of which must continue to evolve and be implemented

Unfortunately, there is no silver bullet or easy road to achieving true interoperability. However, with collaboration among stakeholders, appropriate

Connecting Health and Care for the Nation: A Shared Nationwide Interoperability Roadmap (ONC, 2015b) was released by the Office of the National Coordinator for Health Information Technology in 2015. This document was published as a companion to the *Connecting Health and Care for the Nation: A 10-Year Vision to Achieve an Interoperable Health IT Infrastructure*. The following facts are taken from the Roadmap and its companion infographic, *Shared Nationwide Interoperability Roadmap: The Journey to Better Health and Care*. This outline lists progress toward interoperability since 2009, the current state of health care supporting the need for interoperability, and the future goals and selected payer and outcome milestones for achieving the ultimate in interoperability, "**learning health systems** in which health information flows seamlessly and is available to the right people, at the right place, at the right time" (ONC, 2015a).

Selected Historical Interoperability Achievements

2009	16% of hospitals and 21% of providers adopted basic EHRs.
2011	27% of hospitals and 34% of providers adopted EHRs.
2013	94% of nonfederal acute care hospitals use a certified EHR.
	78% of office-based physicians use an EHR.
	62% of hospitals electronically exchanged health information with providers outside their system.
2014	80% of hospitals can electronically query other organizations for health information.
	14% of office-based providers electronically share patient information with other providers.

Current State of Health Care

- One in three consumers must provide his or her own health information when seeking care for a medical problem.
- A typical Medicare beneficiary sees seven providers annually.
- A typical primary care physician has to coordinate care with 229 other physicians working in 117 practices.
- Eighty to ninety percent of health determinants are *not* related to health care.

- One in eight Americans tracks a health metric using technology.
- It takes seventeen years for evidence to go from research to practice.

Barriers to Interoperability

- States have different laws and regulations making it difficult to share health information across state lines.
- Health information is not sufficiently standardized.
- Payment incentives are not aligned to support interoperability.
- Privacy laws differ and are misinterpreted.
- There is a lack of trust among health care providers and consumers.

2015–2017 Goal and Milestones

Goal: Send, receive, find, and use priority data domains to improve health care quality and outcomes

Roadmap Milestones for a Supportive Payment and Regulatory Environment and Outcomes

> CMS will aim to administer 30 percent of all Medicare payments to providers through alternative payment models that reward quality and value and encourage interoperability by the end of 2016.

> A majority of individuals are able to securely access their electronic health information and direct it to the destination of their choice.

> Providers evolve care processes and information reconciliation to ensure essential health information is sent, found, or received to support safe transitions in care.

> ONC, federal partners, and stakeholders develop a set of measures assessing interoperable exchanges and the impact of interoperability on key processes that enable improved health and health care.

2018–2020 Goal and Milestones

Goal: Expand interoperable health IT and users to improve health and lower cost

Roadmap Milestones for a Supportive Payment and Regulatory Environment and Outcomes

CMS will administer 50 percent of all Medicare payments to providers through alternative payment models that reward quality and value by the end of 2018.

Individuals regularly access and contribute to their longitudinal electronic health information via health IT, send and receive that information through a variety of emerging technologies, and use that information to manage their health and participate in shared decision making with their care, support, and service teams.

Providers routinely and proactively seek outside information about individuals and can use it to coordinate care.

Public and private stakeholders report on progress toward interoperable exchange, including identifying barriers to interoperability, lessons learned, and impacts of interoperability on health outcomes and costs.

incentives, and keeping the patient at the center of our work and efforts, secure and efficient interoperability is certainly within reach.

Usability

In addition to interoperability concerns, clinicians often express frustration with the usability of EHR systems and other clinical information systems. In fact, 55 percent of physicians reported that it was difficult or very difficult to use. Common frustrations include confusing displays, iconography that lacks consistency and intuitive meaning, and the feeling that systems do not support clinicians' cognitive workflow or inhibit them from easily drawing insights or conclusions from the data. Similarly, physicians who participated in a Rand study (Friedberg et al., 2013) felt that EHR data entry was time-consuming, interfered with face-to-face patient care, and was overall inefficient. They also reported that inability to exchange health information and the degradation of clinical documentation were of concern. Others argue that poor usability of EHR systems not only contributes to clinician frustration but also can lead to errors and patient safety concerns (Meeks, Smith, Taylor, Sittig,

2020–2024 Goal and Milestones

Goal: Achieve nationwide interoperability to enable a learning health system

Roadmap Milestones for a Supportive Payment and Regulatory Environment and Outcomes

> The federal government will use value-based payment models as the dominant mode of payment for providers.

> Individuals are able to seamlessly integrate and compile longitudinal electronic health information across online tools, mobile platforms, and devices to participate in shared decision making with their care, support, and service teams.

> Providers routinely use relevant info from a variety of sources, including environmental, occupational, genetic, human service, and cutting-edge research evidence, to tailor care to the individual.

> Public and private stakeholders report on progress on key metrics identified to achieve a learning health system.

Source: ONC (2015a).

Scott, & Singh, 2014; Sittig & Singh, 2011). In essence, usability refers to "the effectiveness, efficiency, and satisfaction with which the intended users can achieve their tasks in the intended context of produce use" (Bevan, 2001). Smartphones are typically viewed as having high usability, because they require little training and are intuitive to use. In fact, we often see young children navigating them before they can even talk!

Given the importance of system usability, a task force was formed by the American Medical Informatics Association (Middleton et al., 2013) to study the issue. They identified key recommendations on critical usability issues, particularly those that may adversely affect patient safety and the quality of care. The recommendations fall into four categories: (1) usability and human factors research, (2) policy recommendations, (3) industry recommendations, and (4) clinical end user recommendations. (See the Perspective.)

As one can discern from AMIA's task force recommendations, usability is a multifaceted issue and one that requires thoughtful research, standardization and interoperability, a common user interface style guide, and systems for identifying best practices and monitoring use as well as adverse events that may affect patient safety.

1. Usability and human factors research agenda in health IT

    a. Prioritize standardized use cases.

    b. Develop a core set of measures for adverse events related to health IT use.

    c. Research and promote best practices for safe implementation of EHR.

2. Policy recommendations

    d. Standardization and interoperability across EHR systems should take account of usability concerns.

    e. Establish an adverse event reporting system for health IT and voluntary health IT event reporting.

    f. Develop and disseminate an educational campaign on the safe and effective use of EHR.

3. Industry recommendations

    g. Develop a common user interface style guide for select EHR functionalities.

    h. Perform formal usability assessments on patient-safety sensitive EHR functionalities.

4. Clinical end user recommendations

    i. Adopt best practices for EHR implementation and ongoing management.

    j. Monitor how IT systems are used and report IT-related adverse events.

Source: Middleton et al. (2013). Reproduced with permission of Oxford University Press.

Health IT Safety

In 2011, the Institute of Medicine published a report titled *Health IT and Patient Safety: Building Safer Systems for Better Care* in which they outlined a number of recommendations to ensure health IT systems are safe. In brief, they suggest that safety is a shared responsibility between vendors and health care organizations and requires the following:

- Building systems using user-centered design principles with adequate testing and simulation
- Embedding safety considerations throughout the implementation process
- Developing and publishing best practices
- Having accreditation agencies (such as the Joint Commission) assume a significant role in testing as part of their accreditation criteria
- Focusing on shared learning and transparency
- Creating a nonpunitive environment for reporting (IOM, 2011)

Since then, the topic of health IT safety has grown in importance as more EHR systems have been deployed. Health IT patient safety concerns include adverse events that reached the patient, near misses that did not reach the patient, or unsafe conditions that increased the likelihood of a safety event (Meeks et al., 2014). Such events are often difficult to define and detect. Consequently, Singh and Sittig (2016) have developed a health IT safety measurement framework that takes into account eight technological and nontechnological dimensions or sociotechnical dimensions (see Table 3.3).

The Health IT Safety Framework provides a conceptual framework for defining and measuring health IT–related patient safety issues. The framework is also built on continuous quality improvement methods that require stakeholders to ask themselves, How are we doing? Can we do better? How can we do better (Singh & Sittig, 2016)? In fact, Singh and Sittig (2016) argue that it is essential that clinicians and leaders make health IT patient safety an organizational priority by ensuring that the governance structure facilitates measuring and monitoring and creating an environment that is conducive to detecting, fixing, and learning from system vulnerabilities. Meeks and colleagues (2014) used a variation of the Health IT Safety Framework in analyzing one hundred different EHR-related safety concerns reported to and investigated by the VA's Informatics Patient Safety Office, which is a voluntary reporting system. The major categories of errors were because of (1) unmet display needs (mismatch between information needs and content

Table 3.3 Sociotechnical dimensions

Dimension	Description
Hardware and software	Computing infrastructure used to support and operate clinical applications and devices
Clinical content	The text, numeric data, and images that constitute the "language" of clinical applications, including clinical decision support
Human-computer interface	All aspects of technology that users can see, touch, or hear as they interact with it
People	Everyone who is involved with patient care and/or interacts in some way with health care delivery (including technology). This would include patients, clinicians and other health care personnel, IT developers and other IT personnel, informaticians
Workflow and communication	Processes to ensure that patient care is carried out effectively, efficiently, and safely
Internal organizational features	Policies, procedures, the physical work environment, and the organizational culture that govern how the system is configured, who uses it, and where and how it is used
External rules and regulations	Federal or state rules (e.g., CMS's Physician Quality Reporting Initiative, HIPAA, and Meaningful Use program) and billing requirements that facilitate or constrain the other dimensions
Measurement and monitoring	Evaluating both intended and unintended consequences through a variety of prospective and retrospective, quantitative, and qualitative methods

Source: Reproduced from *Measuring and Improving Patient Safety through Health Information Technology: The Health IT Safety Framework,* Singh and Sittig, 25: p.228, 2016. With permission from BMJ Publishing Group Ltd.

display; (2) software modifications (concerns about upgrades, modifications, or configurations); (3) system-to-system interfacing (concerns about failure of interfacing between systems); and (4) hidden dependencies on distributed systems (one component of the EHR is unexpectedly or unknowingly affected by the state or condition of another component) (Meeks et al., 2014). They concluded that because EHR-related safety concerns have sociotechnical origins and are multifaceted, health care organizations should build a robust infrastructure to monitor and learn from them.

Numerous factors can affect the safety and effective use of health care information systems—everything from poor usability to software glitches to unexpected downtime or cyber attacks. Health care executives should be aware of these issues and vulnerabilities and ensure their organizations have in place mechanisms to prevent, detect, monitor, and address adverse events that may affect patient safety and quality of care.

SUMMARY

This chapter provided an overview of health care information systems including administrative and clinical information systems. We gave a brief history of the evolution of the use of information systems in health care. Special attention was given to the adoption, use, and features of EHR systems, patient portals, and PHR systems. We also summarized recent literature on the value of EHR systems, which may be categorized into three main areas: (1) quality, outcomes, and safety; (2) efficiency, improved revenues, and cost reduction; and (3) provider and patient satisfaction. Limitations to research findings were noted along with the need for future research. Key issues related to the use of health care information systems were discussed including interoperability, usability, and health IT safety. The chapter concludes with a discussion of a health IT safety framework that may be useful to health care leaders in preventing, detecting, and monitoring health IT–related patient safety issues.

KEY TERMS

Administrative information system

Best of breed

Clinical information systems

Computerized provider order entry (CPOE)

Electronic health record (EHR)

Health IT safety

HIMSS Analytics EMR Adoption Model (EMRAM)

Information blocking

Interoperability

Learning health systems

Mainframe computers

Microcomputer

Minicomputers

Patient portals

Personal health record (PHR)

Usability

LEARNING ACTIVITIES

1. Search the literature and find at least one article describing the adoption and use of one administrative or clinical information system. Summarize the article for your classmates and discuss it with them. What are the key points of the article? What learned lessons does it describe?

2. Visit a health care organization that uses one of the clinical applications described in this chapter. Find out how the application's value is measured or assessed. What do the providers think of it? Health care executives? Nurses? Support staff members? What impact has it had on quality? Patient safety? Efficiency? Satisfaction?

3. Conduct a literature review on interoperability in health care. What progress has been made to date? What challenges lie ahead? How do you think we may overcome these challenges?

4. Interview a CIO or health IT professional in your community regarding interoperability and health information exchange. To what extent is the organization exchanging health information electronically with others? What are the barriers and facilitators to the exchange?

5. Visit a health care organization (outside of a hospital or physician practice) to examine the types and use of information systems used. What are the major management issues related to the use of information systems in this setting? Discuss strategies for addressing these issues.

6. Interview a CMIO or other health care executive to investigate how health IT safety events are detected, monitored, and addressed in his or her organization. How does the organization's approach take into consideration the factors described in the Singh and Sittig's Health IT Safety Framework?

REFERENCES

Abramson, E. L., Edwards, A., Silver, M., & Kaushal, R. (2014). Trending health information technology adoption among New York nursing homes. *The American Journal of Managed Care, 20*(Special Issue), eSP53–eSP59.

Banger, A., & Graber, M. L. (2015). *Recent evidence that health IT improves patient safety: Issue brief.* RTI International. Retrieved July 28, 2016, from https://psnet.ahrq.gov/resources/resource/28967

Barlow, S., Johnson, J., & Steck, J. (2004). The economic effect of implementing an EMR in an outpatient clinical setting. *Journal of Healthcare Information Management, 18*(1), 46–51.

Bercovitz, A. R., Park-Lee, E., & Jamoom, E. (2013). Adoption and use of electronic health records and mobile technology by home health and hospice care agencies. *National health statistics report, no 66.* Hyattsville, MD: National Center for Health Statistics.

Bevan, N. (2001). International standards for HCI and usability. *International Journal of Human-Computer Studies, 55,* 533–552.

Blumenthal, D. (2011). Wiring the health system—origins and provisions of a new federal program: Part one of two. *New England Journal of Medicine, 365*(24), 2323–2329.

Buntin, M. B., Burke, M. F., Hoaglin, M. C., & Blumenthal, D. (2011). The benefits of health information technology: A review of the recent literature shows predominantly positive results. *Health Affairs, 30*(3), 464–471.

Burnum, J. (1989). The misinformation era: The fall of the medical record. *Annals of Internal Medicine, 110,* 482–484.

Chaudhry, B., Wang, J., Wu, S., Maglione, M., Mojica, W., Roth, E., . . . & Shekelle, P. G. (2006). Systematic review: Impact of health information technology on quality, efficiency, and costs of medical care. *Annals of Internal Medicine, 144*(10), 742–752.

Cherry, B. J., Ford, E. W., & Peterson, L. T. (2011). Experiences with electronic health records: Early adopters in long term care facilities. *Health Care Management Review, 36*(3), 265–274.

Classen, D., Resar, R., Griffin, F., Federico, F., Frankel, T, . . . & James, B. C. (2011). Global "trigger tool" shows that adverse events in hospitals may be ten times greater than previously measured. *Health Affairs, 30*(4), 581–589.

Del Beccaro, M. A., Jeffries, H. E., Eisenberg, M. A., & Harry, E. D. (2006). Computerized provider order entry implementation: No association with increased mortality rates in an intensive care unit. *Pediatrics, 118,* 290–295.

DesRoches, C. M., Campbell, E. G., Rao, S. R., Donelan, K., Ferris, T. G., Jha, A., . . . & Blumenthal, D. (2008). Electronic health records in ambulatory care: A national survey of physicians. *New England Journal of Medicine, 359*(1), 50–60.

Emont, S. (2011). *Measuring the impact of patient portals: What the literature tells us.* Oakland, CA: California HealthCare Foundation.

Ford, E. W., Hesse, B. W., & Huerta, T. R. (2016). Personal health record use in the United States: Forecasting future adoption levels. *Journal of Medical Internet Research, 18*(3), e73.

Friedberg, M. W., Chen, P. G., Van Busum, K. R., Aunon, F., Pham, C., Caloyeras, J. P. Mattke, S., Pitchforth, E., . . . & Tutty, P. (2013). *Factors affecting physician professional satisfaction and their implications for patient care, health systems, and health policy.* Santa Monica, CA: Rand Corporation. Retrieved August 3, 2016, from http://www.rand.org/pubs/research_reports/RR439.html

Glaser, J. (2015, April 14). Interoperability: A promise unfulfilled. *Hospitals and Health Networks.*

Goldzweig, C. L., Towfigh, A., Maglione, M., & Shekelle, P. G. (2009). Costs and benefits of health information technology: New trends from the literature. *Health Affairs, 28*(2), w282–w293.

Grieger, D. L., Cohen, S. H., & Krusch, D. (2007). A pilot study to document the return on investment for implementing an ambulatory electronic health record at an academic medical center. *Journal of the American College of Surgeons, 205*(1), 89–96.

Han, Y. Y., Carcillo, J. A., Venkataraman, S. T., Clark, R., Watson, R. S., Nguyen, T. C., & Orr, R. A. (2005). Unexpected increased mortality after implementation of a commercially sold computerized physician order entry system. *Pediatrics, 116*(6), 1506–1512.

Heisey-Grove, D., & Patel, V. (2015, Sept.). Any, certified or basic: Quantifying physician EHR adoption. *ONC Data Brief, No. 28.* Washington, DC: Office of the National Coordinator for Health Information Technology.

Henry, J., Pylypchuck, Y., Searcy, Y., & Patel, V. (2016, May). Adoption of electronic health record systems among US non-federal acute care hospitals: 2008–2015. *ONC Data Brief, No. 35.* Washington, DC: Office of the National Coordinator for Health Information Technology.

Hershey, C., McAloon, M., & Bertram, D. (1989). The new medical practice environment: Internists' view of the future. *Archives of Internal Medicine, 149,* 1745–1749.

HIMSS Analytics. (n.d.). *EMR adoption model (EMRAM).* Retrieved from http://www.himssanalytics.org/provider-solutions

Howley, M. J., Chou, E. Y., Hansen, N., & Dalrymple, P. W. (2014). The long-term financial impact of electronic health record implementation. *Journal of the American Medical Informatics Association, 2015*(22), 443–452. Retrieved from http://skateboardingalice.com/papers/2015_Howley.pdf

Hydari, M. Z., Telang, R., & Marella, W. M. (2014). *Saving patient Ryan: Can advanced medical records make patient care safer.* Retrieved from https://papers.ssrn.com/sol3/papers.cfm?abstract_id=2503702

IEEE. (n.d.) Interoperability. *Standards glossary.* Retrieved from http://www.ieee.org/education_careers/education/standards/standards_glossary.html#top

Institute of Medicine (IOM). (1991). *The computer based patient record: An essential technology for health care.* Washington, DC: National Academies Press.

Institute of Medicine (IOM). (2011). *Health IT and patient safety: Building safer systems for better care.* Washington, DC: National Academies Press.

James, J.T.A. (2013). A new evidence-based estimate of patient harm associated with hospital care. *Journal of Patient Safety, 9,* 122–128.

Jang, Y., Lortie, M. A., & Sanche, S. (2014). Return on investment in electronic health records in primary care practices: A mixed-methods study. *Journal of Medical Informatics, 2*(2), e25. Retrieved from http://medinform.jmir.org/2014/2/e25

Jarvis, B., Johnson, T., Butler, P., O'Shaughnessy, K., Fullam, F., Tran, L., & Gupta, R. (2013). Assessing the impact of electronic health records as an enabler of hospital quality and patient satisfaction. *Academic Medicine, 88*(10), 1471–1477.

Johnson, K. B., Patterson, B. L., Ho, Y., Chen, Q., Nian, H., Davison, C. L., Slagle, J., & Mulvaney, S. A. (2016). The feasibility of text reminders to improve medication adherence in adolescents with asthma. *The Journal of the American Medical Informatics Association, 21*(3), 449–455.

Jones, S., Rudin, R., Perry, T., & Shekelle, P. (2014). Health information technology: An updated systematic review with a focus on meaningful use. *Annals of Internal Medicine, 160,* 48–54.

Kazley, A. S., Diana, M. D., Ford, E., & Menachemi, N. (2011). Is EHR use associated with patient satisfaction in hospitals? *Health Care Management Review, 37*(1).

King, J., Patel, V., Jamoom, E. W., & Furukawa, M. F. (2014). Clinical benefits of electronic health record use: National findings. *Health Services Research, 49*(1), 392–404.

Makary, M. A., & Daniel, M. (2016, May 3). Medical error—the third leading cause of death in the US. *British Medical Journal, 353,* i2139. Retrieved August 3, 2016, from http://www.bmj.com/content/353/bmj.i213

Meeks, D. W., Smith, M. W., Taylor, L., Sittig, D. F., Scott, J. M., & Singh, H. (2014). An analysis of electronic health record-related patient safety concerns. *Journal of the American Medical Informatics Association, 21,* 1053–1059.

Menachemi, N., Powers, T, Au, D. W., & Brooks, R. G. (2010). Predictors of physician satisfaction among electronic health record system users. *Journal of Healthcare Quality, 32*(1), 35–41.

Middleton, B., Bloomrosen, M., Dente, M. A., Hashmat, B., Koppel, R., Overhage, J. M., Payne, T. H., Rosenbloom, S. T., Weaver, C., & Zhang, J. (2013, June). Enhancing patient safety and quality of care by improving the usability of electronic health record systems: Recommendations from AMIA. *Journal of the American Medical Informatics Association, 20,* e2–e8.

ONC. (2015a). *Connecting health and care for the nation: A shared nation-wide interoperability roadmap.* Final version 1.0. Retrieved July 11, 2016, from https://www.healthit.gov/policy-researchers-implementers/draft-interoperability-roadmap

ONC. (2015b). *Report to Congress on health information blocking.* Retrieved August 3, 2016, from https://www.healthit.gov/sites/default/files/reports/info_blocking_040915.pdf

Raglan, G. B., Margolis, B., Paulus, R. A., & Schulkin, J. (2014). Electronic health record adoption among obstetricians/gynecologists in the United States:

Physician practices and satisfaction. *Journal for Healthcare Quality*. Retrieved August 3, 2016, from http://onlinelibrary.wiley.com/doi/10.1111/jhq.12072/full

Rosenbloom, S.T. (2016). Personal-generated health and wellness data for health care. *Journal of the American Medical Informatics Association, 23*(3), 438–439.

Shaw, R. J., Steinberg, D. M., Bonnet, J., Modarai, F., George, A., Cunningham, T., Mason, M., Shahsahebi, M., Grambow, S. C., Bennett, G. G., & Bowsorth, H. B. (2016). Mobile health devices: Will patients actually use them? *Journal of the American Medical Informatics Association, 23*(3), 462–466.

Sittig, D. F., & Singh, H. (2011). Defining health information technology-related errors. *Archives in Internal Medicine, 171*(14), 1281–1284.

Singh, H., & Sittig, D. F. (2016). Measuring and improving patient safety through health information technology: The health IT safety framework. *BMJ Quality and Safety, 25,* 226–232.

Tang, P. C., & Lansky, D. (2005). The missing link: Bridging the patient-provider health information gap. *Health Affairs, 24*(5), 1290–1295.

Whitten, J., & Bentley, L. (2007). *Systems analysis and design methods* (7th ed.). New York, NY: McGraw-Hill/Irvin.

CHAPTER 4

Information Systems to Support Population Health Management

LEARNING OBJECTIVES

- To be able to understand the data and information needs of health systems in managing population health effectively under value-based payment models.

- To be able to discuss key health IT tools and strategies for population health management including EHRs, registries, risk stratification, patient engagement, and outreach, care coordination and management, analytics, health information exchange, and telemedicine and telehealth.

- To be able to discuss the application and use of data analytics to monitor, predict, and improve performance.

The enactment of the Affordable Care Act (ACA) brought about sweeping legislation intended to reduce the numbers of uninsured and make health care accessible to all Americans. It also ushered in an era in which changing reimbursement and care delivery models are driving providers from the current fragmented system focused on volume-based services to an outcomes orientation. As a result, the health care system now taking shape is one in which value-based payment models financially reward patient-centered, coordinated, accountable care.

Against this backdrop, providers' increasing use of evidence-based medicine and growing capabilities in managing volumes of clinical evidence through sophisticated health IT systems will mean that treatments can be tailored for the individual and interventions can be made earlier to keep patients well. Furthermore, **patient engagement** is fast becoming a critical component in the care process, particularly in the area of **population health management (PHM).**

Health care providers' interest in improving population health appears to be increasing because of the sudden ubiquity of the phrase, because many are participating in **accountable care organizations (ACOs),** and because even hospitals not participating in an ACO increasingly have incentives to reduce their number of potentially unavoidable admissions, readmissions, and emergency department visits (Casalino, Erb, Joshi, & Shortell, 2015).

In this chapter we'll not only seek a common understanding of PHM but also explore how the advent of shared accountability financial arrangements between providers and purchasers of care has created significant focus on PHM. We'll also review the core processes associated with accountable care and examine the strategic IT investments and data management capabilities required to support population health management and enable a successful transition from volume-based to **value-based care.**

PHM: KEY TO SUCCESS

Although the ACO model is still new and evolving, approximately 750 ACOs are in operation today, covering some 23.5 million lives under Medicare, Medicaid, and private insurers. Although not all ACOs have demonstrated success in delivering better health outcomes at a lower cost, many have achieved promising results (Houston & McGinnis, 2016). As such, significant ACO growth is expected. In fact, it is predicted that upward of 105 million people will be covered by an ACO by 2020 (Leavitt Partners, 2015).

Similarly, although the industry's move to value-based payment is also in its early stages, value-based contracts are expected to substantially increase throughout the next decade. CMS has a stated goal that 50 percent of Medicare payments will be tied to alternative payment models by the end of 2018 (US DHHS, 2015). In fact, the projected impact of MACRA, which we discussed in Chapter One, on the adoption of value-based payment models is expected to rival the impact of Meaningful Use on adoption of EHRs. In addition, the substantial payment reform activity at the federal level is paralleled by private insurers' efforts to support value-based payment and new models of care. For example, Aetna expects that 75 percent of its contracts will be value-based by 2020 (Jaspen, 2015).

These trends will accelerate the demand for services and technology that enable health systems and other organizations (health plans, Medicaid, community-based organizations, employers, and so forth) to jointly manage the health and care of populations—either as an ACO or in an ACO-like fashion. Although diverse, these organizations will all have a common need to improve operational efficiency, drive better patient outcomes while reducing the overall cost of care, and effectively engage consumers in managing their health and care.

Although the new reimbursement system is still taking shape, it's clear that population health management will become a required core competency for provider organizations in a post fee-for-service payment environment (Institute for Health Technology Transformation, 2012).

Understanding Population Health Management

Population health as a concept first appeared in 2003 when David Kindig and Greg Stoddart (2003) defined it as "the health outcomes of a group of individuals, including the distribution of such outcomes within the group" (p. 380).

It is important to note that medical care is only one of many factors that affect those outcomes. Other factors include public health interventions; aspects of the social environment (income, education, employment, social support, and culture); the physical environment (urban design, clean air and water); genetics; and individual behavior (Institute for Health Technology Transformation, 2012). "Improving the health of populations" was later identified as one element in the Institute for Healthcare Improvement's triple aim for improving the US health care system, along with improving the individual experience of care and reducing the per capita cost of care (Berwick, Nolan & Whittington, 2008, p. 759).

Today, *population health management* comprises the proactive application of strategies and interventions to defined groups of individuals (e.g., diabetics, cancer patients with tumor regrowth, the elderly with multiple comorbidities) to improve the health of individuals within the group at the lowest cost. PHM interventions are designed to maintain and improve people's health across the full continuum of care—from low-risk, healthy individuals to high-risk individuals with one or more chronic conditions (Felt-Lisk & Higgins, 2011). PHM also seeks to minimize the need for expensive encounters with the health care system, such as emergency department visits, hospitalizations, imaging tests, and procedures. This not only lowers costs but also redefines health care as an activity that encompasses far more than sick care, because it systematically addresses the preventative and chronic care needs of every patient—not just high-risk patients who generate the majority of health care costs (Institute for Health Technology Transformation, 2012).

Although population health can also mean the health of the entire population in a geographic area, the population health efforts most health systems and ACOs are undertaking are aimed at providing better preventive and medical care for the "population" of patients "attributed" to their organizations by Medicare, Medicaid, or private health insurers (Casalino et al., 2015).

New Care Delivery and Payment Models: The Link to PHM

As we know, historically, there has been a lack of accountability for the total care of patients, the outcomes of their treatment, and the efficiency with which health resources are used. The fact that health care services are paid primarily on a fee-for-service basis has contributed to the fragmentation and lack of accountability. *Fee-for-service* emphasizes the provision of health services by individual hospitals or providers rather than care that is coordinated across providers to address the patient's needs. Providers are rewarded for volume and for conducting procedures that are often more complex, when simpler, lower-cost, better methods may be more appropriate (Guterman & Drake, 2010).

Value-based care is emerging as a solution to address rising health care costs, clinical inefficiency and duplication of services, and to make it easier for people to get the appropriate care they need. As the federal government continues to test and implement several new payment models designed to achieve optimal health outcomes at a sustainable cost, commercial insurers are also partnering with health care providers in various arrangements that similarly seek to reward value rather than volume of services.

As discussed in Chapter One, two popular models of delivery system reform are the **patient-centered medical home (PCMH)** and the ACO. The PCMH emphasizes the central role of primary care and care coordination, with the vision that every person should have the opportunity to easily access high-quality primary care in a place that is familiar and knowledgeable about his or her health care needs and choices. The ACO emphasizes the urgent need to think beyond patients to populations, providing a vision for increased accountability for performance and spending across the health care system (Patient-Centered Primary Care Collaborative, 2011). Both models rely on health care organizations and physicians providing coordinated and integrated care in an evidence-based, cost-effective way. This, of course, has significant implications for an organization's ability to manage information effectively.

In conjunction with new models of care are new or modified forms of payment for health care services, which are being piloted in various communities around the nation. These include bundled payments, pay for performance, shared savings programs, capitation or global payment, and episode-of-care payments.

Bundled payments may take different forms such as making a single payment for hospital and physician services instead of separate payments, bundling payments for inpatient and post-acute care, or paying based on diagnosis instead of treatment. Bundled payments are often applied to surgical procedures such as hip replacements. Pay-for-performance (P4P) programs reward hospitals, physician practices, and other providers with financial and nonfinancial incentives based on performance on select measures. These performance measures can cover various aspects of health care delivery: clinical quality and safety, efficiency, patient experience, and health information technology adoption. Most P4P programs, however, are still a bonus to a fee-for-service model (Miller, 2011). An integral part of the ACA, shared savings programs are intended to reward providers by paying them a bonus that is explicitly connected to the amount by which they reduce the total cost of care compared to expected levels. Capitation or global payment places full risk with the provider organization; the provider is responsible for the costs of all care that a patient receives. An episode-of-care payment system would pay the provider organization a single payment for all of the services associated with a hospitalization or other episode of acute care, such as a heart attack, including inpatient and post-acute care (Miller, 2011).

The revised payments associated with these programs signal the federal government's most all-encompassing effort thus far to distribute risk and hold providers financially accountable for the quality of care they deliver. Although an in-depth discussion of these and other proposed payment reform systems is beyond the scope of this book, the following resources can provide a wealth of detailed information on health care payment reform initiatives:

- Centers for Medicaid & Medicare Services (www.CMS.gov)
- Healthcare Financial Management Association (www.hfma.org)
- American College of Healthcare Executives (www.ache.org)

Progress to Date: PCMHs

Growing support for the PCMH has arisen across the vast majority of the US health care delivery system to include commercial insurance plans, multiple employers, state Medicaid programs, numerous federal agencies, the Department of Defense, hundreds of safety net clinics, and thousands of small and large clinical practices nationwide (Grundy, Hacker, Langner, Nielsen, & Zema, 2012). Private and public payer initiatives together have grown from eighteen states in 2009 to forty-four states in 2013, and they now cover almost twenty-one million patients. These heterogeneous initiatives overall are becoming larger, paying higher fees, and engaging in more risk sharing with practices (NCQA, 2015).

Because the patient-centered medical home is foundational to ACOs—with ACOs often described as the "medical neighborhood"—the PCMH is likely to gain even greater prominence as ACOs continue to develop in the marketplace (Grundy et al., 2012). Moreover, a growing body of scientific evidence shows that PCMHs are saving money by reducing hospital and emergency department visits, mitigating health disparities, and improving patient outcomes. Examples of specific outcomes achieved by various PCMHs include the following:

- Lower Medicare spending
- More effective care management and optimized use of health care services
- Improved care management and preventative screenings for cardiovascular and diabetes patients
- Reduced socioeconomic disparities in cancer screening (NCQA, 2015)

Additionally, more than nine thousand primary care practices and forty-three thousand clinicians (doctors and nurse practitioners) across the country have earned the PCMH designation from the National Committee for Quality Assurance (NCQA), the nation's largest credentialing organization. The designation is earned by demonstrating achievement of goals related to accessible, coordinated, and patient-centered care (Olivero, 2015).

Progress to Date: ACOs

In the value-based care world, ACOs are expected to play a leadership role in improving population health—whether participating in contracts with Medicare, Medicaid, or managed care organizations (MCOs) or health plans. These arrangements are often complex and may differ widely, including elements such as governance requirements, payment structures, quality metrics, reporting requirements, and data sharing (Houston & McGinnis, 2016).

Several different ACO models, including the Pioneer ACO program and the Medicare Shared Savings Program (MSSP), are testing and evaluating various risk-sharing agreements. In December 2011, CMS signed agreements with thirty-two organizations to participate in the Pioneer ACO model, designed to show how particular ACO payment arrangements can best improve care and generate savings for Medicare. As of May 1, 2016, there are nine Pioneer ACOs participating in the model for a fifth and final performance year (CY2016). The MSSP is a key component of the Medicare delivery system reform initiatives included in the Affordable Care Act and is designed to facilitate coordination and cooperation among providers to improve the quality of care for Medicare fee-for-service (FFS) beneficiaries and reduce unnecessary costs. Eligible providers, hospitals, and suppliers may participate in the MSSP by creating or participating in an ACO.

Although there has been considerable debate among policymakers as to the success of the ACO model, some of these ACOs are already reporting positive results for improving patient outcomes and controlling costs, as shown in Table 4.1 (Houston & McGinnis, 2016).

ACO Challenges

Now with years of observation and learnings to draw from, several key challenges facing ACOs have been identified, including difficulties working across organizational boundaries, building the requisite infrastructure for effective data sharing, and truly engaging patients in the care process. One of the more notable challenges currently being worked on is the alignment and consolidation of myriad quality measures being used in public and private programs.

Effective quality measures are imperative to accountability in organized systems of care, especially when performance affects the ability of the provider to share in savings or determines whether a provider avoids penalties or receives bonus payments (Bipartisan Policy Center, 2015). However, the notion of "measurement fatigue" and the increasing administrative burden it places on providers is a legitimate concern (Buelt, Nichols, Nielsen, & Patel, 2016). Another challenge with quality metrics is that although they tend to capture performance on specific outcomes, such as lower avoidable readmissions, or processes, such as screening for depression, they may not accurately measure the overall health of the patient, making it difficult to assess the true impact and efficacy of ACO arrangements (Houston & McGinnis, 2016).

Table 4.1 Key attributes and broad results of current ACO models

Attribute	Medicare		Commercial ACOs	Medicaid ACOs
	MSSP	Pioneer ACO		
ACO prevalence	333 ACOs in 47 states	18 ACOs in 8 states	528 commercial contracts	66 ACOs in 9 active state-based programs
Key model features	Shared savings payment methodology 33 quality metrics	Designed for large hospital systems Shared savings system with higher risk and reward potential than MSSP Same 33 quality metrics as MSSP	Often independent contracts between ACOs and MCOs Many feature narrow provider networks.	Various approaches to payment including shared savings and capitation Various approaches to quality measurement
Results to date	CMS has reported results for different cohorts of MSSP ACOs based on start date, which have shown significant savings, but it is difficult to aggregate these results, though only 26% of ACOs received shared savings payments ACOs consistently improved on 27 of 33 quality metrics. Increases in patient satisfaction relative to patients not enrolled in ACOs	$304 million in savings over three years ACOS consistently improved on 28 of 33 quality metrics. Increases in patient satisfaction relative to patients not enrolled in ACOs Began with 32 participants; 14 have left program	Not many publicly reported results available across programs due to proprietary information and difficulty comparing results	CO, MN, and VT have collectively reported $129.9 million in savings. ED visits in OR decreased by 22%.

Source: R. Houston and T. McGinnis. January 2016. "Accountable Care Organizations: Looking Back and Moving Forward." Center for Health Care Strategies. Used with permission.

Implications for Health Care Leaders

Through the combination of changing health care business models and payment mechanisms, we are witnessing transformational change in the nature of health care delivery. It is evolving from one of reactive care with fragmented accountability and a dependence on full beds to a model of health management, care that extends over time and place and rewards for efficiency and quality. This transformation poses potent challenges for providers and has enormous implications for today's health care leaders, particularly by placing greater emphasis on these issues:

- Keeping patients well and managing and preventing disease
- Establishing more efficient organization and utilization of care teams and venues of care
- Creating a care culture that is comfortable with change and ongoing automation
- Engaging patients in managing their care and overall health
- Ensuring the most cost-effective care is provided and that clinical processes are streamlined and follow the best evidence

More specifically, accountable care and the move to population health management will require industry perspectives and health care delivery practices to shift from

- Care providers working independently to collaborative teams of providers
- Treating individuals when they get sick to keeping groups of people healthy
- Emphasizing volumes to emphasizing outcomes
- Maximizing the use of resources and assets to applying appropriate levels of care at the right place
- Offering care at centralized facilities to providing care at sites convenient to patients
- Treating all patients the same to customizing health care for each patient
- Avoiding the sickest chronically ill patients to providing special chronic care services
- Being responsible for those who seek services to being responsible for the needs of the community
- Putting forth best efforts to becoming high-reliability organizations (Glaser, 2012b)

Additionally, accountability will bring new performance and utilization risks to providers as the focus shifts from optimizing business unit performance to optimizing network performance. At the same time, instead of maximizing the profitability of care, organizations will increase the volume of desired bundled episodes while controlling costs. At an operational level, organizations must change their structure as well as workflows to implement PHM and adopt new types of automation tools and reporting. This will require setting clear goals, the active participation of leadership—including physician leaders, an assessment of technology requirements, and an effective rollout strategy (Institute for Health Technology Transformation, 2012).

Health IT clearly plays a vital role in the success of new models of care and payment reform and should be an integral part of the organization's planning process. Whether participating in an ACO or not, all health care organizations should be thinking about building a population health management strategy and addressing related gaps in their information technology (IT) capabilities. Minimally, this would include acquiring the capabilities and tools to do the following:

- Know, characterize, and predict the health trajectory that will happen within a population.
- Engage members, families, and care providers to take action.
- Manage outcomes to improve health and care.

ACCOUNTABLE CARE CORE PROCESSES

Accountable care frameworks are based on risk and reward, with providers and organizations agreeing to share the financial risk for a population in return for the opportunity to access rewards on meeting health care quality and cost goals. ACOs are responsible for tracking and measuring specific quality metrics to indicate that patient outcomes are improving or evidence-based processes are being used. Some, but not necessarily all, metrics may be tied directly to the payment methodology, meaning that performance on these metrics will trigger either a quality incentive (such as an increased percentage of shared savings) or a disincentive (such as not receiving any shared savings) (Houston & McGinnis, 2016).

To accomplish the goals of PHM, a provider must deliver proactive preventive and chronic care to its attributed patient population. As such, the care team must maintain regular contact with patients and support their efforts to manage their own health. At the same time, care managers must closely monitor high-risk patients to prevent them from deteriorating or developing complications. The use of evidence-based protocols to diagnose and treat patients in a consistent, cost-effective manner is also central to PHM efforts. In many respects, success in population health management depends largely on a provider's ability to manage several core processes in an accountable care environment. We'll review these core processes in the next sections.

Identifying, Assessing, Stratifying, and Selecting Target Populations

To manage population health effectively, an organization must be able to track and monitor the health of individual patients, while also stratifying its population into subgroups that require particular services at specified intervals. ACOs typically *stratify* their patient population by common care needs, conditions, and expenditure levels and then deploy tailored interventions based on these characteristics (Houston & McGinnis, 2016). For example, a high-risk pregnancy may require more frequent interventions (office visits, fetal heart monitoring, etc.) than standard prenatal care warrants.

Stratification also involves the ability to identify a patient or cohort at risk for a negative health event (e.g., myocardial infarction, stroke, mental health crisis) or preventable health care utilization (e.g., surgical procedure or hospitalization) (Gibson, Hunt, Knudson, Powell, Whittington, & Wozney, 2015). The Agency for Healthcare Research and Quality (AHRQ) describes another method of stratification as being able to identify subpopulations of patients who might benefit from additional services. Examples of these groups include patients needing reminders for preventive care or tests, patients overdue for care or not meeting management goals, patients who have failed to receive follow-up after being sent reminders, and patients who might benefit from discussion of risk reduction (Institute for Health Technology Transformation, 2012).

Although there are numerous ways to identify and segment patients, having the ability to identify risk, alert appropriate stakeholders, and intervene in the care process at the right time is a key component of population health management.

Providing High-Quality Care and Care Management Interventions across the Continuum

A key tenet of accountable care is to ensure that the health and wellness of a population is managed, the most cost-effective care is provided, clinical processes are streamlined and follow the best evidence, the necessary reporting is in place, and payments and reimbursement are appropriate. Although this is an obvious goal for all providers, ACOs must facilitate cross-continuum medical management of patients for active episodes and acute disease processes or for any patient outside of the defined goals of a target population. An ACO must demonstrate, in a variety of ways, its commitment to being patient centered and to engaging patients in their care and overall health.

To effectively care for populations, **care management** involves the patient-centered management and coordination of care events and activities in multiple care settings by one or more providers (e.g., fine-tuning coordination among care team members, identifying care gaps and situations requiring additional interventions, as well as managing care transitions). For example, research indicates that poorly executed transitions of care between different locations (e.g., from hospital to primary care) are associated with increased risks of adverse medication events, hospital readmissions, and higher health care costs. Determining which transitions present the greatest risks and targeting care management services to patients undergoing those transitions should conserve resources and lead to better cost and quality outcomes (AHRQ, 2015).

Additionally, lack of follow-up care after hospital discharge can result in complications, worsening of patients' conditions, and a higher chance of readmission (Nielsen & Shaljian, 2013). Therefore, another example of a care management intervention is ensuring that hospitals notify primary care practices when patients are discharged and that primary care teams follow up with patients shortly thereafter.

The overall aim of *care management* is to manage the most complex patients through the health care system, as well as managing the overall health of a select population (e.g., diabetics and elderly), taking their preferences and overall situation into consideration. Care management ensures that all patients from the lowest risk level to high-risk "super users" receive care at the right time, in the right place, and in a manner best suited for the patient. This requires proactive care, communication, education, and outreach.

Managing Contracts and Financial Performance

Under new payment models, proactively understanding patient coverage and financial responsibility will be more critical than ever. Financial teams must have a solid handle on estimating reimbursement and associated payment distributions, carrying out predictive modeling for reimbursement contracts, measuring performance against contracts and predicting profitability, as well as integrating with other key processes to share information.

For example, profit maximization under a shared savings-risk model requires a shift away from revenue-focused strategies to cost-containment strategies (Houston & McGinnis, 2016). To effectively manage costs, health care executives will need tools and data to support different types of financial modeling, such as modeling the implications of moving patient care to settings other than the hospital or physician's office. ACOs will also need actuarial cost and utilization predictors to effectively manage the care of a defined population.

These changes represent a significant cultural shift for provider organizations that must be prepared to handle a complex mix of public and private sector payment mechanisms.

Measuring, Predicting, and Improving Performance

Data analytics is an integral part of PHM. ACOs typically measure quality and outcomes data against national guidelines or peer groups, and they seek to demonstrate longitudinal improvements. They might also measure costs, utilization, and patient experience on a population-wide basis, and they may use these reports as the basis for quality reporting to payers and other outside entities.

With payment so tightly linked to quality and outcomes, predicting, monitoring, and measuring system performance in key areas becomes paramount in an accountable care environment. Under value-based payment programs, there will be real ramifications for poor care and rewards for improved care. In fact, even low-performing areas can qualify for high payments if they demonstrate year-over-year improvement.

Therefore, providers must have the ability to forecast which patients are likely to become high-risk so they can intervene before a patient's condition worsens. They must also understand in real time if they are complying with a certain set of measures and monitor their continual performance. For example, ACOs will want to measure the effectiveness of care protocols, such as exercise compliance, for a population of diabetic patients. Surgical services providers will need to understand the costs and quality of proposed procedure bundles. Understanding what works and what does not is key to ensuring reimbursements, controlling costs, and, most important, providing the best care for patients (Glaser, 2012a).

Equally important is retrospective monitoring—finding out what didn't happen and why. For example, if a care provider failed to respond to an alert in a timely fashion or deviated from a given standard of care process, they can use these data to determine if new care interventions are necessary or if they need to alter an individual's plan of care. Likewise, knowing that a patient failed to keep an appointment or was unexpectedly seen in the emergency room will enable the care team to engage patients in new ways to better manage chronic disease. With providers facing penalties for readmission, it will be more important than ever to understand if it's the treatment that failed, the discharge plan that failed, or the patient who did not follow through on the post-discharge plan (Chopra & Glaser, 2013).

Preparation and Automation Is Key

Overall, the accountable care movement demands that providers be more focused and aggressive in managing their organization and their patients. Among other challenges, changes in reimbursement will require providers to predict which patients will need extra care, more intensively engage and manage high-risk patients, model the financial implications of delivering sub-par care, assess the performance of core organizational processes such as transitions of care, determine conformance to medical evidence, and report quality measures to purchasers of care.

The long-term success of the transition to value-based payment models and PHM relies largely on health care providers investing in the IT tools and infrastructure—as well as acquiring the data management and analysis expertise—needed to automate and support these core processes. In addition, as with any IT endeavor, expertise in change management and workflow redesign is also a core requirement.

Even for providers that may not be participating in an ACO, building the organizational and IT competencies to support accountable care is critical to staying competitive. Organizations that fail to develop and demonstrate accountable care capabilities may not fulfill their obligations to the community they serve—in fact, they may not survive.

Yet, organizations embracing the transformation from traditional fee-for-service to value-based PHM are finding significant gaps in their IT capabilities (Gibson et al., 2015). In the following section we examine the core IT building blocks and capabilities necessary to support accountable care and the move to PHM.

DATA, ANALYTICS, AND HEALTH IT CAPABILITIES AND TOOLS

As more providers and health systems evolve into ACOs, they are becoming increasingly aware of what it takes to manage care from a population health perspective. As we know, this includes establishing new partner networks, targeting populations, aligning providers and contracts, developing cross-continuum protocols for care management, and enabling efficient data sharing.

It's All about the Data

For a PHM program to be effective there is a critical need to focus on the data and information that will increasingly power clinical decisions. This includes aggregating and normalizing clinical data, claims data, administrative data, and self-reported patient data to create a holistic view of the patients within a health care network. These data enable the network to identify populations of patients whose conditions can be managed through evidence-based care plans that are coordinated across care settings.

For example, the risk of progression from glucose intolerance to diabetes mellitus can be influenced by diet and exercise. Individuals within this "rising risk" population are at different stages of readiness to change and consequently at different stages of modifiable risk. Having this insight enables providers to offer services at the appropriate level and time (AHRQ, 2015).

However, for many organizations, obtaining population health data can be difficult because it must be collected and organized from many disparate sources (e.g., laboratory information systems, EHRs, practice management systems, and home-monitoring devices). Data types that require aggregation and normalization include labs, radiology reports, medications, vital signs, diagnoses, demographic information, and more. Returning to our diabetes example, although a diabetic's blood glucose result is discrete data that can be found in an EHR, the results of the same patient's foot or eye exam may be found only in text format within a practice management system.

Data management for PHM purposes is also challenging because there's no guarantee the various IT systems talk to each other, and each provider and health plan may have a different system for patient identification and provider attribution. An important first step in connecting patient data across different care settings is to establish master patient indices (Glaser & Salzberg, 2011). Patient indices can serve as a crosswalk among the different medical record numbers and identifiers that may be used by various provider organizations to correctly identify patients. In addition, a record locator service may be used to determine which patient records exist for a member and where the source data is located. The key concept behind having a record locator service is that a patient's health information is housed on computers at the various sites of his or her care and this information is queried and aggregated from these sites at the time of a request.

Beyond the EHR: Core PHM Solution Components

Although a certified EHR certainly provides the necessary foundation for effectively responding to new payment models, population health requires a range of IT applications, PHM solution components, and analytical capabilities. In fact, early adopters of PHM solutions are already seeing the need for next-generation capabilities to support the following transitions:

- From management of the sickest patients to management of all patients
- Static risk categorization to risk categorization that follows a patient's evolving risk
- Focus on a single disease or condition based on simple data values and events to a focus on multi-disease or condition using evidence-based care plans
- "List" generation with significant manual work for care managers to significant process automation
- Loosely connected care "actors" to a care team that includes the patient and family
- Retrospective analysis to concurrent analysis (Glaser, 2016a)

As organizations look to enhance their population health management strategies, they should make investments that enable the IT platform to do the following:

- Collect data from multiple, disparate sources in near–real time, including any EHR, devices used in the home and at work, and other data sources, such as pharmacy benefit managers or insurance claims.
- Support organizations in not only aggregating but also transforming and reconciling data to establish a longitudinal record for each individual within a population.
- Identify and stratify populations to pinpoint gaps in care, enabling providers to act on information and match the right care programs to the right individuals (Glaser, 2016a).

In addition to having an EHR that spans the continuum of care, providers pursuing PHM might invest in a PHM platform that sits above the EHR and other sources of data and must be EHR agnostic. In general, the following key technologies will enable the core accountable care processes.

Revenue Cycle Systems and Contract Management Applications

One could argue that the *revenue cycle system* forms the foundation of a provider's response to accountable care and payment reform. As the reimbursement environment becomes more complex, revenue cycle systems must evolve to support payments based on quality and performance, requiring new capabilities such as these:

- Aggregating charges to form bundles and episodes, with the aggregation logic enabling different groupings for different payers
- Managing the distribution of payment for a bundle to the physicians, hospitals, and non-acute facilities that delivered the care
- Streamlining transitions between disparate reimbursement methodologies and contracts when billing and collecting
- Providing tools for retrospective analysis of clinical and administrative data to identify areas for improving the quality of care and reducing the cost of care delivered

These new capabilities must complement routine activities such as registering patients, scheduling appointments, and administering patient billing.

Care Management Systems

Used by care managers and discussed previously, *care management systems* enable proactive surveillance, automation, coordination, and facilitation of services for many different subpopulations across the care continuum. Specific capabilities might include helping to facilitate transitions of care more efficiently, use of automated campaigns (e-mail, text, phone) to better manage high-risk patients, and supporting care teams in delivering evidence-based interventions to reduce high-cost utilization.

According to time-motion studies published in the journal *Population Health Management* by Prevea Health, automation of routine care management tasks enables care managers to manage two to three times as many patients as they can with manual methods (Handmaker & Hart, 2015).

Rules Engines and Workflow Engines

Processes that are efficient, predictable, and robust enable an organization to thrive in an accountable care environment. *Workflow and rules engines* can monitor process performance, alerting staff members to missed steps, sequence issues, or delays.

Workflow engines specialize in executing a business process, not just decisions made at a discrete point in time. The technology can greatly assist in clinical decision making by not only presenting clinicians with alerts and reminders, such as a rules engine, but also by encouraging teamwork in clinical decisions, assisting with the time management and task allocation in process delivery, stating changes in patient or operational conditions, and creating behind-the-scenes automation of process steps.

In a value-based purchasing world where each core measure needs to be associated with what's happening today, performance improvement interventions must occur in real time—that is, while the patient is still in the acute care cycle. Therefore, sophisticated IT tools such as workflow and rules engines that push information to the front lines, guiding decisions at the point of highest possible impact, will be required.

Data Warehouse, Analytics, and Business Intelligence

Analytics will facilitate proactive management of key performance metrics, because accountable care creates a greater need to assess care quality and costs, examine variations in practice, and compare outcomes.

An *enterprise data warehouse* will fuel a wide range of analytic needs and provide intelligence to enable continual care process improvement initiatives. For example, it will be imperative that an organization can compare a hypertensive patient's total cost of care relative to its peers and national benchmarks, and perhaps even more important, predict if those costs will significantly increase because of comorbidities, complications, or gaps in care.

Applied to the data in registries or warehouses, predictive analytics tools can also help caregivers identify patients who are likely to present in the ER or be readmitted so they can tailor appropriate interventions and avoid penalties for excessive readmissions.

Although most providers lack experience with the tools and techniques associated with advanced data analysis, the application of **business intelligence (BI)** in health care will become the platform on which the organization not only monitors performance but also makes critical decisions to uncover new revenue opportunities, reduce costs, reallocate resources, and improve care quality and operational efficiency. Thus, enhancing an organization's competency in data analytics and BI will become essential for success in population health management.

Health Information Exchange (HIE)

Essential to successful implementation of new models of care and payment reform is the exchange of clinical and administration information among different health care entities and between providers and patients. Although there has been some success in the regional **health information exchange (HIE)** movement, much of the focus now is on HIE capabilities at the integrated delivery system or ACO level. This enables providers to obtain a composite clinical picture of the patient regardless of where that patient was seen. By participating in an HIE or sharing health information, a number of potential important benefits may be realized:

- Serves as a building block for improved patient care, quality, and safety
- Makes relevant health care information readily available when and where it is needed
- Provides the means to reduce duplication of services that can lead to reduced health care costs
- Enables automation of administrative tasks
- Provides governance and management over the data exchange process
- Facilitates achievement of meaningful use requirements (HIMSS, 2010)

The concept of HIE is not new. For nearly two decades organizations and collaborators have tried to facilitate HIE, but unfortunately a number of HIE initiatives have failed to be sustainable over the long term (Vest & Gamm, 2010). The HITECH Act placed renewed interest in the success of HIE by providing incentive payments to eligible providers for Meaningful Use of electronic health records, which includes having the ability to exchange information electronically with others in order to have a comprehensive view of the patient's health and care (Rudin, Salzberg, Szolovitis, Volk, Simon, & Bates, 2011). However, despite investment at the national, state, and local levels, the increase in HIE utilization remains modest.

In fact, a recent survey of organizations facilitating health information exchange found that 30 percent of hospitals and 10 percent of ambulatory practices now participate in one of the 119 operational health information exchange efforts across the United States (Adler-Milstein, Bates, & Jha, 2013). Although this is substantial growth from prior surveys, the researchers also found that 74 percent of HIE efforts report struggling to develop a sustainable business model. These findings suggest that despite progress, there is a substantial risk that many current efforts to promote health information exchange will fail when public funds supporting these initiatives are depleted. Adding to the challenge, HIE efforts have struggled to engage payers,

Figure 4.1 Percent of nonfederal acute care hospitals that electronically exchanged laboratory results, radiology reports, clinical care summaries, or medication lists with ambulatory care providers or hospitals outside their organization: 2008–2015

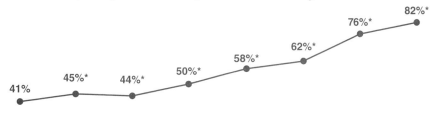

| 2008 | 2009 | 2010 | 2011 | 2012 | 2013 | 2014 | 2015 |

Source: Henry, Patel, Pylypchuk, and Searcy (2016).

and only 40 percent of HIE efforts in the country have one or more payers providing financial support (Adler-Milstein, Cross, & Lin, 2016).

Still, there is reason to remain optimistic, with more recent data showing that hospitals' rates of electronically exchanging laboratory results, radiology reports, clinical care summaries, or medication lists with ambulatory care providers or hospitals outside their organization has doubled since 2008 (see Figure 4.1). Moreover, this exchange has significantly increased annually since 2011 (Henry, Patel, Pylypchuk, & Searcy, 2016).

Although there is still significant progress to be made to improve the use of exchanged information and to address barriers to interoperability, HIE is critically important to the success of care transformation efforts nationwide. Thus, the industry must continue its efforts toward achieving sustainable HIE approaches to ensure that the massive national investment in health IT throughout the past decade delivers its intended return—higher-quality care, improved outcomes, and lower cost.

Registries and Scorecards

Serving as a kind of central database for PHM, registries can be used for patient monitoring, care gap assessment, point-of-care reminders, care management, and public health and quality reporting, among other uses. By integrating clinical, financial, and operational data across disparate sources into a single chronic condition and wellness registry solution, data can be normalized and turned into meaningful, actionable information.

For example, registries and scorecards enable providers to identify, score, and predict risks of individuals or populations to allow targeted interventions to be implemented. When applied to a population, the registry can show, for example, how all of a particular provider's patients with type 2 diabetes are doing, which diabetic patients are out of control, or how well an entire organization is treating patients with that condition (Nielsen & Shaljian, 2013).

Longitudinal Record and Care Plan

As we know, even if a provider is diligently capturing patient information in an EHR, the data are valuable only in the world of collaborative, accountable care if the information can be integrated with patient data from other sources and harmonized to produce a single, consolidated record at the member level. The longitudinal record presents a complete picture of the patient's medical history in an organized, coherent view.

Serving as the sister solution to the longitudinal record, a longitudinal care plan provides a consolidated, normalized view of indicators to be monitored, events due to happen, and actions to be taken to ensure that a patient maintains and improves his or her level of health.

Patient Engagement Tools

Medical interventions that occur solely through office-based patient-provider interactions will no longer provide the level of monitoring and scrutiny needed to manage the health of individuals and populations. As such, providers must continue to harness the power of technology to engage patients in their care via tools such as home-monitoring devices, patient portals, and personal health records (PHRs), as well as through the use of social media, texting, and e-mail.

Portals and PHRs

Although patient portal use is still considered modest at best, given later-stage meaningful-use requirements and the anticipated benefits of patient engagement in the value-based care world, many providers are ramping up their portal efforts and seeing adoption rates well above 20 percent (Buckley, 2015). Another recent study predicts that PHR adoption will exceed 75 percent by 2020, an optimistic projection that outpaces the PHR goals set under the Meaningful Use incentive program (Ford, Hesse, & Huerta, 2016). These consumer-centric technologies are designed to help patients and consumers better manage their own health and care, securely communicate with providers, pay bills, obtain test results, view doctors' notes, refill prescriptions, schedule appointments, and so on.

Despite the fact that the environment for building, creating, and developing an HIE organization has never been better, the concerns about long-term sustainability and the impact and value of exchanging health information persist. The National eHealth Collaborative (NeHC) conducted a comprehensive study of twelve fully operationally HIEs across the nation to find out from their leaders what factors have led to their success (NeHC, 2011). In-depth structured interviews were conducted with senior executives representing the business, clinical, and technical areas of each HIE. The key critical success factors these leaders identified in sustaining an HIE are as follows:

- Aligning stakeholders with HIE priorities in an intensive and ongoing effort. Create a shared vision that all stakeholders can embrace and that serves as the cornerstone to success. Foster an environment that is built on trust and that promotes learning and resolves differences when they arise. Make ongoing and effective stakeholder engagement a priority.
- Establishing and maintaining consistent brand identity and role as a trusted, neutral entity dedicated to protecting the interests of participants. Data use and data integrity are two critical elements. The culture, policies, and procedures regarding the use of data must ensure that no entity will gain competitive advantage at the expense of others. Consent and security policies must meet the requirements of various stakeholders and regions or

Some patient portals and PHRs are integrated into a provider's existing website, and others are extensions of the organization's EHR system. For example, New York-Presbyterian (NYP) Hospital's award-winning patient portal, myNYP.org, was built to expand on its existing EHR. Use of the portal led to a 42 percent increase of appointments scheduled using myNYP.org, and it lowered the no-show rated from 20 percent to 12 percent over a period of six months after it was made available in January 2012 (Glaser, 2013). Additional applications of the same appointment-alert technology can provide customized patient education material and personalized reminders to patients who fit a specific clinical profile, such as patients who missed an immunization.

Social Media

Additionally, with one-third of consumers using online forums and social media sites such as Facebook, Twitter, and YouTube for health-related matters states. The HIE infrastructure must ensure that patient data are accurate, reliable, and trustworthy.

- Ensuring alignment with vision in making strategic choices. Assess the stakeholders' alignment with the initiative and congruence with the vision before deciding to pursue them. Regardless of how promising a source of funding may have initially appeared, some HIEs chose not to pursue it because the funding source did not have the full support of all stakeholders.

- Considering structural characteristics and dynamics of the HIE market. The geographic location, composition of stakeholders, and resource capabilities are all factors to consider.

- Understanding clinical workflow and managing change. The implementation of an HIE requires that clinicians and administrative staff members understand the impact of HIE applications on workflow and identify opportunities to improve efficiencies.

Different business models, governance structures, and strategies may be used to create value for the HIE participants.

Source: NeHC (2011).

(PwC, 2012), many providers are actively engaged in using social media to communicate with patients and disseminate information on everything from emergency department wait times to new clinical offerings and research endeavors. They might also use social media channels to provide useful links to self-management tools and invitations to chronic care management programs. In fact, nearly 95 percent of hospitals have a Facebook page and just over 50 percent have a Twitter account (Griffis et al., 2014).

Automated Messaging

Similar to social media, the use of automated messaging tools (via text, e-mail, or phone) can be equally beneficial in urging patients to schedule necessary appointments, fill their prescriptions, and comply with discharge orders. For example, one study showed that diabetic and hypertensive patients were two to three times more likely to attend a chronic care visit if

Given the modest adoption rates of PHRs and patient portals to date, research firm KLAS asked providers what best practices for patient portal adoption they would pass along to other providers trying to improve their rates. The following are their suggestions:

1. Educate patients.
"What contributes to adoption is educating our patients about the portal, helping them sign up, and encouraging them to use it. But education is key. Patients have embraced the portal and use it for much of our communication, bill pay, results review, and more."

2. Educate patients—again and again.
"We ask patients on the phone whether they have signed up for the portal, and at their appointments we check to see whether they have filled things out on the portal. Then the medical assistants who greet the patients ask whether they have put their information on the portal. We promote the portal five or six times. On their way out, the doctors tell the patients that they are going to send their results to the portal."

3. Educate staff members as if they were patients.
"The patients get inundated and get tired of hearing it, but it was the kickoff that got everybody in the practice used to pushing the portal. We also made everyone here register on the portal to see what the patients would go through and so we could make changes and adjustments to fit our needs. It is an ongoing process, and we try to do contests every quarter. That is what contributes to our success, and it is pretty impressive."

4. Give patients a reason to use the portal.
"We are apparently doing something right in encouraging patients to come to our portal. They come to the portal to fill out the patient history and

successfully contacted using automated provider communications (Nielsen & Shaljian, 2013).

PHM is most effective when a symbiotic relationship exists between human interventions and automation tools. Patient engagement tools and outreach programs enable providers to correspond with each person in their patient populations, with the goal of raising the percentages of patients receiving the recommended care as reflected in the quality measures payers use to evaluate provider and health system performance. More important, the medication list. I think that is because of the way our front desk staff members make new-patient appointments and the way they present the portal to the patients. They tell them that we can give them less waiting time when they come in if they get on the portal. We have an aggressive sign-up process. We give patients a Chromebook in the waiting room and help them sign up for the portal right away. We have a similar process in the ED and inpatient areas. We try to push as much content to the portal as possible."

5. Talk to your vendor and physicians.
"We drove adoption from the top down. In our initial phase, the adoption didn't go well because we thought we knew what we were doing and could do it ourselves. We went back and listened to Medfusion. We took the portal to the doctors who understand technology. They came back from a CMS meeting and said we had to do the portal. They said we might not like it, but we have to do it."

6. Hold your vendor accountable.
"When we started to deploy Empower in our ambulatory area, we hit challenges and barriers with the physician group. The physicians really wanted to yank the product out; they didn't want anything to do with it. They were beyond frustrated. We worked with MEDSEEK and the physicians, and in the last year and a half, we went from having a handful of patients on the portal to having sixty-five thousand. We were finally able to leverage the solution in the ambulatory space after we made changes to the product and the interface. There were deal breakers in how the product looked and felt from a patient perspective, and we worked through those."

Source: Buckley (2015). Used with permission.

such programs assist providers in keeping patients as healthy as possible for as long as possible, a core tenant of PHM.

Telemedicine and Telehealth

The growing use of *telemedicine* can make patient interactions more convenient, expand geographic horizons particularly where needed medical specialists are few in number, and make care more accessible to those with mobility issues.

With an abundance of patient-generated health information now available through online patient communities, social media can play a vital role in improving our understanding of disease and accelerating new approaches to treatment. Consider the following ways patient and consumer use of social media is benefiting health care.

Creates a Sense of Community

For those seeking emotional support and tips for coping with a disease, social media delivers on many fronts. It can enable the formation of communities regardless of member locations and enable members to communicate asynchronously.

Sites such as PatientsLikeMe and Inspire provide virtual medical communities focused on chronic diseases where patients can discuss their conditions, track key health information, share side effects of medications and therapies, and bond with others as they chronicle the highs and lows of their health care journeys.

In fact, a 2014 survey of PatientsLikeMe members found that the vast majority of adult social media users with health conditions embrace the idea of sharing their health information online if it helps clinicians improve care, assists other patients, or advances medical research.

Users of online health communities also frequently cite as reasons for their membership the accountability the sites provide them in managing their own health and reaching their health-related goals, as well as the motivation, support, and advice they receive from others. Online communities can also lessen the feeling of isolation that often accompanies those with rare conditions or parents with a critically ill child.

Delivers New Clinical Research Insights

As more and more patients use social media to track their health conditions and actively participate in their care, there is a greater opportunity to use this real-world data to better inform new treatments and treatment decisions, enhance symptom management, and ultimately improve outcomes.

For example, in analyzing the results of observational data housed on PatientsLikeMe, researchers found that lithium therapy had no impact on ALS disease progression, which was later confirmed by subsequent randomized trials (Chretien & Kind, 2013).

Although PatientsLikeMe began as a social network enabling people to crowdsource the collective wisdom of others, it has developed into a powerful analytical platform for clinicians and researchers. In fact, the network is quite transparent with its members about how it makes money—by sharing the information members provide about their experience with diseases and selling it to their partners (companies that are developing or selling products to patients). This may include drugs, devices, equipment insurance, or medical services.

In addition to helping patients find and take advantage of clinical trials, health care social networks also provide an opportunity for participant-led research, in which members initiate new fields of study. For instance, Inspire members with spontaneous coronary artery dissection (SCAD) persuaded researchers at the Mayo Clinic to launch new research about their condition, which led to the creation of a SCAD registry, a key step in the further study of this rare disease (Tweet, Gulati, Aase, & Hayes, 2011). Indeed, there is tremendous potential for online patient communities to contribute to the notion of a continuously learning health system.

Builds Awareness of Cause-Related Issues or Personal Health Care Crises
Social media can also serve as the birthplace for beneficial social movements, as well as hubs for galvanizing emotional and financial support for a personal health care crisis.

The ALS Ice Bucket Challenge is a terrific example of social media's power to deliver on the fund-raising aspect of the campaign and on the equally important goal of helping the public become more aware of ALS and efforts to find a cure.

The simple act of pouring ice on one's head, capturing it on video, and calling out another person to do the same spread across social media channels like wildfire. With everyone from schoolchildren to celebrities getting in on the act, the ALS Association raised $115 million in 2014, a staggering increase from its $23.5 million intake in 2013 (ALS Association, 2015).

On a smaller scale, sites such as GoFundMe and My Cancer Circle can help keep family and friends abreast of a loved one's illness and treatment status, provide tools to coordinate meal deliveries and rides to medical appointments, as well as enable financial contributions to help offset personal health care expenses.

Provides Assistance with Treatment, Physician, or Hospital Selection
Although physician rating sites have been around for many years, social media has given health care consumers a more active voice and an ever-present tool set for broadcasting opinions on all things health care–related—from physicians and hospitals to medications, devices, and insurance plans.

Like it or not, social media is proving to be a vehicle that can help scale positive and negative attitudes about one's health care experience at Internet speed. In fact, a 2012 survey by Demi & Cooper Advertising and DC Interactive found that 41 percent of people said social media would affect their choice of a specific doctor, hospital, or medical facility.

Of course, the downside here is that the negative opinions of a vocal minority could cause unjust reputation management issues for providers.

With the viewpoints of those in online social networks playing such a key role in influencing health care decisions, providers ought to ensure they are optimizing their social media channels and actively participating in helping consumers share positive opinions online.

Complements Traditional Approaches to Measuring Patient Satisfaction
Beyond just randomly monitoring opinions shared on social media, savvy providers may want to turn to social media to supplement their

The American Telemedicine Association defines telemedicine or tele-health as exchanging medical information via electronic communications to improve a patient's clinical health status. Health care providers are embracing telemedicine because they see it as an efficient and cost-effective way to deliver quality care and improve patient satisfaction (Glaser, 2015a). Today's telehealth framework spans the continuum of care and can include services such as the following:

- Telepsychiatry
- Remote image interpretation (teleradiology, teledermatology)
- e-Visits or televisits between providers and their patients
- Video visits for semi-urgent care
- Clinician-to-clinician consultations
- Critical care (virtual ICU, telestroke)
- Remote monitoring of a patient with a chronic disease
- Cybersurgery or telesurgery

traditional means of capturing patient satisfaction and feedback on inpatient experience.

In fact, researchers at Boston Children's Hospital conducted a study to determine if Twitter could provide a reasonable form of complementary quality measurement, given the real-time nature of tweets. The team amassed unsolicited knowledge (versus data gleaned from very targeted survey questions) about what pleased or angered consumers by collecting more than 400,000 tweets directed at the Twitter handles of nearly 2,400 US hospitals between 2012 and 2013 (Ulrich, 2015).

Although certainly no replacement for patient satisfaction surveys, according to the researchers the data are suggestive and provide proof of principle that Twitter and the right analytical tools may provide a valuable means for complementing standard approaches to measuring quality. Moreover, the ability to correlate social media data points such as tweets with actual outcomes measures (e.g., patient length of stay in the emergency department or readmission rates) provides an interesting avenue for further exploration.

Source: Glaser (2016b). Reprinted from *H&HN Daily* by permission, April 11, 2016, Copyright 2016, by Health Forum, Inc.

Let's take a closer look at some of the more popular applications of **telemedicine and telehealth.** Two-way interactive video-conferencing or other web-based technologies can be used when a face-to-face consultation is necessary. In addition, a number of peripheral devices can be linked to computers to aid in interactive examination. For example, a stethoscope can be linked to a computer, enabling the consulting physician to hear the patient's heartbeat from a distance. Electronic monitoring of physiological vital signs can be done through electronic intensive care unit (eICU) patient-monitoring systems, and telesurgery can enable a surgeon in one location to remotely control a robotic arm to perform surgery in another location.

Telehealth is also being used to capture and monitor data from patients at home. Examples include monitoring patient blood sugar levels through glucometers attached to cell phones and conducting teledermatology visits with the aid of cell phone cameras.

According to the American Hospital Association (AHA), 52 percent of hospitals used some form of telehealth in 2013, and another 10 percent were beginning to implement such services (AHA, 2015). Its growth potential is also notable. Business information provider IHS predicts the US telehealth market will grow from $240 million in revenue in 2013 to $1.9 billion in 2018—an annual growth rate of more than 50 percent (EY, 2014).

In addition to the growing demand for access and convenience, the need for telemedicine is driven by other factors such as the following:

- Significant increase in the US population
- Shortage of licensed health care professionals
- Increasing incidence of chronic diseases
- Need for efficient care of the elderly, homebound, and physically challenged patients
- Lack of specialists and health facilities in rural areas and in many urban areas
- Avoidance of adverse events, injuries, and illnesses that can occur within the health care system

These factors become increasingly important as new health care delivery and payment models evolve and providers are challenged to better manage chronic diseases, avoid readmissions, improve quality, and remove low acuity care from high-cost venues. As we know, the long-term benefits of population health programs are predicated in large part on managing high-cost, chronically ill patient populations more effectively. Furthermore, the rapid deployment of high deductible health plans, which make consumers more conscious and accountable for their health care consumption and spending, has added to the pressure on providers to provide low-cost, convenient options.

Despite all its promise, several major barriers must be addressed if telemedicine is to be used more widely and become available. Concerns about provider acceptance, interstate licensure, overall confidentiality and liability, data standards, and lack of universal reimbursement for telemedicine services from public and private payers are among the complex and evolving issues affecting the widespread use of telemedicine. Furthermore, its cost-effectiveness has yet to be fully demonstrated.

Nonetheless, the barriers are beginning to erode under mounting pressure from all health care constituents. Licensure portability will further ease the barriers to accessing services, whereas regulatory and payment policy changes in support of telehealth are widely expected in the coming years. For instance, on the private payer side, telemedicine use has been bolstered by a growing number of states enacting parity laws, which require health insurers to treat telehealth services the same way they would in-person services.

TRANSITIONING FROM THE RECORD TO THE PLAN

As we reviewed in this chapter, the profound changes in reimbursement and care models are altering the structure of care provision, requiring providers to make investments in a comprehensive IT portfolio—beyond the EHR—to support PHM and enable the core processes associated with accountable care. These changing business and payment models are leading not only to significant changes in organization and practice but also to changes in the fundamental nature and design of the EHR itself. These changes can be characterized as a transition from the electronic health record to the electronic health plan (Glaser, 2015b).

The EHR does not disappear as a result of this shift. We will still need traditional EHR capabilities: providers need to review a radiology report and document a patient's history and the care delivered. Problems must be recorded and medications reconciled. However, the strategic emphasis will move to technologies and applications that assist the care team (including the patient) in developing and managing the longitudinal, cross-venue health plan and assessing the outcomes of that plan.

For example, evidence-based pathways and decision-support logic have been embedded into EHRs to guide provider decisions according to a plan based on patient condition. EHRs can now include or be enhanced by the specific PHM technologies we discussed that enable the organization to understand its aggregate performance in undertaking disease-specific plans for multiple patients.

Provider organizations will not thrive in an era of health reform because they have a superb and interoperable EHR. They will thrive because the care they deliver consistently follows a plan designed to ensure desired outcomes. The EHR must evolve so it focuses on individual patients' care plans—the steps required to maintain or create health.

Every patient's EHR should clearly display the master care plan—a long-term care plan to maintain health integrated with short-term plans for transient conditions. The EHR should be organized according to this master plan: it should highlight the steps needed to recover or maintain health, list the expectations of every caregiver the patient interacts with, and include tools such as decision support and a library of standard care plans. Interoperability is a necessity, because various providers must be able to use the plan-based EHR.

Care Plan Attributes

The care health plan has attributes that need to be present to ensure health and should be based on some fundamental ideas.

First, all people have a foundational plan. If the person is a healthy young man, the plan may be simple: establishing health behaviors such as exercise. If the person is a middle-aged man with high cholesterol and sleep apnea, the plan may be annual physicals, statins, a CPAP machine, and a periodic colonoscopy. If a person is frail and elderly with multiple chronic diseases, the plan may be merging the care for each chronic condition, ensuring proper diet, and providing transportation for clinic visits.

Second, plans are a combination of medical care strategies with goals to maintain health (such as losing weight) along with public health campaigns (such as immunizations).

Third, on top of foundational plans there may be transient plans. For the patient undergoing a hip replacement there is a time-bounded plan beginning with presurgery testing and ending when rehabilitation has been completed. A patient undergoing a bad case of the flu has a time-bounded plan.

Fourth, people who have a common plan are members of the same population. These populations may be all patients undergoing a coronary artery bypass graft in a hospital, all patients with a certain chronic disease, or all patients at high risk of coronary artery disease. Moreover, a particular person may be a member of multiple populations at the same time.

Fifth, risk is the likelihood that the plan will not be followed or will not result in desired outcomes. A patient motivated to manage his or her blood pressure has a lower risk than a patient who is not motivated. A frail person with multiple chronic diseases is at greater risk that the plans will not keep him or her out of the hospital than a person whose health is generally good despite having multiple chronic diseases.

Sixth, not all care will be amenable to a predefined patient plan. Life-threatening trauma, diseases of mysterious origin, sudden complications—all require skilled caregivers to make the best decisions possible at the moment.

Seventh, plans should be based on the evidence of best care and health practices. And the effectiveness of a plan should be measurable, either in terms of plan steps being completed or desired outcomes being achieved (Glaser, 2015a).

The Plan-Centric EHR

The EHR needs to evolve into plan-centric applications. Among others, these applications will have several key characteristics.

A Library of Plans That Cover a Wide Range of Situations

This library will include, for instance, plans for managing hypertension, removing an appendix, losing weight, and treating cervical cancer. There will be variations in plans that reflect variations in patient circumstances and preferences, for example, plans that depend on whether the patient is a well-managed diabetic or plans that reflect the slower surgical recovery time of an elderly person.

Algorithms to Form a Patient's Master Plan

A master plan will combine, for example, the patient's asthma, hysterectomy, depression, and weight-reduction plans into a single plan. These algorithms will identify conflicts and redundancies among the plans and highlight the care steps that optimize a patient's health for all plans. For example, if each of the five plans has six care steps, the algorithms can determine which steps are the most important.

Team-Based

The master plan will cover the steps to be carried out by a patient's primary care provider, specialists, nurse practitioners, pharmacists, case managers, and the patient. Each team member can see the master plan and his or her specific portion of the plan. Team members can assign tasks to each other (Glaser, 2015a).

Business Models in Other Industries

Major changes in an industry's business model invariably lead to major changes in the focus and form of the core applications used by that industry. For example, financial services, retailers, and music distributors, along with many other industries, have also experienced massive shifts in their business models.

Several decades ago, financial deregulation enabled banks to offer brokerage services. The business model of many banks shifted from banking (offering mortgages as well as checking and savings accounts) to wealth management. As banks shifted from transaction-oriented services to services that optimized a customer's financial assets, their core applications broadened to include an additional set of transactions (buying and selling stocks) and new services (financial advisory services).

Prior to the web, most retailers' business models focused on establishing a brand, offering an appropriate set of well-priced products, and building attractive stores in convenient locations. The web enabled retailers to gather significantly richer data about a customer's buying patterns and interests (and to use real-time logic to guide purchasing decisions). Retailers' core applications broadened to include well-designed e-commerce sites and analytics of customer behavior.

In both examples, even though there was a significant shift in the business model, applications needed for the previous model continued to be necessary. Banks still had to handle savings account and mortgage payment transactions. Retailers still needed to manage inventory. And advances in these legacy applications—expanding inventory breadth and reducing inventory-carrying costs—continue to be important. In each case, a critical new set of applications were added to the legacy applications. Often, these new applications were more important than legacy applications.

The business model changes in health care will lead to a shift from applications focused on the patient's record to applications focused on the patient's plan for health. This evolution in the nature of the EHR is a key component to achieving success in population health management.

SUMMARY

As the health care industry continues its transition from a fragmented, volume-based system toward one that embraces the notion of patient-centered, accountable care driven by value-based payment models, providers must consider what new relationships, processes, and IT assets and skills will be required to succeed—particularly when it comes to managing the health and care of attributed populations.

By implementing a PHM strategy, organizations have enormous opportunity to use data and analytics to improve inefficiency and waste, thereby reducing costs, and monitor adherence to evidence-based protocols to drive better outcomes. Several PCMHs and ACOs are already showing promising performance in the emerging world of value-based payment and population health management.

In addition to having a robust EHR, organizations looking to enhance their PHM strategies should consider several key solution components. PHM technologies can help providers stratify and select target populations, identify gaps in care, predict outcomes and apply early interventions, and actively engage patients in their care. Moreover, they can enable an organization to understand its aggregate performance in undertaking disease-specific plans for multiple patients and better manage contracts and financial performance.

Additionally, because value-based payment is based on conformance to chronic disease protocols, providers must have the ability to aggregate and normalize real-time, accurate, cross-continuum data from disparate sources illustrating how well the data conform to those protocols. As we know, many hospitals and health systems do not operate from a position of excess revenue, and as outcomes become increasingly tied to the reimbursement stream, it will become critical that providers can rely on their data and IT tools to detect and remedy variations in care.

Population health management solutions are intended to complement—not replace—the traditional EHR. They represent a shift from applications focused on documenting the patient's record of care to applications focused on developing the patient's plan for health.

KEY TERMS

Accountable care organizations
(ACOs)

Analytics

Business intelligence (BI)

Care management

Health information exchange (HIE)

Patient engagement

Patient-centered medical home
(PCMH)

Population health management
(PHM)

Stratification

Telemedicine and telehealth

Value-based care

LEARNING ACTIVITIES

1. Interview a health care executive or CEO in your local community. To what extent is the organization involved in population health management? How is that person using health IT to further his or her PHM initiatives? To what extent does the organization's health IT capabilities facilitate PHM? What other capabilities are needed?

2. Investigate the adoption and use of telemedicine and telehealth in your state. How is it being used? What benefits have been realized? What challenges or obstacles still exist? How important is telemedicine and telehealth in providing access to care? In improving quality of care? And in reducing costs?

3. Explore the health IT products on the market that are designed to facilitate care management. What are their key features and functions? In what specific ways do these tools facilitate communication among providers and patients and families?

4. Conduct a literature review on the use of social media in health care. How are consumers using social media to learn more about their health or health conditions? How are health care organizations using social media to connect with consumers? Where do you see the future of social media in health care evolving?

5. Evaluate different models of care within your local community or state. Did you find any examples of accountable care organizations or

patient-centered medical homes? Explain. Working as a team, visit or interview a leader from a site that uses an innovative model of care. Describe the model, its uses, challenges, and the degree of patient coordination and integration. How is health IT used to support the delivery of care and the reporting of outcomes?

6. Explore the extent to which health information exchange is occurring within your community, region, or state. Who are the key players? To what extent is information being exchanged across organizations for patient care purposes? What challenges have they faced? How have they overcome them, if at all?

7. Visit a health care organization that uses an EHR system and provides patients access to their information via a patient portal. To what extent are patients using the portal? For what purposes are they using them? What are the demographic characteristics of the portal users and nonusers? What strategies might you employ to promote greater usage?

REFERENCES

Adler-Milstein, J., Bates, D. W., & Jha, A. K. (2013). Operational health information exchanges show substantial growth, but long-term funding remains a concern. *Health Affairs, 32*(8), 1486–1492.

Adler-Milstein, J., Cross, D., & Lin, S. (2016). Assessing payer perspectives on health information exchange. *Journal of the American Medical Informatics Association, 23*(2), 297–303.

AHRQ. (2015, April). Issue brief: Care management; Implications for medical practice, health policy, and health services research. *AHRQ Publication No. 15-0018-EF.* Retrieved May 2016 from http://www.ahrq.gov/professionals/ preventionchroniccare/improve/coordination/caremanagement/index.html

ALS Association. (2015). *ALS ice bucket challenge—FAQ.* Retrieved February 2016 from http://www.alsa.org/about-us/ice-bucket-challenge-faq.html

American Hospital Association (AHA). (2015, Jan.). *Trendwatch: The promise of tele-health for hospitals, health systems and their communities.* Retrieved October 2015 from http://www.aha.org/research/reports/tw/15jan-tw-telehealth.pdf

Berwick, D., Nolan, T., & Whittington, J. (2008). The triple aim: Care, health, and cost. *Health Affairs, 27*(3), 759–769.

Bipartisan Policy Center. (2015, July). *Transitioning from volume to value: Accelerating the shift to alternative payment models.* Retrieved May 2016 from http://bipartisanpolicy.org/wp-content/uploads/2015/07/BPC-Health-Alternative-Payment-Models.pdf

Buckley, C. (2015, May). *Patient portals adoption: From 5% to 20% and beyond.* KLAS. Retrieved May 2016 from http://www.klasresearch.com/resources/klas-blog/klas-blog/2015/08/17/patient-portal-adoption-from-5-to-20-and-beyond

Buelt, L., Nichols, L., Nielsen, M., & Patel, K. (2016, Feb.). *The patient-centered medical home's impact on cost and quality annual review of evidence 2014–2015.* Patient-Centered Primary Care Collaborative. Retrieved May 2016 from https://www.pcpcc.org/resource/patient-centered-medical-homes-impact-cost-and-quality-2014-2015

Chopra, N., & Glaser, J. (2013, April 9). Ready, set, go: Performance-based reimbursement. *H&HN Daily.*

Chretien, K. C., & Kind, T. (2013). Social media and clinical care: Ethical, professional, and social implications. *Circulation, 127,* 1413–1421.

Casalino, L., Erb, N., Joshi, M., & Shortell, S. (2015, Aug.). Accountable care organizations and population health organizations. *Journal of Health Politics, Policy and Law, 40(4),* 821–837.

EY. (2014). *Shaping your telehealth strategy.* Health Care Industry Post. Retrieved October 2015 from http://www.ey.com/Publication/vwLUAssets/EY-shaping-your-telehealth-strategy/$FILE/EY-shaping-your-telehealth-strategy.pdf

Felt-Lisk, S., & Higgins, T. (2011, Aug.). Exploring the promise of population health management programs to improve health. *Mathematica Policy Research Issue Brief.* Retrieved May 2016 from https://www.mathematica-mpr.com/our-publications-and-findings/publications/exploring-the-promise-of-population-health-management-programs-to-improve-health

Ford, E., Hesse, B., & Huerta, T. (2016). Personal health record use in the United States: Forecasting future adoption levels. *Journal of Medical Internet Research, 18*(3).

Gibson, R., Hunt, J., Knudson, S., Powell, K., Whittington, J., & Wozney, B. (2015). Guide for developing and information technology investment road map for population health management. *Population Health Management, 18*(3), 159–171.

Glaser, J. (2012a, Oct. 9). The growing role of analytics and business intelligence. *H&HN Daily.*

Glaser, J. (2012b, April 10). Six key technologies to support accountable care. *H&HN Weekly.*

Glaser, J. (2013, June). Expanding patients' role in their care. *H&HN Daily.*

Glaser, J. (2015a, Dec.). Telemedicine hits its stride. *H&HN Daily.*

Glaser, J. (2015b, Aug. 11). From the electronic health record to the electronic health plan. *H&HN Daily.*

Glaser, J. (2016a, June 13). All roads lead to population health management. *H&HN Daily.*

Glaser, J. (2016b, April 11). Five reasons to "like" patients' use of social media. *H&HN Daily.*

Glaser, J., & Salzberg, C. (2011). *The strategic application of information technology in health care organizations* (3rd ed.). San Francisco, CA: Jossey-Bass.

Griffis, H. M., Kilaru, A. S., Werner, R. M., Asch, D. A., Hershey, J. C., Hill, S., Ha, Y. P., Sellers, A., Mahoney, K., & Merchant, R. M. (2014). Use of social media across US hospitals: Descriptive analysis of adoption and utilization. *Journal of Medical Internet Research, 16*(11), e264.

Grundy, P., Hacker, T., Langner, B., Nielsen, M., & Zema, C. (2012, Sept.). *Benefits of implementing the primary care patient-centered medical home: A review of cost & quality results, 2012.* Patient-Centered Primary Care Collaborative. Retrieved May 2016 from https://www.pcpcc.org/guide/benefits-implementing-primary-care-medical-home

Guterman, S., & Drake, H. (2010, May). *Developing innovative payment approaches: Finding the path to high performance.* New York, NY: The Commonwealth Fund.

Handmaker, K., & Hart, J. (2015). 9 steps to effective population health management. *Healthcare Financial Management, 69*(4), 70–76.

Health Information Management and Systems Society (HIMSS). (2010). *Overview of HIE in era of meaningful use.* Retrieved February 2013 from http://www.himss.org/content/files/12_21_2010_HIE%20OverView%20in%20HITECH.pdf

Henry, J., Patel, V., Pylypchuk, Y., & Searcy, T. (2016, May). Interoperability among US non-federal acute care hospitals in 2015. *ONC Data Brief, No. 36.* Washington, DC: Office of the National Coordinator for Health Information Technology.

Houston, R., & McGinnis, T. (2016, Jan.). *Accountable care organizations: Looking back and moving forward.* Center for Health Care Strategies. Retrieved May 2016 from http://www.chcs.org/resources/?fwp_paged=4

Institute for Health Technology Transformation. (2012). *Population health management: A Roadmap for provider-based automation in a new era of healthcare.* Retrieved May 2016 from http://iht2.ihealthtran.com/blast372.html

Jaspen, B. (2015, May). Value-based care will drive Aetna's future goals. *Forbes.* Retrieved May 2016 from http://www.forbes.com/sites/brucejapsen/2015/05/15/value-based-care-may-drive-aetna-bid-for-cigna-or-humana/#3a9f829e6512

Kindig, D., & Stoddart, G. (2003). What is population health? *American Journal of Public Health, 93*(3), 380–383.

Leavitt Partners. (2015, Dec.). *Projected growth of accountable care organizations.* Retrieved May 2016 from http://leavittpartners.com/2015/12/projected-growth-of-accountable-care-organizations-2/

Miller, H. D. (2011). *Transitioning to accountable care: Incremental payment reforms to support higher quality, more affordable health care.* Pittsburgh, PA: Center for Healthcare Quality and Payment Reform.

The National Committee for Quality Assurance (NCQA). (2015, June). *Latest evidence: Benefits of the patient-centered medical home.* Retrieved May 2016

from https://www.ncqa.org/Portals/0/Programs/Recognition/
PCMHEvidenceReportJune2015_Web.pdf?ver=2016-02-24-143948-347

National eHealth Collaborative (NeHC). (2011, July). *Secrets of HIE success revealed: Lessons from the leaders.* Washington, DC: Author.

Nielsen, M., & Shaljian, M. (2013, Oct.). *Managing populations, maximizing technology: PHM in the medical neighborhood.* Patient-Centered Primary Care Collaborative. Retrieved May 2016 from https://www.pcpcc.org/resource/managing-populations-maximizing-technology

Olivero, M. (2015, March). Is a "medical home" in your future? *US News & World Report.* Retrieved May 2016 from http://health.usnews.com/health-news/patient-advice/articles/2015/03/09/is-a-medical-home-in-your-future

Patient-Centered Primary Care Collaborative. (2011, March). *Better to best: Value-driving elements of the patient centered medical home and accountable care organizations.* Retrieved May 2016 from https://www.pcpcc.org/guide/better-best

PwC. (2012, April). *Social media likes healthcare: From marketing to social business.* Retrieved February 2016 from http://download.pwc.com/ie/pubs/2012_social_media_likes_healthcare.pdf

Rudin, R. S., Salzberg, C. A., Szolovitis, P., Volk, L. A., Simon, S. R., & Bates, D. W. (2011). Care transitions as opportunities for clinicians to use data exchange services: How often do they occur? *Journal of the American Medical Informatics Association, 18*(6), 853–859.

Tweet, M. S., Gulati, R., Aase, L. A., & Hayes, S. N. (2011). Spontaneous coronary artery dissection: A disease-specific, social networking community–initiated study. *Mayo Clinic Proceedings, 86*(9), 845–850.

US Department of Health & Human Services (US DHHS). (2015, Jan.). *Better, smarter, healthier: In historic announcement, HHS sets clear goals and timeline for shifting Medicare reimbursements from volume to value.* Retrieved May 2016 from http://www.hhs.gov/about/news/2015/01/26/better-smarter-healthier-in-historic-announcement-hhs-sets-clear-goals-and-timeline-for-shifting-medicare-reimbursements-from-volume-to-value.html

Ulrich, T. (2015, October). *What can patients' tweets teach us about their health care experiences?* Boston Children's Hospital Notes. Retrieved February 2016 from http://notes.childrenshospital.org/twitter-as-a-patient-experience-measurement-tool/

Vest, J. R., & Gamm, L. D. (2010). Health information exchange: Persistent challenges and new strategies. *Journal of the American Medical Informatics Association, 17,* 288–294.

PART TWO

Selection, Implementation, Evaluation, and Management of Health Care Information Systems

CHAPTER 5

System Acquisition

LEARNING OBJECTIVES

- To be able to explain the process a health care organization generally goes through in selecting a health care information system.

- To be able to describe the systems development life cycle and its four major stages.

- To be able to discuss the various options for acquiring a health care information system (for example, purchasing, leasing, contracting with vendor for cloud computing services, or building a system in-house) and the pros and cons of each option.

- To be able to discuss the purpose and content of a request for information and request for proposal in the system acquisition process.

- To gain insight into the problems that may occur during the system acquisition process.

- To gain an understanding of the health care IT industry and the resources available for identifying health care IT vendors

and learning about their history, products, services, and reputation.
* To gain insight into the importance of understanding IT architecture.

By now you should have an understanding of the various types of health care information systems and the value they can bring to health care organizations and the patients they serve. This chapter describes the typical process a health care organization goes through in acquiring or selecting a new clinical or administrative application. Acquiring an information system (IS) application can be an enormous investment for health care organizations. In addition to the initial cost, there are a host of long-term costs associated with maintaining, supporting, and enhancing the system. Health care professionals need access to reliable, complete, and accurate information in order to provide effective and efficient health care services and to achieve the strategic goals of the organization. Selecting the right application, one that meets the organization's needs, is a critical step. Too often information systems are acquired without exploring all options, without evaluating costs and benefits, and without gaining sufficient input from key constituent user groups. The results can be disastrous.

This chapter describes the people who should be involved, the activities that should occur, and the questions that should be addressed in acquiring any new information system. The suggested methods are based on the authors' years of experience and on countless case studies of system acquisition successes and failures published in the health care literature.

SYSTEM ACQUISITION: A DEFINITION

In this book *system acquisition* refers to the process that occurs from the time the decision is made to select a new system (or replace an existing system) until the time a contract has been negotiated and signed. System implementation is a separate process described in the next chapter, but both are part of the systems development life cycle. The actual system selection, or acquisition, process can take anywhere from a few days to a couple of years, depending on the organization's size, structure, complexity, and needs. Factors such as whether the system is deemed a priority and whether adequate resources (time, people, and funds) are available can also directly affect the time and methods used to acquire a new system (Jones, Koppel, Ridgley, Palen, Wu, & Harrison, 2011).

Prior to arriving at the decision to select a new system, the health care executive team should engage in a strategic IS planning process in which the strategic goals of the organization are formulated and the ways in which information technology (IT) will be employed to aid the organization in achieving its strategic goals and objectives are discussed. We discuss the need for aligning IT plans with the strategic goals of the organization and for determining IT priorities in Chapter Twelve. In this chapter, we assume that a strategic IT plan exists, IT priorities have been established, the new system has been adequately budgeted, and the organization is ready to move forward with the selection process. We also assume that the organization has conducted a readiness assessment and is well equipped to move forward with the health IT project or initiative. The AHRQ National Resource Center for Health IT has available a number of tools publicly available that can be helpful to health care organizations in assessing their readiness for health IT projects such as EHR implementations and for ensuring that they have in place the personnel, technical, and financial resources to embark on the initiative. These tools can be found at https://healthit.ahrq.gov/health-it-tools-and-resources. Additionally, the Office of the National Coordinator for Health Information Technology (ONC) has readiness tools available and implementation blueprints that serve as excellent resources at https://www.healthit.gov/providers-professionals/ehr-implementation-steps.

SYSTEMS DEVELOPMENT LIFE CYCLE

No board of directors would recommend building a new health care facility without an architect's blueprint and a comprehensive assessment of the organization's and the community's needs and resources. The architect's blueprint helps ensure that the new facility has a strong foundation, is well designed, fosters the provision of high-quality care, and has the potential for growth and expansion. Similarly, the health care organization needs a blueprint to aid in the planning, selection, implementation, and support of a new health care information system. The decision to invest in a health care information system should be well aligned with the organization's overall strategic goals and should be made after careful thought and deliberation. Information systems are an investment in the organization's infrastructure, not a one-time purchase. Health care information systems require not only up-front costs and resources but also ongoing maintenance, support, upgrades, and eventually, replacement.

The process an organization generally goes through in planning, selecting, implementing, and evaluating a health care information system is known as the **systems development life cycle (SDLC).** Although the SDLC is most commonly described in the context of software development, the process also applies when systems are purchased from a vendor or leased through **cloud-based computing** services. Cloud computing is a general term that refers to a broad range of application, software, and hardware services delivered over the Internet. Regardless of how the system is acquired, most health care organizations follow a structured process for selecting and implementing a new computer-based system. The systems development process itself involves participation from individuals with different backgrounds and areas of expertise. The specific mix of individuals depends on the nature and scope of the new system.

Many SDLC frameworks exist, some of which employ an incremental approach, but most have four general phases, or stages: planning and analysis, design, implementation, and support and evaluation (Wager & Lee, 2006) (see Figure 5.1). Each phase has a number of tasks that need to be performed. In this chapter we focus on the first two phases; Chapter Six focuses on the last two.

The SDLC approach assumes that this four-phase life of an IS starts with a need and ends when the benefits of the system no longer outweigh its maintenance costs, at which point the life of a new system begins (Oz, 2012). Hence, the entire project is called a *life cycle*. After the decision has been made to explore further the need for a new information system, the feasibility of the system is assessed and the scope of the project defined (in actuality it is at times difficult to tell when this decision making ends and analysis begins). The primary focus of this **planning and analysis phase**

Figure 5.1 Systems development life cycle

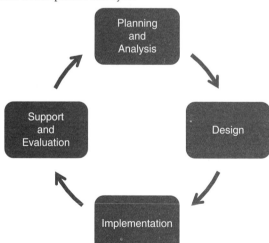

is on the business problem, or the organization's strategy, independent of any technology that can or will be used. During this phase, it is important to examine current systems and problems in order to identify opportunities for improvement. The organization should assess the feasibility of the new system—is it technologically, financially, and operationally feasible? Furthermore, sometimes it is easy to think that implementing a new IS will solve all information management problems. Rarely, if ever, is this the case. But by critically evaluating existing systems and workflow processes, the health care team might find that current problems are rooted in ineffective procedures or lack of sufficient training. Not always is a new system needed or *the* answer to a problem.

Once it is clear that a new IS is needed, the next step is to assess the information needs of users and define the functional requirements: What functions must the system have to fulfill the need? This process can be very time-consuming. However, it is vital to solicit widespread participation from end users during this early stage—to solicit and achieve buy-in. As part of the needs assessment, it is also helpful to gather, organize, and evaluate information about the organization in which the new system is to operate. Through defining system requirements, the organization specifies what the system should be able to do and the means by which it will fulfill its stated goals.

Once the team knows what the organization needs, it enters the second stage, the **design phase,** when it considers all its options. Will the new system be designed in-house? Will the organization contract with an outside developer? Or will the organization purchase a system from a health information systems vendor or contract with a vendor for cloud-based services? A large majority of health care organizations purchase a system from a vendor or at least look first at the systems available on the market. Contracting with the vendor to host the applications, software, hardware, and infrastructure via cloud computing is also growing in popularity in health care (Griebel et al., 2015). System design is the evaluation of alternative solutions to address the business problem. It is generally in this phase that all alternatives are considered, a **cost-benefit analysis** is done, a system is selected, and vendor negotiations are finalized.

After the contract has been finalized or the system has been chosen, the third phase, *implementation,* begins. The **implementation phase** requires significant allocation of resources in completing tasks, such as conducting work-flow and process analyses, installing the new system, testing the system, training staff members, converting data, and preparing the organization and staff members for the go-live of the new system. Finally, once the system is put into operation, the **support and evaluation phase** begins. It is common to underestimate the number of staff and resources needed to effectively keep new and existing information systems functioning properly. No matter how much time and energy were spent on the design and build of the application, you can count on the fact that changes will need to be made, glitches fixed, and upgrades installed. Likewise, most mission-critical systems need to be functioning 99.99 percent of the time—that is, with little downtime. Sufficient resources (people, technology, infrastructure, and upgrades) need to be allocated to maintain and support the new system. Moreover, maintaining and supporting the new system is not enough. Health care executives and boards often want to know the value of the IT investment, thus the degree to which the new system has achieved its goals and objectives should be assessed. Eventually, the system will be replaced and the SDLC process begins again.

With this general explanation of the SDLC established, we begin by focusing on the first two phases—the planning and analysis phase and the design phase. Together they constitute what we refer to as the *system acquisition process.*

SYSTEM ACQUISITION PROCESS

To gain an understanding of and appreciation for the activities that occur during the system acquisition process, we will follow a health care facility through the selection process for a new information system—specifically, an electronic health record (EHR) system. In this case the organization, which we will call Valley Practice, is a multiphysician primary care practice.

What process should the practice use to select the EHR? Should it purchase a system from a vendor, contract with a vendor for cloud-based services, or seek the assistance of a system developer? Who should lead the effort? Who should be involved in the process? What EHR products are available on the market? How reputable are the vendors who develop these products? These are just a few of the many questions that should be asked in selecting a new IS.

Although the time and resources needed to select an EHR (or any health care information system) may vary considerably from one setting to another, some fundamental issues should be addressed in any system acquisition initiative. The sections that follow the case study describe in more detail the major activities that should occur (see Exhibit 5.1), relating them to the multiphysician practice scenario. We assume that the practice wishes to purchase (rather than develop) an EHR system. However, we briefly describe other options and point out how the process may differ when the EHR acquisition process occurs in a larger health care setting, such as integrated health systems.

Exhibit 5.1 Overview of system acquisition process

- Establish **project steering committee** and appoint project manager.
- Define project objectives and scope of analysis.
- Screen the marketplace and review vendor profiles.
- Determine system goals.
- Determine and prioritize system requirements.
- Develop and distribute a **request for proposal (RFP)** or a **request for information (RFI).**
- Explore other options for acquiring system (e.g., leasing, hiring system designer, building in-house).
- Evaluate vendor proposals.
  - Develop evaluation criteria.
  - Hold vendor demonstrations.
  - Make site visits and check references.
  - Prepare vendor analysis.
- Conduct cost-benefit analysis.
- Prepare summary report and recommendations.
- Conduct contract negotiations.

Establish a Project Steering Committee

One of the first steps in any major project such as an EHR acquisition effort is to create a *project steering committee.* This committee's primary function is to plan, organize, coordinate, and manage all aspects of the acquisition process. Appointing a project manager with strong communication skills, organizational skills, and leadership abilities is critical to the project. In our Valley Practice case, the project manager was a physician partner. In larger health care organizations such as hospitals, it would likely be a CIO involved in the effort and that person might also be asked to lead it.

Increasingly, clinicians such as physicians and nurses with training in informatics are being called on to lead clinical system acquisition and implementation projects. Known as *chief medical informatics officers (CMIOs)* or *chief nursing informatics officers (CNIOs),* these individuals bring to the

CASE STUDY

Replacing an EHR System

Valley Practice provides patient care services at three locations, all within a fifteen-mile radius, and serves nearly one hundred thousand patients. Valley Practice is owned and operated by seven physicians; each physician has an equal partnership. In addition to the physicians, the practice employs nine nurses, fifteen support staff members, a business officer manager, an accountant, and a chief executive officer (CEO).

During a two-day strategic planning session, the physicians and management team created a mission, vision, and set of strategic goals for Valley Practice. The mission of the facility is to serve as the primary care "medical home" of individuals within the community, regardless of the patients' ability to pay. Valley Practice wishes to be recognized as a "high-tech, high-touch" practice that provides high-quality, cost- effective patient care using evidence-based standards of care. Consistent with its mission, one of the practice's strategic goals is to replace its legacy EHR with an EHR system that adheres to industry standards for security and interoperability and that fosters patient engagement, with the long-term goal of supporting health fitness applications.

Dr. John Marcus, the lead physician at Valley Practice, asked Dr. Julie Brown, the newest partner in the group, to lead the EHR project initiative. Dr. Brown joined the practice two years ago after completing an internal medicine residency at an academic medical center that had a fully integrated EHR system available in the hospital and its ambulatory care clinics. Of all the physicians at Valley Practice, Dr. Brown has had the most experience using EHR applications via portable devices. She has been a vocal advocate for migrating to a new EHR and believes it is essential to enabling the facility to achieve its strategic goals.

Dr. Brown agreed to chair the project steering committee. She invited other key individuals to serve on the committee, including Dr. Renee Ward, a senior physician in the practice; Mr. James Rowls, the CEO; Ms. Mary Matthews, RN, a nurse; and Ms. Sandy Raymond, the business officer manager.

After the project steering committee was formed, Dr. Marcus met with the committee to outline its charge and deliverables. Dr. Marcus expressed his appreciation to Dr. Brown and all of the members of the committee for their willingness to participate in this important initiative. He assured them that they had his full support and the support of the entire physician team.

Dr. Marcus reviewed with the committee the mission, vision, and strategic goals of the practice as well as the committee's charge. The committee was asked to fully investigate and recommend the top three EHR products available in the vendor community. He stressed his desire that the committee members would focus on EHR vendors that have experience and a solid track record in implementing systems in physician practices similar to theirs and that have Office of the National Coordinator for Health Information Technology (ONC)–certified EHR products. He is intrigued with the idea of cloud-based EHR systems provided they can ensure safety, security, and confidentiality of data; are reliable and scalable; and have the capacity to convert data easily from the current system into the new system. The vendor must also be willing to sign a business associates' agreement ensuring compliance with HIPAA security and privacy regulations.

Dr. Marcus is also interested in exploring what opportunities are available for health information exchange within the region. He envisions that the practice will likely partner with specialists, hospitals, and other key stakeholders in the community to provide coordinated care across the continuum under value-based reimbursement models. Under the leadership of Dr. Brown, the members of the project steering committee established five project goals and the methods they would use to guide their activities. Ms. Moore, the consultant, assisted them in clearly defining these goals and discussing the various options for moving forward. They agreed to consider EHR products only from those vendors that had five or more years of experience in the industry and had a solid track record of implementations (which they defined as having done twenty-five or more). Dr. Ward, Mr. Rowls, and Ms. Matthews assumed leadership roles in verifying and prioritizing the requirements expressed by the various user groups.

The five project goals were based on Valley Practice's strategic goals. These project goals were circulated for discussion and approved by the CEO and the physician partners. Once the goals were agreed on, the project steering committee appointed a small task group of committee members to carry out the process of defining system functionality and requirements. Because staff time was limited, the task group conducted three separate focus groups during the lunch period—one with the nurses, one with the support staff members, and a third with the physicians. Ms. Moore, the consultant, conducted the focus groups, using a semi-structured nominal group technique.

Concurrently with the requirements definition phase of the project, Mr. Rowls and Dr. Brown, with assistance from Ms. Moore, screened the EHR vendor marketplace. They reviewed the literature, consulted with colleagues in the state medical association, and surveyed practices in the state that they knew used state-of-the-art EHR systems. Mr. Rowls made a few phone calls to chief information officers (CIOs) in surrounding hospitals who had experience with ambulatory care EHR to get their advice. This initial screening resulted in the identification of eight EHR vendors whose products and services seemed to meet Valley Practice's needs.

Given the fairly manageable number of vendors, Ms. Moore suggested that the project steering committee use a short-form RFP. This form had been developed by her consulting firm and had been used successfully

project a clinical perspective as well as an understanding of IT and information management processes. (The roles of CMIOs and CNIOs are described more fully in Chapter Eight.) Regardless of the discipline or background of the project manager (for example, IT, clinical, or administrative), he or she should bring to the project passion, interest, time, strong interpersonal and communication skills, and project management skills and should be someone who is well respected by the organization's leadership team and who has the political clout to lead the effort effectively.

Pulling together a strong team of individuals to serve on the project steering committee is also important. These individuals should include representatives from key constituent groups in the practice. At Valley Practice, a physician partner, a nurse, the business officer manager, and the CEO agreed to serve on the committee. Gaining project buy-in from the various user groups should begin early. This is a key reason for inviting representatives from key constituent groups to serve on the project steering committee. They should be individuals who will use the EHR system directly or whose jobs will be affected by it.

Consideration should also be given to the size of the committee; typically, having five to six members is ideal. In a large facility, however, this may not be possible. The committee for a hospital or health systems might have fifteen to twenty members, with representatives from key clinical areas such as laboratory medicine, pharmacy, and radiology in addition to representatives from the administrative, IT, nursing, and medical staffs.

by other physician practices to identify top contenders. The short-form RFPs were sent to the eight vendors; six responded. Each of these six presented an initial demonstration of its EHR system on site. Following the demonstrations, the practice staff members completed evaluation forms and ranked the various vendors. After reviewing the completed RFPs and getting feedback on the vendor presentations, the committee determined that three vendors had risen to the top of the list.

Dr. Brown and Dr. Ward visited four physician practices that used EHR systems from these three finalists. Mr. Rowls checked references and prepared the final vendor analysis. A detailed cost-benefit analysis was conducted, and the three vendors were ranked. All three vendors, in rank order, were presented in the final report given to Dr. Marcus and the other physician partners. Dr. Marcus, Dr. Brown, and Mr. Rowls spent four weeks negotiating a contract with the top contender. It was finalized and approved after legal review and after all the partners agreed to it.

It is important to have someone knowledgeable about IT serving on the project steering committee. This may be a physician, a nurse, the CEO, or an outside consultant. In a physician group practice, having an in-house IT professional is not always possible. The committee chair might look internally to see if someone has the requisite IT knowledge, skills, interests, and also the time to devote to the project, but the chair also might look externally for a health care IT professional who might serve in a consultative role and help the committee direct its activities appropriately.

Define Project Objectives and Scope of Analysis

Once the project steering committee has been established, its first order of business is to clarify the charge to the committee and to define project goals. The charge describes the scope and nature of the committee's activities. The charge usually comes from senior leadership or a lead physician in the practice. Project goals should also be established and communicated in well-defined, measurable terms. What does the committee expect to achieve? What process will be used to ensure the committee's success? How will milestones be acknowledged? How will the committee communicate progress and resolve problems? What resources (such as time, personnel, and travel expenses) will the committee need to carry out its charge? What method will be used to evaluate system options? Will the committee consider contracting with a system developer to build a system or outsourcing the system to an application service provider? Or is the committee only considering systems available for purchase from a health care information systems vendor?

Once project goals are formulated, they can guide the committee's activities and also clarify the resources needed and the likely completion date for the project. Here are some examples of typical project goals:

- Assess the practice's information management needs and establish goals and objectives for the new system based on these needs.
- Conduct a review of the literature on EHR products and the market resources for these products.
- Investigate the top-ten EHR system products for the ambulatory care arena.
- Visit two to four health care organizations similar to ours that have implemented an EHR system.
- Schedule vendor demonstrations for times when physicians, nurses, and others can observe and evaluate without interruptions.

As part of the goal-setting process, the committee should determine the extent to which various options will be explored. For example, the Valley Practice project steering committee decided at the onset that it was going to consider only EHR products available in the vendor community and ONC-certified. Users can be assured that certified EHR products meet certain standards for content, functionality, and interoperability.

The committee further stipulated that it would consider only vendors with experience (for example, five or more years in the industry) and those with a solid track record of system installations (for example, twenty-five or more installations). The committee members felt the practice should contract with a system developer only if they were unable to find a suitable product from the vendor community—their rationale being that the practice wanted to be known as high-tech, high-touch. They also believed it was important to invest in IT personnel who could customize the application to meet practice needs and who would be able to assist the practice in achieving project and practice goals.

Screen the Marketplace and Review Vendor Profiles

Concurrently with the establishment of project goals, the project steering committee should conduct its first, cursory review of the EHR marketplace and begin investigating vendor profiles. Many resources are available to aid the committee in this effort. For example, the Valley Practice committee might obtain copies of recent market analysis reports—from research firms such as Gartner or KLAS—listing and describing the vendors that provide EHR systems for ambulatory care facilities. The committee might also attend trade shows at conferences of professional associations such as the Healthcare Information and Management Systems Society (HIMSS) and the American Medical Informatics Association (AMIA). (Appendix A provides an overview of the health care IT industry and describes a variety of resources available to health care organizations interested in learning about health care IT products, such as EHR systems, available in the vendor community.)

Determine System Goals

Besides identifying project goals, the project steering committee should define system goals. System goals can be derived by answering questions such as, What does the organization hope to accomplish by implementing an EHR system? What is it looking for in a system? If the organization intends to transform existing care processes, can the system support the new processes? Such goals often emerge during the initial strategic planning process when the decision is made to move forward with the selection of the new system. At this point, however, the committee should state its goals and needs for a new EHR system in clearly defined, specific, and measurable terms. For example, a system goal such as "select a new EHR system" is very broad and not specific. Here are some examples of specific and measurable goals for a physician practice.

Our EHR system should do the following:

- Enable the practice to provide service to patients using evidence-based standards of care.

- Aid the practice in monitoring the quality and costs of care provided to the patients served.

- Provide clinicians with access to accurate, complete, relevant patient information, on-site and remotely.

- Improve staff member efficiency and effectiveness.

- More fully engage patients in their own care by providing patients with ready access to their test results, immunization records, patient education materials, and other aids.

- Enable the practice to manage chronic disease patient care more effectively.

These are just a few of the types of system goals the project steering committee might establish as it investigates a new EHR for the organization. The system goals should be aligned with the strategic goals of the organization and should serve as measures of success throughout the system acquisition process.

Determine and Prioritize System Requirements

Once the goals of the new system have been established, the project steering committee should begin to determine system requirements. These requirements may address everything from what information should be available to the provider at the point of care to how the information will be secured to what type of response time is expected. The committee may use any of a variety of ways to identify system requirements. One approach is to have a subgroup of the committee conduct focus-group sessions or small-group interviews with the various user groups (physicians, nurses, billing personnel, and support staff members). A second approach is to develop and administer a written or an electronic survey, customized for each user group, asking individuals to identify their information needs in light of their job role or function. A third is to assign a representative from each specific area to obtain input from users in that area. For example, the nurse on the Valley Practice project steering committee might interview the other nurses; the business office manager might interview the support staff members. System requirements may also emerge as the committee examines templates provided by consultants or peer institutions, looks at vendor demonstrations and sales material, or considers new regulatory requirements the organization must meet.

The committee may also use a combination of these or other approaches. At times, however, users do not know what they want or will need. Hence, it can be extremely helpful to hold product demonstrations, meet with consultants, or visit sites already using EHR systems so that those who will use or be affected by the EHR can see and hear what is possible. Whatever methods are chosen to seek users' information system needs, the end result should be a list of requirements and specifications that can be prioritized or ranked. This ranking should directly reflect the specific strategic goals and circumstances of the organization.

The system requirements and priorities will eventually be shared with vendors or the system developer; therefore, it is important that they be clearly defined and presented in an organized, easy-to-understand format. For example, it may be helpful to organize the requirements into categories such as *software* (system functionality, software upgrades); *technical infrastructure* (hardware requirements, network specifications, backup, disaster recovery, security); and *training and support* (initial and ongoing training, technical support). These requirements will eventually become a major component of the RFP submitted to vendors or other third parties (discussed next).

Develop and Distribute the RFP or RFI

Once the organization has defined its system requirements, the next step in the acquisition process is to package these requirements into a structure that a third party can respond to, whether that third party be a development partner or a health information systems vendor. Many health care organizations package the requirements into a *request for proposal.* The RFP provides the vendor with a comprehensive list of system requirements, features, and functions and asks the vendor to indicate whether its product or service meets each need. Vendors responding to an RFP are also generally required to submit a detailed and binding price quotation for the applications and services being sought.

RFPs tend to be highly detailed and are therefore time-consuming and costly to develop and complete. However, they provide the health care organization and each vendor with a comprehensive view of the system needed. Health care IT consultants can be extremely resourceful in assisting the organization with developing and packaging the RFP. An RFP for a major health care information system acquisition generally contains the following information (sections marked with an asterisk [*] are completed by the vendor; the other sections are completed by the organization issuing the RFP):

- Instructions for vendors:
  - o Proposal deadline and contact information: where and when the RFP is due; whom to contact with questions
  - o Confidentiality statement and instructions: a statement that the RFP and the responses provided by the vendor are confidential and are proprietary information
  - o Specific instructions for completing the RFP and any stipulations with which the vendor must comply in order to be considered
- Organizational objectives: type of system or application being sought; information management needs and plans
- Background of the organization:

- o Overview of the facility: size, types of patient services, patient volume, staff composition, strategic goals of organization
- o Application and technical inventory: current systems in use, hardware, software, network infrastructure
- System goals and requirements: goals for the system and functional requirements (may be categorized as mandatory or desirable and listed in priority order). Typically this section includes application, technical, and integration requirements. Increasingly, health care providers are interested in assessing and testing system usability. Incorporating scripted scenarios in the requirements section of the RFP that are based on existing workflow and business processes can provide meaningful information during the selection process (Corrao, Robinson, Swiernik, & Naeim, 2010; Eisenstein, Jurwishin, Kushniruk, & Nahm, 2011; IOM, 2011).
- Vendor qualifications: *general background of vendor, experience, number of installations, financial stability, list of current clients, standard contract, and implementation plan
- Proposed solutions: *how vendor believes its product meets the goals and needs of the health care organization. Vendor may include case studies, results from system analysis projects, and other evidence of the benefits of its proposed solution.
- Criteria for evaluating proposals: how the health care organization will make its final decisions on product selection
- General contractual requirements: *warranties, payment schedule, penalties for failure to meet schedules specified in contract, vendor responsibilities, and so forth
- Pricing and support: *quote on cost of system, using standardized terms and forms

The RFP may become the basis for a legally binding contract or obligation between the vendor and the solicitor, so it is important for both parties to carefully consider the wording of questions and the corresponding responses (AHIMA, 2007).

RFPs are not the only means by which to solicit information from vendors. A second approach that is often used is the *request for information.* An RFI is less formal, considerably shorter than an RFP, and less time-consuming to develop. It is often used as part of the fact-finding process to obtain basic information on the vendor's background, product descriptions, and service capabilities. Some health care organizations send out an RFI before distributing the RFP in order to screen out vendors whose products or services are not consistent with the organization's needs or to narrow the field of vendors to a manageable number. The RFI can serve as a tool in gathering background information on vendors' products and services and providing the project steering committee with a better sense of the health IT marketplace. How does one decide whether to use an RFP, an RFI, both, or neither during the system acquisition process? Several factors should be considered. Although time-consuming to develop, the RFP is useful in forcing a health care organization to define its system goals and requirements and prioritize its needs. The RFP also creates a structure for objectively evaluating vendor responses and provides a record of documentation throughout the acquisition process. System acquisition can be a highly political process; by using an RFP the organization can introduce a higher degree of objectivity into that process. RFPs are also useful data collection tools when the technology being selected is established and fully developed, when there is little variability between vendor products and services, when the organization has the time to fully evaluate all options, and when the organization needs strong contract protection from the selected vendor (DeLuca & Enmark, 2002). However, not all vendors may wish to submit a response to an RFI or RFP because of costs or suitability.

There are also drawbacks to RFPs. In addition to taking considerable time to develop and review, they can become cumbersome and so detail oriented that they lose their effectiveness. For instance, it is not unusual to receive three binders full of product and service information from one vendor. If ten vendors respond to an RFP (about five is ideal), the project steering committee may be overwhelmed and find it difficult to wade through and differentiate among vendor responses. Having too much information to summarize can be as crippling to a committee in its deliberations as having too little.

Therefore a scaled-back RFP or an RFI might be a desirable alternative. An RFI might be used when the health care organization is considering only a small group of vendors or products or when it is still in the exploratory stages and has not yet established its requirements. Some facilities use an even less formal process consisting primarily of site visits and system demonstrations.

Regardless of the tool(s) used, it is important for the health care organization to provide sufficient detail about its current structure, strategic IT goals, and future plans so that the vendor can respond appropriately to its needs. Additionally, the RFP or RFI (or variation of either) should result in enough specific detail that the organization gets a good sense of the vendor—its services, history, vision, stability in the marketplace, and system or product functionality. The organization should be able to easily screen out vendors whose products are undeveloped or not yet fully tested (DeLuca & Enmark, 2002).

Explore Other Acquisition Options

In our Valley Practice case, the physicians and staff members opted to acquire an EHR system from the vendor community. Organizations such as Valley Practice often turn to the market for products that they will run on their own IT infrastructure. But there are times when they do not go to the market—they choose to leverage someone else's infrastructure (by contracting with an application service provider or vendor who offers cloud computing services) or they build the application (by contracting with a system developer or using in-house staff members).

Option to Contract with Vendor for Cloud Computing Services

In recent years, there has been a wider availability of high-speed or broadband Internet connections, more sophisticated vendor solutions, and a growing number of options for hosting software, hardware, and infrastructure via the Internet. These services are generally referred to as *cloud computing*, a general term that refers to the applications delivered as services over the Internet and the hardware and software in the data centers that provide those services. Vendors and companies may use different terms to describe cloud-based services. Common options include application service provider (ASP), software as a service (SaaS), infrastructure as a service, and platform as a service. The scope of services and payment methods also can vary considerably. However, cloud computing options generally require less upfront capital expenses, fewer IT staff members and resources, and greater scalability and access to analytic capabilities (Armbrust et al., 2010). Essentially the health care provider contracts with the vendor to host and maintain the clinical or administrative application and related hardware; the health care organization or provider simply accesses the system remotely over a network connection and pays the monthly or negotiated fees.

Why might a health care organization consider contracting with a vendor in a cloud-based service arrangement rather than purchasing an EHR system (or other application) from a vendor? There are several reasons. First, the facility may not have the IT staff members needed to run or support the desired system. Hiring qualified personnel at the salaries they demand may be difficult, and retaining them may be equally challenging. Second, cloud-based options enable health care organizations to use clinical or administrative applications with fewer up-front costs and less capital. For a small physician practice, these financial arrangements can be particularly appealing. Because many vendors offer cloud-based services on fixed monthly fees or fees based on use, organizations are better able to predict costs. Third, by contracting with a vendor to host, manage, or support IT, the health care organization can focus on its core business and not get bogged down in IT support issues, although it may still have to deal with issues of system enhancements, user needs, and the selection of new systems. Other advantages are rapid deployment and 24/7 technical support. They also offer scalability and flexibility, so as the practice or organization grows or shrinks in size or volume, they pay only for the services used. Other benefits include upgrades that can be made once and applied across a network of users instantaneously; users can access services from any standardized device no matter their location; and a cloud-based network can easily accommodate changes in use (increase and decrease during certain periods).

However, cloud computing services have some disadvantages and limitations that the health care organization should consider in its deliberations. Although rapid deployment of the application can be a tremendous advantage to an organization, the downside is the fact that the application will likely be a standard, off-the-shelf product, with little if any customization. This means that the organization has to adapt or mold its operations to the application rather than tailoring the application to meet the operational needs of the organization. A second drawback deals with technical support. Although technical support is generally available, it is unrealistic to think that the vendor's support personnel will have intimate knowledge of the organization and its operations. Frustrations can mount when one lacks in-house IT technical staff members when and where they are needed. Third, health care providers have long been concerned about data ownership, security, and privacy—worries that increase when another organization hosts their clinical data and applications. How the vendor will secure data and maintain patient privacy should be clearly specified in the contract. Likewise, to minimize downtime, the vendor should have clear plans for backing up data, preventing disasters, and recovering data.

As the industry matures, we will likely see different variations and greater choices among organizations offering cloud-based services. A recent review of the literature found cloud computing used in six primary domains: (1) telemedicine and teleconsultation, (2) medical imaging, (3) public health and patients' self-management, (4) clinical information systems, (5) therapy, and (6) secondary use of data (Griebel et al., 2015). Additionally, cloud computing is designed to support cooperation, care coordination, and information sharing.

The health care executive considering a move to cloud computing should carefully consider the type of application moving to the cloud (clinical, administrative) and the cloud service model that will be the most attractive economic option (Cloud Standards Customer Council, 2012). Health care executives should also thoroughly research the company and its products and consider factors such as company viability, target market, functionality, integration, implementation and training help desk support, security, pricing, and service levels. It is important to be able to trust the vendor and products and to choose systems and services wisely.

Option to Contract with a System Developer or Build In-House

An alternative to purchasing or leasing a system from a vendor is to contract with a developer to design a system for your organization. The developer may be employed in-house or by an outside firm. Working with a system developer can be a good option when the health care organization's needs are highly uncertain or unique and the products available on the market do not adequately meet these needs. Developing a new or innovative application can also give the organization a significant competitive advantage. The costs and time needed to develop the application can be significant, however. It is also important to consider the long-term costs. If the developer leaves, how difficult would it be to hire and retain someone to support and maintain the system? How will problems with the system be addressed? How will the application be upgraded? What long-term value will it bring the organization? These are a few of the many questions that should be addressed in considering this option. It is rare for a health care organization to develop its own major clinical information system.

Evaluate Vendor Proposals

In the Valley Practice case, the project steering committee decided to focus its efforts at first on considering only EHR products available for purchase or lease in the vendor community. The committee came to this conclusion after its initial review of the EHR marketplace. Committee members felt there were a number of vendors whose products appeared to meet practice needs. They also felt strongly that in-house control of the EHR system was important to achieving the practice goal of becoming a high-tech, high-touch organization, because they wanted to be able to customize the application. Realizing this, the committee had budgeted for an IT director and an IT support staff member. Members felt that the long-term cost savings from implementing an EHR would justify these two new positions.

Develop Evaluation Criteria

The project steering committee at Valley Practice decided to go through the RFP process. It developed criteria by which it would review and evaluate vendor proposals. Criteria were used to grade each vendor's response to the RFP. Grading scales were established so the committee could accurately compare vendors' responses. These grading scales involved assigning more weight to required items and less weight to those deemed merely desirable. Categories of "does not meet requirement," "partially meets requirement," and "meets requirement" were also used. RFP documents were compared item by item and side by side, using the grading scales established by the committee (see Table 5.1 for sample criteria). To avoid information overload, a common condition in the RFP review process, the project steering committee focused on direct responses to requirements and referred to supplemental information only as needed. Summary reports of each vendor's response to the RFP were then prepared by a small group of committee members and distributed to the committee at large.

Hold Vendor Demonstrations

During the vendor review process, it is important to host vendor system demonstrations. The purpose of these demonstrations is to give the members

Table 5.1 Sample criteria for evaluation of RFP responses

Type of Application: Electronic Health Record System

Vendor Name: The EHR Company

Criteria	Meets Requirement	Partially Meets Requirement	Does Not Meet Requirement
1. Alerts user to possible drug interactions	x		
2. Provides user with list of alternate drugs	x		
3. Advises user on dosage based on patient's weight	x		
4. Allows user to enter over-the-counter medications		x (on different screen)	
5. Allows easy printout of prescriptions	x		

of the health care organization an opportunity to (1) evaluate the look and feel of the system from a user's point of view, (2) validate how much the vendor can deliver of what has been proposed, (3) conduct system **usability testing,** and (4) narrow the field of potential vendors. It is often a good idea to develop demonstration scripts and require all vendors to present their systems in accordance with these scripts. Scripts generally reflect the requirements outlined in the RFP and contain a moderate level of detail. For example, a script might require demonstrating the process of registering a patient or renewing a prescription. The use of scripts can ensure that all vendors are evaluated on the same basis or functionality. At the same time, it is important to allow vendors some creativity in presenting their product and services. When scripts are used, they need to be provided to vendors at least one month in advance of the demonstration, and vendors and health care organization must adhere to them. It is also important to have end users carry out certain functions or procedures that they would usually do in the course of the day using the vendor's system. You might ask them to complete a system usability survey after they have had a chance to use the system and practice on several records. Figure 5.2 is an example of a system usability scale questionnaire in which end users are asked to respond to each item using a Likert scale of 1 to 5, from strongly disagree to strongly agree. Criteria should be developed and used in evaluating vendor demonstrations, just as they are for reviewing vendor responses to the RFP.

Make Site Visits and Check References

After reviewing the vendors' RFPs and evaluating their product demonstrations, it is advisable to make site visits and check references. By visiting other facilities that use a vendor's products, the health care organization should gain additional insight into what the vendor would be like as a potential partner. It can be extremely beneficial to visit organizations similar to yours. For instance, in the Valley Practice case, representatives from key practice constituencies decided to visit other ambulatory care practices to see how a specific system was being used, the problems that had been encountered, and how these problems had been addressed.

How satisfied are the staff members with the system? How responsive has the vendor been to problems? How quickly have problems been resolved? To what degree has the vendor delivered on its promises? Hearing answers to such questions firsthand from a variety of users can be extremely helpful in the vendor review process.

Figure 5.2 System usability scale questionnaire

	Strongly disagree				Strongly agree

1. I think that I would like to use this system frequently

1	2	3	4	5

2. I found the system unnecessarily complex

1	2	3	4	5

3. I thought the system was easy to use

1	2	3	4	5

4. I think that I would need the support of a technical person to be able to use this system

1	2	3	4	5

5. I found the various functions in this system were well integrated

1	2	3	4	5

6. I thought there was too much inconsistency in this system

1	2	3	4	5

7. I would imagine that most people would learn to use this system very quickly

1	2	3	4	5

8. I found the system very cumbersome to use

1	2	3	4	5

9. I felt very confident using the system

1	2	3	4	5

10. I needed to learn a lot of things before I could get going with this system

1	2	3	4	5

Source: Brooke (1996); Lewis and Sauro (2009).

Other Strategies for Evaluating Vendors

A host of other strategies can be used to evaluate a vendor's reputation and product and service quality. Organizational representatives might attend vendor user group conferences, review the latest market reports, consult with colleagues in the field, seek advice from consultants, and request an extensive list of system users.

Prepare a Vendor Analysis

Throughout the vendor review process, the project steering committee members should have evaluation tools in place to document their impressions and the views of others in the organization who participate in any or all of the review activities (review of RFPs, system demonstrations, site visits, reference checks, and so forth). The committee should then prepare vendor

Figure 5.3 Cost-benefit analysis

Vendor	50 MDs	10 MDs	5 MDs	1 MD	Fin.	Tech.	Interop.	Dec. Support	Clin./ Oper. Rank	Clin./ Oper. Points
Vendor 1	$5,588	$6,178	$6,806	$13,449	3	4	4.4	3.8	2	68
Vendor 2	$6,413	$6,594	$7,413	$13,373	3	4	3.4	2.9	5	27
Vendor 3	$3,378	$4,360	$5,130	$8,842	3	4	1.9	4.2	4	28
Vendor 4	$6,899	$6,086	$7,678	$15,437	5	4	4.1	4.3	1	70
Vendor 5	$5,945	$8,494	$9,543	$34,308	4	3	3.5	3.9	6	25
Vendor 6	$4,468	$4,580	$5,654	$12,927	3	3	2.4	4.1	3	46

analysis reports that summarize the major findings from each of the review activities. How do the vendors compare in reputation? In quality of their product? In quality of service? How do the systems compare in terms of their initial and ongoing costs? To what degree is the vendor's vision for product development aligned with the organization's strategic IT goals?

Conduct a Cost-Benefit Analysis

The final analysis should include an evaluation of the cost and benefits of each proposed system. Figure 5.3 shows a comparison of six vendor products. Criteria were developed to score and rank each vendor's system. As the figure illustrates, the selection committee ranked vendor 4 the top choice.

The capital cost analysis may include software, hardware, network or infrastructure, third-party, and internal capital costs. The total cost of ownership should factor in support costs and the costs of the resources needed (including personnel) to implement and support the system. Once the initial and ongoing costs are identified, it is important to weigh them against the benefits of the systems being considered. Can the benefits be quantified? Should they be included in the final analysis?

Prepare a Summary Report and Recommendations

Assuming the capital cost analysis supports the organization in moving forward with the project, the project steering committee should compile a final report that summarizes the process and results from each major activity or event. The report may include these elements:

- System goals and criteria
- Process used
- Results of each activity and conclusions
- Cost-benefit analysis
- Final recommendation and ranking of vendors

It is generally advisable to have two or three vendors in the final ranking, in the event that problems arise with the first choice during contract negotiations, the final step in the system acquisition process.

Conduct Contract Negotiations

The final step of the system acquisition process is to negotiate a contract with the vendor. This, too, can be time-consuming, and therefore it is helpful to seek expert advice from business or legal advisors. The contract outlines expectations and performance requirements, who is responsible for what (for example, training, interfaces, support), when the product is to be delivered (and vendor financial liability for failing to deliver on time), how much customization can be performed by the organization purchasing the system, how confidentiality of patient information will be handled, and when payment is due. The devil is in the details, and although most technical terms are common among vendors, other language and nuances are not. Establish a schedule and a pre-implementation plan that includes a timeline for implementation of the applications and an understanding of the resource requirements for all aspects of the implementation, including cultural change management, workflow redesign, application implementation, integration requirements, and infrastructure development and upgrades, all of which can consume substantial resources.

PROJECT MANAGEMENT TOOLS

Throughout the course of the system acquisition project, a lot of materials will be generated, many of which should be maintained in a project repository. A **project repository** serves as a record of the project steering committee's progress and activities. It includes such information and documents as minutes of meetings, correspondence with vendors, the RFP or RFI, evaluation forms, and summary reports. This repository can be extremely useful when there are changes in staff members or in the composition of the committee and when the organization is planning for future projects. The project manager should assume a leadership role in ensuring that the project repository is established and maintained. Following is a sample of the typical contents of a project repository.

PERSPECTIVE
Sample Contents of a Project Repository

- Committee charge and membership (including contact information)
- Project objectives (including method that will be used to select system)
- System goals
- Timeline of committee activities (for example, Gantt chart)
- System requirements (mandatory and desirable)
- RFP
- RFI
- Evaluation forms for
  - o Responses to RFPs
  - o Vendor demonstrations
  - o Site visits
  - o Reference checks
- Summary report and recommendations
- Project budget and resources

Managing the various aspects of the project and coordinating activities can be a challenging task, particularly in large organizations or when a lot of people are involved and many activities are occurring simultaneously. It is important that the project manager helps those involved to establish clear roles and responsibilities for individual committee members, set target dates, and agree on methods for communicating progress and problems. Many project management tools exist that can be useful here. For example, a simple Gantt chart (Figure 5.4) can document project objectives, tasks and activities, responsible parties, and target dates and milestones. A Gantt chart can also display a graphical representation of all project tasks and activities, showing which ones may occur simultaneously and which ones must be completed before another task can begin. Other tools enable one to allocate time, staff members, and financial resources to each activity. (Gantt charts and other timelines can be created with software programs such as Visio or Microsoft Project. A discussion of these tools is beyond the scope of this book but can be found in most introductory project management textbooks.)

Figure 5.4 Example of a simple Gantt chart

ID	EMR	Start	End	Jan 2017				Feb 2017				Mar 2017			
				1/16	1/23	1/30	2/6	2/13	2/20	2/27	3/6	3/13	3/20	3/27	4/3
1	Define project objectives	1/17/2017	1/17/2017	▬											
2	Conduct preliminary review of vendors	1/21/2017	2/8/2017		▬▬▬▬										
3	Determine system requirements	1/21/2017	3/15/2017		▬▬▬▬▬▬▬▬▬▬▬▬										
4	Conduct focus groups	2/1/2017	2/28/2017				▬▬▬								
5	Survey key user groups	2/1/2017	3/10/2017				▬▬▬▬▬▬								
6	Develop and administer RFP	3/15/2017	4/15/2017										▬▬▬		
7	Hold vendor demonstrations	4/15/2017	4/29/2017												
8	Conduct cost-benefit analysis	5/2/2017	5/13/2017												

It is important to clearly communicate progress within the project steering committee and to individuals outside the committee. Senior management should be kept apprised of project progress, budget needs, and committee activities. Regular updates should be provided to senior management as well as other user groups involved in the process. Communication can be formal and informal—everything from periodic update reports at executive meetings to facility newsletter briefings to informal discussions at lunch.

THINGS THAT CAN GO WRONG

Managing the system acquisition process successfully requires strong and effective leadership, planning, organizational, and communication skills. Things can and do go wrong. Upholding a high level of objectivity and fairness throughout the acquisition process is important to all parties involved. Failing to do so can hamper the overall success of the project. Following is a list of some common pitfalls in the system acquisition process, along with strategies for avoiding them.

Failing to manage vendor access to organizational leadership. The vendor may schedule private time with the CEO or a board member in the hope of influencing the decision and bypassing the project steering committee entirely. It is not unusual to hear that processes or decisions have been altered after the CEO has been on a golf outing or taken a trip to the Super Bowl with a vendor. The vendor may persuade the CEO or a board member to overturn or question the decisions of the project steering committee, crippling the decision process. Hence, it should be clearly communicated to all parties (senior management, board, and vendor) that all vendor requests and communication should be channeled through the project steering committee.

Failing to keep the process objective (getting caught up in vendor razzle-dazzle). Related to the need to manage vendor access to decision makers is the need to keep the process objective. The project steering committee should assume a leadership role in ensuring that there are clearly defined criteria and methods for selecting the vendor. These criteria and methods should be known to all the parties involved and should be adhered to. In addition, it is important that the committee and other organizational representatives remain unbiased and not get so impressed with the vendor's razzle-dazzle (in the form, for example, of exquisite dinners or fancy gadgets) that they fail to assess the vendor or the product objectively. Consider the politics of a situation but do not allow the vendor to drive the result—take the high road to avoid the appearance of favoritism.

Overdoing or underdoing the RFP. Striking a balance between too much and too little information and detail in the RFP and also determining how much weight to give to the vendors' responses to the RFP can be challenging. The project steering committee should err on the side of being *reasonable*—that is, the committee should include enough information and detail that the vendor can appropriately respond to the organization's needs and should give the vendor responses to the RFP appropriate consideration in the final decision. Organizations should also be careful that they do not assign either too much or too little weight to the RFP process.

Failing to involve the leadership team and users extensively during the selection process. A sure way to disenchant the leadership team and end users is to fail to involve them adequately in the system acquisition process. There should be ample opportunity for people at all levels of the organization who will use or be affected by the new information system to have input into its selection. Involvement can include everything from being invited and encouraged to attend vendor presentations during uninterrupted time to being asked to join a focus group in which user input is sought. It is important that the project steering committee seek input and involvement throughout the acquisition process, not simply at the end when the decision is nearly final. Far too often information system projects fail because the leadership team and end users were not actively involved in the selection of the new system. Involving people from the very beginning helps them to be an integral part of the process and the solution.

Turning negotiations into a blood sport. You want to negotiate a fair deal with the vendor and not leave the vendor's people feeling as though they have just been "beaten" in a contest. A lopsided deal results in a disenchanted partner and can create a bad climate. Understand what is required from all parties and establish

performance criteria for payments and remedies for nonperformance.
It is important to form a healthy, respectful long-term relationship with
the vendor.

These are just a few of the many issues that can arise during the system
acquisition process that the health care executive should be aware of. Failing
to appropriately address these issues can interfere with the organization's
ability to successfully select and implement a system that will be adopted
and widely used.

INFORMATION TECHNOLOGY ARCHITECTURE

Congruent with the selection process, it is important for health care executives to have an understanding of the underlying **IT architecture.** In other
words, how does the organization choose among different technologies and
ultimately bring them together into a cohesive set of health care information
systems? This section addresses this important question by examining health
care information system architecture.

An organization's information systems require that a series of core
technologies come together, or work together as whole, to meet the IT goals
of the organization. The way that core technologies, along with the application software, come together should be the result of decisions about what
information systems are implemented and used within the organization and
how they are implemented and used. For example, the EHR system or the
patient accounting system with which users ultimately interact involves not
just the application software but also the network, servers, security systems,
and so forth that all come together to make the system work effectively.
This coming together should never be a haphazard process. It should be
engineered.

In discussing IT architecture, we will cover several topics:

- A definition of architecture
- Architecture perspectives
- Architecture examples
- Observations about architecture

A Definition of Architecture

A design and a blueprint guide the coming together of a house. The coming
together of information systems is guided by information technology

architecture. For the house, the development of the blueprint and the design is influenced by the builder's objectives for the house (is it to be a single-family house or an apartment building, for example) and the desired properties of the house (energy efficient or handicap accessible, for example). For an organization's information systems, the development of an architecture is influenced by the organization's objectives (EHRs that span multiple hospitals, for example) and the systems' desired properties (efficient to support and having a high degree of application integration, for example).

Following the design and the blueprints, the general contractor, plumbers, carpenters, and electricians use building materials to create the house. Following the architecture for the organization's information systems, the IT staff members and the organization's vendors implement the core technologies and application software and integrate them to create the information systems.

IT architecture consists of concepts, strategies, and principles that guide an organization's technology choices and the manner in which the organization integrates and manages these choices. For example, an organization's architecture discussion concludes that the organization should use industry standard technology. This decision reflects an organizational belief that standard technology will have a lower risk of obsolescence, be easier to support, and be available from a large number of IT vendors that use standard technology. Guided by its architecture decision, the organization chooses to implement networks that conform to a specific standard network protocol and decides to use the Windows operating system for its workstations.

Two additional terms are sometimes used either as synonyms for or in describing architecture: *platform* and *infrastructure.* In this text, however, we adhere to accepted distinctions among these three terms. For example, you might hear IT personnel say that "our systems run on a Microsoft, HP, and Cisco platform." Platforms are the specific vendors and technologies that an organization chooses for its information systems. You might hear of a Windows platform or web-based platform. Platform choices should be guided by architecture discussions. You might also hear IT personnel talk about the infrastructure of the health care information system. Infrastructure refers to the entire base of IT that an organization uses—its networks, servers, workstations, and so on. Organizations choose specific platforms from specific vendors to implement their infrastructure. An organization's infrastructure can have several platforms—CISCO for networks, Microsoft for workstations, and so on. Although infrastructure is not vendor or technology specific, it is not quite as broad a term as architecture, which encompasses much more than specific technologies and networks.

In creating an infrastructure, an organization will implement platforms and be guided by its IT architecture.

Architecture Perspectives

Organizations adopt various frames of reference as they approach the topic of architecture. This section will illustrate two approaches, one based on the characteristics and capabilities of the desired architecture and the other based on application integration.

Characteristics and Capabilities

Glaser (2002, p. 62) defines architecture as "the set of organizational, management, and technical strategies and tactics used to ensure that the organization's information systems have critical, organizationally defined characteristics and capabilities." For example, an organization can decide that it wants an information system that has characteristics such as being agile, efficient to support, and highly reliable.

In addition, the organization can decide that its information systems should have capabilities such as being accessible by patients from their homes or being able to incorporate clinical decision support. If it wants high reliability, it will need to make decisions about fault-tolerant computers and network redundancy. If it wants users to be able to customize their clinical information screens, this will influence its choice of a clinical information system vendor. If it wants providers to be able to structure clinical documentation, it will need to make choices about natural language processing, voice recognition, and templates in its electronic medical record.

Architecture choices are guided by organizational decisions about the capabilities and characteristics that are desired of its information systems.

Application Integration

Another way of looking at information systems architecture is to look at how applications are integrated across the organization. One often hears vendors talk about architectures such as best of breed, monolithic, and visual integration. *Best of breed* describes an architecture that enables each department to pick the best application it can find and that then attempts to integrate these applications by means of an interface engine that manages the transfer of data between these applications—for example, it can send a transaction with registration information on a new patient from the admitting system to the laboratory system.

Monolithic describes the architecture of a set of applications that all come from one vendor and that all use a common database management system and common user interface.

Visual integration architecture wraps a common browser user interface around a set of diverse applications. This interface enables the user, for example, a physician, to use one set of screens to access clinical data even though those data may come from several different applications.

This view of architecture is focused on the various approaches to the integration of applications: integration by sharing data between applications, integration by having all applications use one database, and integration by having an integrated access to data. This view does not address other aspects of architecture, for example, the means by which the organization might get information to mobile workers.

Architecture Examples

A few examples will help illustrate how architecture can guide IT choices. Each example begins with an architecture statement and then shows some choices about core technologies and applications and the approach to implementing them that might result from this statement.

Statement. We would like to deliver an EHR to our small physician practices that is inexpensive, reliable, and easy to support. To do this we will

- Run the application from our computer room, reducing the need for practice staff members to manage their own servers and do tasks such as backups and applying application enhancements
- Run several practices on one server to reduce the cost
- Obtain a high-speed network connection, and a backup connection, from our local telephone company to provide good application performance and improve reliability

Statement. We would like to have decision-support capabilities in our clinical information systems. To do this we will

- Purchase our applications from a vendor whose product includes a very robust rules engine
- Make sure that the rules engine has the tools necessary to author new decision support and maintain existing clinical logic
- Ensure that the clinical information systems use a single database with codified clinical data

Statement. We want all of our systems to be easy and efficient to support. To do this we will

- Adopt industry standard technology, making it easier to hire support staff members
- Implement proven technology—technology that has had most of the bugs worked out
- Purchase our application systems from one vendor, reducing the support problems and the finger-pointing that can occur between vendors when problems arise

Observations about Architecture

Organizations will often bypass the architecture discussion in their haste to "get the IT show on the road and begin implementing stuff." Haste makes waste, as people say. It is terribly important to have thoughtful architecture discussions. There are many organizations, for example, that never took the time to develop thoughtful plans for integrating applications and that then discovered, after millions of dollars of IT investments, that this oversight meant that they could not integrate these applications or that the integration would be expensive and limited.

As we will see in Chapter Thirteen, the organizations that have been very effective in their applications of IT over many years have had a significant focus on architecture. They have realized that thoughtful approaches to agility, cost efficiency, and reliability have a significant impact on their ability to continue to apply technology to improve organizational performance. For example, information systems that are not agile can be difficult (or impossible) to change as the organization's needs evolve. This ossification can strangle an organization's progress. In addition, information systems that have reliability problems can lead an organization to be hesitant to implement new, strategically important applications—how can they be sure that this new application will not go down too often and impair their operations?

Organizational leadership must take time to engage in the architecture discussion. The health care executive does not need to be involved in deciding which vendor to choose to provide network switches. But he or she does need a basic understanding of the core technologies in order to help guide the formation of the principles and strategies that will direct that decision. In the following example, the application integration perspective on architecture (choosing among best of breed, monolithic, and visual integration) illustrates a typical architecture challenge that a hospital might face.

A hospital has adopted a best-of-breed approach and, over the course of several years, has implemented separate applications that support the registration, laboratory, pharmacy, and radiology departments and the transcription of operative notes and discharge summaries. An interface engine has been implemented that enables registration transactions to flow from the registration system to the other systems.

However, the physicians and nurses have started to complain. To retrieve a patient's laboratory, pharmacy, and radiology records and transcribed materials, they have to sign into each of these systems, using a separate user name and password. To obtain an overall view of a patient's condition, they have to print out the results from each of these systems and assemble the different printouts. All of this takes too much time, and there are too many passwords to remember.

Moreover, the hospital would like to analyze its care, in an effort to improve care quality, but the current architecture does not include an integrated database of patient results.

The hospital has two emerging architectural objectives that the current architecture cannot meet:

1. Provide an integrated view of a patient's results for caregivers.
2. Efficiently support the analysis of care patterns.

SUMMARY

Acquiring or selecting a new clinical or administrative information system is a major undertaking for a health care organization. It is important that the process be managed effectively. Although the time and resources needed to select a new system will vary depending on the size, complexity, and needs of the organization, certain fundamental issues should be addressed in any system acquisition project.

This chapter discussed the various activities that occur in the system acquisition process. These activities were presented in the context of a multiphysician group practice that wishes to replace its current paper record with an EHR system by acquiring a system from a reputable vendor. Key activities in the system selection process are (1) establishing a project steering

· PERSPECTIVE
Choosing the System Architecture

To address these objectives, the hospital decides to implement a browser-based application that will do the following:

- Gathers clinical data from each application and presents it in a unified view for the caregivers
- Supports the entry of one user ID and password that is synchronized with the user ID and password for each application

In addition, the hospital decides to implement a database that receives clinical results from each of the applications and stores these data for access by query tools and analysis software.

To achieve its emerging objectives, the hospital has migrated from best-of-breed architecture to visual integration architecture. The hospital has also extended to visual integration architecture by adding an integrated database for analysis purposes.

In analyzing what would be the best architecture to meet its new objectives, the hospital considered monolithic architecture. It could meet its objectives by replacing all applications with one integrated suite of applications from one vendor. However, the hospital decided that this approach would be too expensive and time-consuming. Besides, the current applications (laboratory, pharmacy, and radiology) worked well; they just weren't integrated. The monolithic architecture approach to integration was examined and discarded.

committee and appointing a strong project manager to lead the effort, (2) defining project objectives, (3) screening the vendor marketplace, (4) determining system goals, (5) establishing system requirements, (6) developing and administering an RFP or RFI, (7) evaluating vendor proposals, and (8) conducting a cost-benefit analysis on the various options. Other options such as contracting with a vendor for cloud computing service arrangements or a system developer were also discussed. This chapter presented some of the issues that can arise during the system selection process and outlined the importance of documenting and communicating project activities and progress. Finally, the chapter concluded with a general overview of IT architecture and its relevance in making IT investment decisions.

KEY TERMS

Acquisition process

Cloud-based computing

Cost-benefit analysis

Design phase

Implementation phase

Planning and analysis phase

Project repository

Project steering committee

Request for information (RFI)

Request for proposal (RFP)

Support and evaluation phase

Systems development life cycle (SDLC)

Usability testing

IT architecture

LEARNING ACTIVITIES

1. Interview a health care executive regarding the process last used by his or her organization to acquire a new information system. How did that process compare with the system acquisition process described in this chapter?

2. Assume you are part of a project steering committee in a rural nonprofit hospital. The hospital is interested in replacing its legacy EHR system. You offer to screen the marketplace to see what types of EHRs are available. Prepare a fifteen-minute summary report of your findings to the committee at large.

3. Conduct a literature review (including an Internet search) on various cloud-based computing services available in health care. What criteria might you use to compare them? How do they differ in terms of service, support, and financing arrangements?

4. Find and critique a sample RFP for a health care organization. What did you like about it? What aspects of it did you feel could be improved? Explain.

5. This chapter described a typical physician practice that wishes to select an EHR system. Using the information in the Valley Practice scenario, draft a script for vendors to use in demonstrating their products and services to Valley Practice staff members. Include a description of the process you used to arrive at the script.

6. Working with your classmates in small groups, assume that you are a Valley Practice committee member interested in obtaining user feedback on the EHR vendor demonstrations. Develop a survey instrument that might be used to solicit and summarize participants' responses to each vendor demonstration. Swap the survey your group designed with another group's survey; critique each other's work.

REFERENCES

American Health Information Management Association (AHIMA). (2007). *The RFP process for EHR systems* (updated). Retrieved February 2013 from http://library .ahima.org/xpedio/groups/public/documents/ahima/bok1_047961. hcsp?dDocName=bok1_047961

Armbrust, M., Fox, A., Griffith, R. Joseph, A. D., Katz, R., Konwinski, A., . . . & Zaharia, M. (2010). A view of cloud computing. *Communications of the ACM, 53*(4), 50–58.

Brooke, J. (1996). SUS: A "quick and dirty" usability scale. In P. W. Jordan, B. Thomas, I. L. McClelland, & B. A. Weerdmeester (Eds.), *Usability evaluation in industry* (pp. 189–194). London, UK: Taylor & Francis.

Cloud Standards Customer Council. (2012). *Impact of cloud computing on healthcare.* Retrieved from http://www.cloud-council.org/deliverables/CSCC-Impact-of-Cloud-Computing-on-Healthcare.pdf

Corrao, N. J., Robinson, A. G., Swiernik, M. A., & Naeim, A. (2010). Importance of testing for usability when selecting and implementing an electronic health or medical record system. *Journal of Oncology Practice, 6*(3), 120–124.

DeLuca, J., & Enmark, R. (2002). *The CEO's guide to health care information systems* (2nd ed.). San Francisco, CA: Jossey-Bass.

Eisenstein, E. L., Jurwishin, D., Kushniruk, A. W., & Nahm, M. (2011). Defining a framework for health information technology evaluation. *Studies in Health Technology and Informatics, 164,* 94–99.

Glaser, J. (2002). *The strategic application of information technology in health care organizations* (2nd ed.) San Francisco, CA: Jossey-Bass.

Griebel, L., Prokosch, H., Kopcke, F., Toddenroth, D., Christoph, J., Leb, I., Engel, I., & Sedlmayr, M. (2015). A scoping review of cloud computing in healthcare. *BMC Medical Informatics and Decision Making, 15,* 17, 1–16.

Institute of Medicine (IOM). (2011). *Health IT and patient privacy: Building safer systems for better care.* Washington, DC: National Academies Press.

Jones, S. S., Koppel, R., Ridgley, M. S., Palen, T., Wu, S., & Harrison, M. I. (2011, Aug.). *Guide to reducing unintended consequences of electronic health records.* Rockville, MD: Agency for Healthcare Research and Quality.

Lewis, J. R., & Sauro, J. (2009). The factor structure of the system usability scale. In *Proceedings of the Human Computer Interaction International Conference* (HCII 2009), San Diego, CA.

Oz, E. (2012). *Management information systems: Instructor edition* (6th ed.). Boston, MA: Course Technology.

Wager, K. A., & Lee, F. W. (2006). Introduction to healthcare information systems. In M. Johns (Ed.), *Health information management technology: An applied approach* (2nd ed.). Chicago, IL: American Health Information Management Association.

CHAPTER 6

System Implementation and Support

LEARNING OBJECTIVES

- To be able to discuss the process that a health care organization typically goes through in implementing a health care information system.

- To be able to assess the organizational and behavioral factors that can affect system acceptance and use and strategies for managing change.

- To be able to develop a sample system implementation plan for a health care information system project, including the types of individuals who should be involved.

- To gain insight into many of the things that can go wrong during system implementations and strategies that health care manager can employ to alleviate potential problems.

- To be able to discuss the importance of training, technical support, infrastructure, and ongoing maintenance and evaluation of any health care information system project.

Once a health care organization has finalized its contract with the vendor to acquire an information system, the **system implementation** process begins. Selecting the right system does not ensure user acceptance and success; the system must also be incorporated effectively into the day-to-day operations of the health care organization and adequately supported or maintained. Whether the system is built in-house, designed by an outside consultant, or leased or purchased from a vendor, it will take a substantial amount of planning and work to get the system up and running smoothly and integrated into operations.

This chapter focuses on the two final stages of the system development life cycle: implementation and then support and evaluation. It describes the planning and activities that should occur when implementing a new system. Our discussion focuses on a vendor-acquired system; however, many of the activities described also apply to systems designed in-house, by an outside developer, or acquired or leased through cloud-based computing services.

Implementing a new system (or replacing an old system) can be a massive undertaking for a health care organization. Not only are there workstations to install, databases to build, and networks to test but also there are processes to redesign, users to train, data to convert, and procedures to write. There are countless tasks and details that must be appropriately coordinated and completed if the system is to be implemented on time and within budget— and widely accepted by users. Essential to the process is ensuring that the introduction of any new health care information system or workflow change results in improved organizational performance, such as a reduction in medication errors, an improvement in care coordination, and more effective utilization of tests and procedures.

Concerns have been raised about the potential for EHRs to result in risk to patient safety. Health care information systems such as EHRs are enormously complex and involve not only the technology (hardware and software) but also people, processes, workflow, organizational culture, politics, and the external environment (licensure, accreditation, regulatory agencies). The Institute of Medicine published a report that offers health care organizations and vendors suggestions on how to work collaboratively to make health IT safer (IOM, 2011). Poor user-interface designs, ineffective workflow, and lack of interoperability are all considered threats to patient safety. Several of the suggested strategies for ensuring system safety are discussed in this chapter.

Along with attending to the many activities or tasks associated with system implementation, it is equally important to manage change effectively and address organizational and behavioral issues. Studies have shown that over half of all information system projects fail. Numerous political, cultural, behavioral, and ethical factors can affect the successful implementation and use of the new system (Ash, Anderson, & Tarczy-Hornoch, 2008; Ash, Sittig, Poon, Guappone, Campbell, & Dykstra, 2007; McAlearney, Hefner, Sieck, & Huerta, 2015; Sittig & Singh, 2011). We devote a section of this chapter to strategies for **managing change** and the organizational and behavioral issues that can arise during the system implementation process. The chapter concludes by describing the importance of supporting and maintaining information systems.

SYSTEM IMPLEMENTATION PROCESS

System implementation begins once the organization has acquired the system and continues through the early stages following the go-live date (the date when the system is put into general use for everyone). Similar to the system acquisition process, the system implementation process must have a high degree of support from the senior executive team and be viewed as an organizational priority. Sufficient staff, time, and resources must be devoted to the project. Individuals involved in rolling out the new system should have sufficient resources available to them to ensure a smooth transition.

The time and resources needed to implement a new health care information system can vary considerably depending on the scope of the project, the needs and complexity of the organization, the number of applications being installed, and the number of user groups involved. There are, however, some fundamental activities that should occur during any system implementation, regardless of its size or scope:

- Organize the implementation team and identify a system champion.
- Clearly define the project scope and goals.
- Identify accountability for the successful completion of the project.
- Establish and institute a project plan.

Failing to appropriately plan for and manage these activities can lead to cost overruns, dissatisfied users, project delays, and even system sabotage. In fact, during the industry rush to take advantage of CMS incentive dollars, a flurry of EHR stories hit the news—with everything from CIOs and CEOs losing their jobs as a result of "failed" EHR implementations, to hospital operations screeching to a halt, to significant financial problems arising from glitches in the revenue cycle. These high-profile cases brought national attention to the consequences of a failed implementation. During system implementation, facilities often see their days in accounts receivable and denials increase while cash flow slows. By organizations anticipating risks to the revenue cycle prior to go-live and as part of EHR workflow, they are in a much better position to stay on track and maintain positive financial performance during the transition (Daly, 2016). In today's environment, in which capital is scarce and resources are limited, health care organizations cannot afford to mismanage implementation projects of this magnitude and importance. Examining lessons learned from others can be helpful.

Organize the Implementation Team and Identify a Champion

One of the first steps in planning for the implementation of a new system is to organize an **implementation team.** The primary role and function of the team is to plan, coordinate, budget, and manage all aspects of the new system implementation. Although the exact team composition will depend on the scope and nature of the new system, a team might include a project leader, **system champion**(s), key individuals from the clinical and administrative areas that are the focus of the system being acquired, vendor representatives, and information technology (IT) professionals. For large or complex projects, it is also a good idea to have someone skilled in project management principles on the team. Likewise, having a strong project leader and the right mix of people is critically important.

Implementation teams often include some of the same people involved in selecting the system; however, they may also include other individuals with knowledge and skills important to the successful deployment of the new system. For example, the implementation team will likely need at least one IT professional with technical database and network administration expertise. This person may have had some role in the selection process but is now being called on to assume a larger role in installing the software, setting up the data tables, and customizing the network infrastructure to adequately support the system and the organization's needs.

The implementation team should also include at least one system champion. A system champion is someone who is well respected in the organization, sees the new system as necessary to the organization's achievement of its strategic goals, and is passionate about implementing it. In many health care settings the system champion is a physician, particularly when the organization is implementing a system that will directly or indirectly affect how physicians spend their time. The physician champion serves as an advocate of the system, assumes a leadership role in gaining buy-in from other physicians and user groups, and makes sure that physicians have adequate input into the decision-making process. Other important qualities of system champions are strong communication, interpersonal, and listening skills. The system champion should be willing to assist with pilot testing, to train and coach others, and to build consensus among user groups (Miller & Sim, 2004). Numerous studies have demonstrated the importance of the system champion throughout the implementation process (Ash, Stavri, Dykstra, & Fournier, 2003; Daly, 2016; Miller, Sim, & Newman, 2003; Wager, Lee, White, Ward, & Ornstein, 2000; Yackanicz, Kerr, & Levick, 2010). When implementing clinical applications that span numerous clinical areas, such as nursing, pharmacy, and physicians, having a system champion from each division can be enormously helpful in gaining buy-in and in facilitating communication among staff members. The various system champions can also assume a pivotal role in ensuring that project milestones are achieved and celebrated.

Clearly Define the Project Scope and Goals

One of the implementation team's first items of business is to determine the scope of the project and develop tactical plans. To set the tone for the project, a senior health care executive should meet with the implementation team to communicate how the project relates to the organization's overall strategic goals and to assure the team of the administration's commitment to the project. The senior executive should also explain what the organization or health system hopes the project will achieve.

The goals of the project and what the organization hopes to achieve by implementing the new system should emerge from early team discussions. The system goals defined during the system selection process (discussed in Chapter Five) should be reviewed by the implementation team. Far too often health care organizations skip this important step and never clearly define the scope of the project or what they hope to gain as a result of the new system. At other times they define the scope of the project too broadly or scope creep occurs. The goals should be specific, measurable, attainable, relevant, and timely. They should also define the organization's criteria for success (Cusack & Poon, 2011).

Let's look at two hypothetical examples from two providers that we will call Rutledge Retirement Community and St. Luke's Medical Center. The implementation team at Rutledge Retirement Community defined its goal and the scope of the project and devised measures for evaluating the extent to which Rutledge achieved this goal. The implementation team at St. Luke's Medical Center was responsible for completing Phase 1 of a three-part project; however, the scope of the team's work was never clearly defined.

CASE STUDY

Rutledge Retirement Community

Rutledge Retirement Community in a Commission on Accreditation of Rehabilitation Facilities (CARF)–accredited continuum of care community offers residential, assisted living, and skilled care to residents in southern Georgia. An implementation team was formed and charged with managing all aspects of the EHR rollout. Rutledge's mission is to be "the premier continuum of care facility in the region providing high-quality, resident-centered care with family engagement." Considering how to achieve this mission, the team identified the EHR as the building block needed to improve care coordination, reduce medication errors, and create communication channels with families of residents by offering a family portal. In addition to establishing this goal, the team went a step further to define what a successful EHR implementation initiative would consist of. Team members then developed a core set of metrics—reduction in medication errors, reduction in duplicate services, and increased communication with family regarding residents' health status. Family and caregiver satisfaction with communication were also assessed.

St. Luke's Medical Center

St. Luke's Medical Center set out to implement a digital medical record, planning to do so in three phases. Phase 1 would involve establishing a clinical data repository, a central database from which all ancillary clinical systems would feed. Phase 2 would consist of the implementation of computerized physician order entry (CPOE) and nursing documentation systems, and Phase 3 would see the elimination of all outside paper reports through the implementation of a document-imaging system. St. Luke's staff members felt that if they could complete all three phases, they would have, in essence, a true electronic or digital patient record. The implementation team did not, however, clearly define the scope of its work. Was it to complete Phase 1 or all three phases? Likewise, the implementation team never defined what it hoped to accomplish or how implementation of the digital record fit into the medical center's overall mission or organizational goals. It never answered the question, How will we know if we are successful? Some project team members argued that a digital record was not the same as an EHR and questioned whether the team was headed down the right path. The ambiguity of the implementation team's scope of work led to disillusionment and a sense of failing to ever finish the project.

Identify Accountability for the Successful Completion of the Project

Four roles are important in the management of large health care information system projects:

- Business sponsor
- Business owner
- Project manager
- IT manager

Business Sponsor

The **business sponsor** is the individual who holds overall accountability for the project. The sponsor should represent the area of the organization that is the major recipient of the performance improvement that the project intends to deliver. For example, a project that involves implementing a new claims processing system may have the chief financial officer as the business sponsor. A project to improve nursing workflow may ask the chief nursing officer to serve as business sponsor. A project that affects a large portion of the organization may have the CEO as the business sponsor.

The sponsor's management or executive level should be appropriate to the magnitude of the decisions and the support that the project will require. The more significant the undertaking, the higher the organizational level of the sponsor.

The business sponsor has several duties:

- Secures funding and needed business resources—for example, the commitment of people's time to work on the project
- Has final decision-making and sign-off accountability for project scope, resources, and approaches to resolving project problems
- Identifies and supports the business owner(s) (discussed in the next section)
- Promotes the project internally and externally and obtains the buy-in from business constituents
- Chairs the project steering committee and is responsible for steering committee participation during the life of the project
- Helps define deliverables, objectives, scope, and success criteria with identified business owners and the project manager
- Helps remove business obstacles to meeting the project timeline and producing deliverables, as appropriate

Business Owner

A **business owner** generally has day-to-day responsibility for running a function or a department; for example, a business owner might be the director of the clinical laboratories. A project may need the involvement of several business owners. For example, the success of a new patient accounting system may depend on processes that occur during registration and scheduling (and hence the director of outpatient clinics and the director of the admitting department will both be business owners) and may also depend on adequate physician documentation of the care provided (and hence the administrator of the medical group will be another business owner).

Business owners often work on the project team. Among their several responsibilities are the following:

- Representing their department or function at steering committee and project team meetings
- Securing and coordinating necessary business and departmental resources
- Removing business obstacles to meeting the project timeline and producing deliverables, as appropriate
- Working jointly with the project manager on several tasks (as described in the next section)

Project Manager

The **project manager** does just that—manages the project. He or she is the person who provides the day-to-day direction setting, conflict resolution, and communication needed by the project team. The project manager may be an IT staffer or a person in the business, or function, benefiting from the project. Among their several responsibilities, project managers accomplish the following:

- Identify and obtain needed resources.
- Deliver the project on time, on budget, and according to specification.
- Communicate progress to sponsors, stakeholders, and team members.
- Ensure that diligent risk monitoring is in place and appropriate risk mitigation plans have been developed.
- Identify and manage the resolution of issues and problems.
- Maintain the project plan.
- Manage project scope.

The project manager works closely with the business owners and business sponsor in performing these tasks. Together they set meeting agendas, manage the meetings, track project progress, communicate project status, escalate issues as appropriate, and resolve deviations and issues related to the project plan.

IT Manager

The **IT manager** is the senior IT person assigned to the project. In performing his or her responsibilities, the IT manager does the following:

- Represents the IT department
- Has final IT decision-making authority and sign-off accountability
- Helps remove IT obstacles to meeting project timelines and producing deliverables
- Promotes the project internally and externally and obtains buy-in from IT constituents

Establish and Institute a Project Plan

Once the implementation team has agreed on its goals and objectives and has identified key individuals responsible for managing the project, the next major step is to develop and implement a project plan. The project plan should have the following components:

- Major activities (also called *tasks*)
- Major milestones
- Estimated duration of each activity
- Any dependencies among activities (so that, for example, one task must be completed before another can begin)
- Resources and budget available (including staff members whose time will be allocated to the project)
- Individuals or team members responsible for completing each activity
- Target dates
- Measures for evaluating completion and success

These are the same components one would find in most major projects. What are the major activities or tasks that are unique to system implementation projects? Which tasks must be completed first, second, and so forth? How should time estimates be determined and milestones defined?

System implementation projects tend to be quite large, and therefore it can be helpful to break the project into manageable components. One approach to defining components is to have the implementation team brainstorm and identify the major activities that need to be done before the go-live date. Once these tasks have been identified, they can be grouped and sequenced based on what must be done first, second, and so forth. Those tasks that can occur concurrently should also be identified (see Figure 6.1.). A team may find it helpful to use a consultant to guide it through the implementation process. Or the health care IT vendor may have a suggested implementation plan; the team must make sure, however, that this plan is tailored to suit the unique needs of the organization in which the new system is to be introduced.

The subsequent sections describe the major activities common to most information system implementation projects (outlined in the "Typical Components of an Implementation Plan" box) and may serve as a guide. These activities are not necessarily in sequential order; the order used should be determined by the institution in accordance with its needs and resources.

Workflow and Process Analysis

One of the first activities necessary in implementing any new system is to review and evaluate the existing workflow or business processes. Members of the implementation team might also observe the current information system in use (if there is one). Does it work as described? Where are the problem areas? What are the goals and expectations of the new system? How do organizational processes need to change in order to optimize the new system's value and achieve its goals? Too often organizations never critically evaluate current business processes but plunge forward implementing the new system while still using old procedures. The result is that they simply automate their outdated and inefficient processes.

Before implementing any new system, the organization should evaluate existing procedures and processes and identify ways to improve workflow, simplify tasks, eliminate redundancy, improve quality, and improve user (customer) satisfaction. In complex settings, it can be critically important to have informatics professionals such as CMIOs and CNIOs actively involved in the implementation team in analyzing workflow and information flow (Elias, Barginere, Berry, & Selleck, 2015). Although describing them is beyond the scope of this book, many extremely useful tools and methods are available for analyzing workflow and redesigning business processes (see, for example,

Figure 6.1 Project timeline with project phases

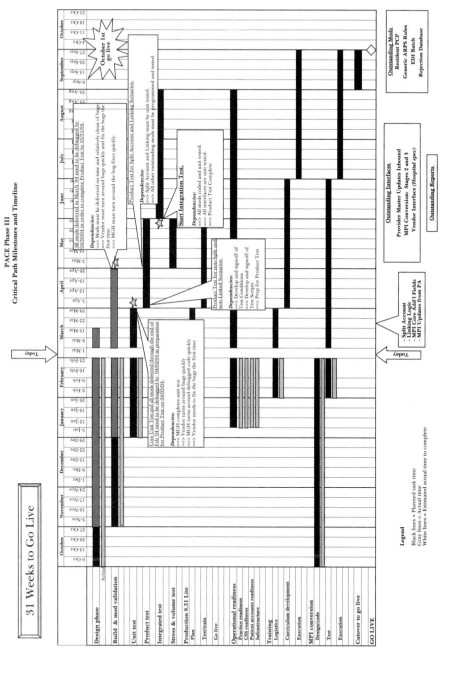

Typical Components of an Implementation Plan

1. Workflow and process analysis

- Analyze or evaluate current process and procedures.
- Identify opportunities for improvement and, as appropriate, effect those changes.
- Identify sources of data, including interfaces to other systems.
- Determine location and number of workstations needed.
- Redesign physical location as needed.

2. System installation

- Determine system configuration.
- Order and install hardware.
- Prepare data center.
- Upgrade or implement IT infrastructure.
- Install software and interfaces.
- Customize software.
- Test, retest, and test again . . .

3. Staff training

- Identify appropriate training method(s) to be used for each major user group.
- Prepare training materials.

Guide to Reducing Unintended Consequences of Electronic Health Records, by Jones, Koppel, Ridgley, Palen, Wu, & Harrison, 2011). Observing the old system in use, listening to users' concerns, and evaluating information workflow can identify many of the changes needed. In addition, the vendor generally works with the organization to map its future workflow using flow-charts or flow diagrams. It is critical that all key areas affected by the new system participate in the workflow analysis process so that potential problems can be identified and addressed *before* the system goes live. For example, if a new CPOE application is to be implemented using a phased-in approach, in which the system will go-live unit by unit over a three-month process, how will the organization ensure orders are not lost or duplicated if a patient is transferred between a unit using CPOE and a unit using handwritten orders? What will downtime procedures entail? If paper orders are generated during

- Train staff members.
- Test staff member proficiency.
- Update procedure manuals.

4. Conversion

- Convert data.
- Test system.

5. Communications

- Establish communication mechanisms for identifying and addressing problems and concerns.
- Communicate regularly with various constituent groups.

6. Preparation for go-live date

- Select date when patient volume is relatively low.
- Ensure sufficient staff members are on hand.
- Set up mechanism for reporting and correcting problems and issues.
- Review and effect process reengineering.

7. System downtime procedures

- Develop downtime procedures.
- Train staff members on downtime procedures.

downtime, how will these orders be stored or become part of the patient's permanent medical record?

Involving users at this early stage of the implementation process can gain initial buy-in to the idea and the scope of the process redesign. In all likelihood, the organization will need to institute a series of process changes as a result of the new system. Workflow and processes should be evaluated critically and redesigned as needed. For example, the organization may find that it needs to do away with old forms or work steps, change job descriptions or job responsibilities, or add to or subtract from the work responsibilities of particular departments. Getting users involved in this reengineering process can lead to greater user acceptance of the new system.

Let's consider an example. Suppose a multiphysician clinic is implementing a new practice management system that includes a patient portal for appointment scheduling, prescription refills, and paying bills. The clinic might wish to begin by appointing a small team of individuals knowledgeable about analyzing workflow and processes to work with staff members in studying the existing process for scheduling patient appointments, refilling prescriptions, and patient billing. This team might conduct a series of individual focus groups with schedulers, physicians and nurses, and patients, and ask questions such as these:

- Who can schedule patient appointments?
- How are patient appointments made, updated, or deleted?
- Who has access to scheduling information? From what locations?
- How well does the current system work? How efficient is the process?
- What are the major problems with the current scheduling system and process? In what ways might it be improved?

The team should tailor the focus questions so they are appropriate for each user group. The answers can then be a guide for reengineering existing processes and workflow to facilitate the new system. A similar set of questions could be asked concerning the refill of prescriptions or patient billing processes.

During the workflow analysis, the team should also examine where the new system's actual workstations will be located, how many workstations will be needed, and how information will flow between manual organizational processes (such as phone calls) and the electronic information system. Here are a few of the many questions that should be addressed in ensuring that physical layouts are conducive to the success of the new system:

- Will the workstations be portable or fixed? If users are given portable units, how will these be tracked and maintained (and protected from loss or theft)? If workstations are fixed, will they be located in safe, secure areas where patient confidentiality can be maintained?
- How will the user interact with the new system?
- Does the physical layout of each work area need to be redesigned to accommodate the new system and the new process?
- Will additional wiring be needed?
- How will the new system affect the workflow within the practice among office staff members, nurses, and physicians?
- Will the e-prescribing function with local pharmacies be affected by the change?

System Installation

The next step, which may be done concurrently with the workflow analysis, is to install the hardware, software, and network infrastructure to support the new information system and build the necessary interfaces. IT staff members play a crucial role in this phase of the project. They will need to work closely with the vendor in determining system specifications and configurations and in preparing the computer center for installation. It may be, for example, that the organization's current computer network will need to be replaced or upgraded. During implementation, having adequate numbers of computer workstations placed in readily accessible locations is critical. Those involved in the planning need to determine beforehand the maximum number of individuals likely to be using the system at the same time and accommodate this scenario. Vendors may recommend a certain number of workstations or use of hand-held devices; however, the organization must ensure the recommendations are appropriate.

Typically when a health care organization acquires a system from a vendor, quite a bit of customization is needed. IT personnel will likely work with the vendor in setting up and loading data tables, building interfaces, and running pilot tests of the hardware and software using actual patient and administrative data. It is not unlikely when purchasing a clinical application such as order entry from a vendor, for example, that the health care organization is provided a shell or basic framework from which to build the order sets or electronic forms. A great deal of customization and building of templates occurs. Thus, it is a good idea to pay physicians for their time involved in the project. For instance, if you need a physician's time to assist in building or reviewing order sets for the cardiology division, factor that into the resources needed for the project, perhaps by allocating two hours per week to the project for a certain period of time. Otherwise, you may be pulling physicians away from seeing patients and revenue-generating activities. It demonstrates the value placed on the physician's time and commitment to the project.

We recommend piloting the system in a unit or area before rolling out the system enterprise-wide. This test enables the implementation team to evaluate the system's effectiveness, address issues and concerns, fix bugs, and then apply the lessons learned to other units in the organization before most people even start using the system. Vendors will often offer guiding principles and strategies that they have found effective in implementing systems.

Consideration should be given to choosing an appropriate area (for example, a department or a location) or set of users to pilot the system.

Following are some of the questions the implementation team should consider in identifying potential pilot sites:

- Which units or areas are willing and equipped to serve as a pilot site? Do they have sufficient interest, administrative support, and commitment?
- Are the staff and management teams in each of these units or areas comfortable with being system guinea pigs?
- Do staff members have the time and resources needed to serve in this capacity?
- Is there a system champion in each unit or area who will lead the effort?

In migrating from one electronic system to another, such as from a legacy EHR to a new EHR, it may be more appropriate to go-live at once, instead of a more staggered or phased approach. For example, when Bon Secours Health System embarked on the implementation of an EHR system among fourteen hospitals, they decided after the second hospital EHR implementation to adopt the EHR vendor's revenue cycle system along with the clinical application, and go-live with both systems at once (Daly, 2016). This enabled them to monitor clinical and financial indicators at the same time and ensure that the charge master and revenue cycle teams worked collaboratively prior to and following implementation.

Staff Training

Training is an essential component of any new system implementation. Although no one would argue with this statement, the implementation team will want to consider many issues as it develops and implements a training program:

- How much training is needed? Do different user groups have different training needs?
- Who should conduct the training?
- When should the training occur? What intervals of training are ideal?
- What training format is best: for example, formal, classroom-style training; one-on-one or small-group training; computer-based training; or a combination of methods?
- What is the role of the vendor in training?

- Who in the organization will manage or oversee the training? How will training be documented?

- What criteria and methods will be used to monitor training and ensure that staff members are adequately trained? Will staff members be tested on proficiency?

- What additional training and support are available to physicians and others after go-live?

There are various methods of training. One approach, commonly known as **train the trainer,** relies on the vendor to train selected members of the organization who will then serve as super-users and train others in their respective departments, units, or areas. These super-users should be individuals who work directly in the areas in which the system is to be used; they should know the staff members in the area and have a good rapport with them. They will also serve as resources to other users once the vendor representatives have left. They may do a lot of one-on-one training, hand-holding, and other work with people in their areas until these individuals achieve a certain comfort level with the system. The main concern with this approach is that the organization may devote a great deal of time and resources to training the trainers only to have these trainers leave the institution (often because they've been lured away by career opportunities with the vendor).

Another method is to have the vendor train a pool of trainers who are knowledgeable about the entire system and who can rotate through the different areas of the organization working with staff members. The trainer pool might include IT professionals (including clinical analysts) and clinical or administrative staff members such as nurses, physicians, lab managers, and business managers.

Regardless of who conducts the training, it is important to introduce fundamental or basic concepts first and enable people to master these concepts before moving on to new ones. Studies among health care organizations that have implemented clinical applications such as CPOE systems have shown that classroom training is not nearly as effective as one-on-one coaching, particularly among physicians (Holden, 2011; Metzger & Fortin, 2003). Most systems can track physician use; physicians identified as low-volume users may be targeted for additional training.

Timing of the training is also important. Users should have ample opportunity to practice *before* the system goes live. For instance, when a nursing documentation system is being installed, nurses should have the chance to practice with it at the bedside of a typical patient. Likewise, when a CPOE system is going in, physicians should get to practice ordering a set of tests during their morning rounds. This *just-in-time training* might occur several times, for example, three months, two months, one month, and one week before the go-live date. Its purpose is to enable users to practice on the system multiple times before go-live. Training might be supplemented with computer-based training modules that enable users to review concepts and functions at their own pace. Training has to be a priority and at least some of training should be in an environment free of distractions. Eventually staff members will want to use the system in a near-live or simulated environment. Additional staff members should be on hand during the go-live period to assist users as needed during the transition to the new system. In general, the implementation team should work with the vendor to produce a thoughtful and creative training program.

Once the details of how the new system is to work have been determined, it is important to update procedure manuals and make the updated manuals available to the staff members. Designated managers or representatives from the various areas may assume a leadership role in updating procedure manuals for their respective areas. When people must learn specific IT procedures such as how to log in, change passwords, and read common error messages, the IT department should ensure that this information appears in the procedure manuals and that the information is routinely updated and widely disseminated to the users. Procedure manuals serve as reference guides and resources for users and can be particularly useful when training new employees.

Effective training is important. Staff members need to be relatively comfortable with the application and need to know to whom they should turn if they have questions or concerns. We recommend having the users evaluate the training prior to go-live.

Conversion

Another important task is to convert the data from the old system to the new system and then adequately test the new system. Staff members involved in the data conversion must determine the sources of the data required for the new system and construct new files. It is particularly important that data be complete, accurate, and current before being converted to the new system. Data should be *cleaned* before being converted. Once converted, the data should run through a series of validation checkpoints or procedures to ensure the accuracy of the conversion.

IT staff members who are knowledgeable in data conversion procedures should lead the effort and verify the results with key managers from the appropriate clinical and administrative areas. The specific conversion procedures used will depend on the nature of the old system and its structure as well as on the configuration of the new system.

Finally, the new system will need to be tested. The main purpose of the testing is to simulate the live environment as closely as possible and determine how well the system and accompanying procedures work. Are there programming glitches or other problems that need to be fixed? How well are the interfaces working? How does response time compare to what was expected? The system should be populated with live data and tested again. Vendors, IT staff members, and user staff members should all participate in the testing process. As with training, one can never test too much. A good portion of this work has to be done for the pilot testing. It may need to be repeated before going live. And the pilot lessons will guide any additional testing or conversion that needs to be done. In some cases, it may be advisable to run the old and new systems in tandem (parallel conversion) for a period of time until it is evident that the new system is operating effectively. This can reduce organizational risk. Again, running parallel systems is not always feasible or appropriate. Instead, organizations may opt to implement the system using a phased approach over a period of time.

Communications

Equally as important as successfully carrying out the activities discussed so far is having an effective plan for communicating the project's progress. This plan serves two primary purposes. First, it identifies how the members of the implementation team will communicate and coordinate their activities and progress. Second, it defines how progress will be communicated to key constituent groups, including but not limited to the board, the senior administrative team, the departments, and the staff members at all levels of the organization affected by the new system. The communication plan may set up formal and informal mechanisms. Formal communication may include everything from regular updates at board and administrative meetings to written briefings and articles in the facility newsletter. The purpose should be to use as many channels and mechanisms as possible to ensure that the people who need to know are fully informed and aware of the implementation plans. Informal communication is less structured but can be equally important. Implementing a new health care information system is a major undertaking, and it is important that all staff members (day, evening, and night shifts) be made aware of what is happening. The methods for communication may be varied, but the message should be consistent and the information presented up-to-date and timely. For example, do not rely on e-mail communication as your primary method only to discover later that your organization's nurses do not regularly check their e-mail or have little time to read your type of message.

Preparation for System Go-Live

A great deal of work goes into preparing for the go-live date, the day the organization transitions from the old system to the new. Assuming the implementation team has done all it can to ensure that the system is ready, the staff members are well trained, and appropriate procedures are in place, the transition should be a smooth one. Additional staff members should be on hand and equipped to assist users as needed. It is best to plan for the system to go-live on a day when the patient census is typically low or fewer patients than usual are scheduled to be seen. Disaster recovery plans should also be in place, and staff members should be well trained on what to do should the system go down or fail. Designated IT staff members should monitor and assess system problems and errors.

System Downtime Procedures

One thing that you can count on is that systems will go down. Both scheduled and unscheduled downtime exist, and downtime procedures need to be developed and communicated well before go-live. Any negative impact will be minimized if the organization has invested in a stable and secure technical IT infrastructure and backup procedures and fail-safe systems are in place. But everyone needs to know what to do if the system is down, from the registration staff members to the nursing staff members to the medical staff members and the transport team. How will orders be placed? If a paper record is kept during downtime, what is the procedure for getting the documentation in electronic form when the system is up again? How will scheduled downtime be communicated to units? And all staff members? If an organization relies heavily on computerized systems to care for patients, downtime should be minimal or near 0 percent. However, business continuity procedures must be in place to ensure patient safety and continuity of care.

MANAGING CHANGE AND THE ORGANIZATIONAL ASPECTS

Implementing an information system in a health care facility can have a profound impact on the organization, the people who work there, and the patients they serve. Individuals may have concerns and apprehensions about the new system: How will the new system affect my job responsibilities or productivity? How will my workload change? Will the new system cause me more or less stress? Even individuals who welcome the new system, see the need for it, and see its potential value may worry: What will I do if the system is down? Will the system impede my relationship with my patients? Who will I turn to if I have problems or questions? Will I be expected to type my notes into the system? With the new system comes change, and change can be difficult if not managed effectively.

Effecting Organizational Change

The management strategies required to manage change depend on the type of change. As one moves from incremental to fundamental change, the magnitude and risk of the change increase enormously, as does the uncertainty about the form and success of the outcome.

Managing change has several necessary aspects:

- Leadership
- Language and vision
- Connection and trust
- Incentives
- Planning, implementing, and iterating (Keen, 1997)

Leadership

Change must be led. Leadership, often in the form of a committee of leaders, will be necessary to accomplish the following:

- Define the nature of the change.
- Communicate the rationale for and approach to the change.
- Identify, procure, and deploy necessary resources.
- Resolve issues and alter direction as needed.
- Monitor the progress of the change initiative.

This leadership committee needs to be chaired by an appropriate senior leader. If the change affects the entire organization, the CEO should chair the committee. If the change is focused on a specific area, the most senior leader who oversees that area should chair the committee.

Language and Vision

The staff members who are experiencing the change must understand the nature of the change. They must know what the world will look like (to the degree that this is clear) when the change has been completed, how their roles and work life will be different, and why making this change is important. The absence of this vision or a failure to communicate the importance of the vision elevates the risk that staff members will resist the change and through subtle and not-so-subtle means cause the change to grind to a halt. Change is hard for people. They must understand the nature of the change and why they should go through with what they will experience as a difficult transition.

Leaders might describe the vision, the desired outcome of efforts to improve the outpatient service experience, in this way:

- Patients should be able to get an appointment for a time that is most convenient for them.
- Patients should not have to wait longer than ten minutes in the reception area before a provider can see them.
- We should communicate clearly with patients about their disease and the treatment that we will provide.
- We should seek to eliminate administrative and insurance busywork from the professional lives of our providers.

These examples illustrate a thoughtful use of language. They first and foremost focus on patients. But the organization also wants to improve the lives of its providers. The examples use the word *should* rather than the word *must* because it is thought that staff members won't believe the organization can pull off 100 percent achievement of these goals, and leaders do not want to establish goals seen as unrealistic. The examples also use the word *we* rather than the word *you*. *We* means that this vision will be achieved through a team effort, rather than implying that those hearing this message have to bear this challenge without leadership's help.

Connection and Trust

Achieving connection means that leadership takes every opportunity to present the vision throughout the organization. Leaders may use department head meetings, medical staff forums, one-on-one conversations in the hallway, internal publications, and e-mail to communicate the vision and to keep communicating the vision. Even when they start to feel ill because they have communicated the vision one thousand times, they have to communicate it another one thousand times. A lot of this communication has to be done in person, where others can see the leaders, rather than hiding behind an e-mail. The communication must invite feedback, criticism, and challenges.

The members of the organization must trust the integrity, intelligence, compassion, and skill of the leadership. Trust is earned or lost by everything that leaders do or don't do. The members must also trust that leaders have thoughtfully come to the conclusion that the difficult change has excellent reasons behind it and represents the best option for the organization. Organizational members are willing to rise to a challenge, often to heroic levels, if they trust their leaders. Trust requires that leaders act in the best interests of the staff and the organization and that leaders listen and respond to the organization's concerns.

Incentives

Organizational members must be motivated to support significant change. At times, excitement with the vision will be sufficient incentive. Alternatively, fear of what will happen if the organization fails to move toward the vision may serve as an incentive. Although important, neither fear nor rapture is necessarily sufficient.

If organizational members will lose their jobs or have their roles changed significantly, education that prepares them for new roles or new jobs must be offered. Bonuses may be offered to key individuals, awarded according to the success of the change and each person's contribution to the change. At times, frankly, support is obtained through old-fashioned horse-trading—if the other person will support the change, you will deliver something that is of interest to him or her (space, extra staff members, a promotion). Incentives may also take the form of awards—for example, plaques and dinners for two—to staff members who go above and beyond the call of duty during the change effort.

Planning, Implementing, and Iterating

Change must be planned. These plans describe the tasks and task sequences necessary to effect the change. Tasks can range from redesigning forms to managing the staged implementation of application systems to retraining staff members. Tasks must be allotted resources, and staff members accountable for task performance must be designated.

Implementation of the plan is obviously necessary. Because few organizational changes of any magnitude will be fully understood beforehand, problems will be encountered during implementation. New forms may fail to capture necessary data. The estimate of the time needed to register a patient may be wrong and long lines may form at the registration desk. The planners may have forgotten to identify how certain information would flow from one department to another.

These problems are in addition to the problems that occur, for example, when task timetables slip and dependent tasks fall idle or are in trouble. The implementation of the application has been delayed and will not be ready when the staff members move to the new building—what do we do? Iteration and adjustment will be necessary as the organization handles problems created when tasks encounter trouble and learns about glitches with the new processes and workflows.

Organizational and Behavioral Factors

The human factors associated with implementing a new system should not be taken lightly. A great deal of change can occur as a result of the new system. Some of the changes may be immediately apparent; others may occur over time as the system is used more fully. Many IT implementation studies have been done in recent years, and they reveal several strategies that may lead to greater organizational acceptance and use of a new system:

- Create an appropriate environment, one in which expectations are defined, met, and managed.
- Know your culture and do not underestimate user resistance.
- Allocate sufficient resources, including technical support staff members and IT infrastructure.
- Provide adequate initial and ongoing training.
- Manage unintended consequences, especially those known to affect implementations such as CPOE and EHR systems.
- Establish strong working relationships with vendors.

Each of these strategies is described in the following sections.

Create an Appropriate Environment

If you ask a roomful of health care executives, physicians, nurses, pharmacists, or laboratory managers if they have ever experienced an IT system failure, chances are over half of the hands in the room will go up. In all likelihood the people in the room would have a much easier time describing a system failure than a system success. If you probed a little further and asked why the system was a failure, you might hear comments such as these: "the system was too slow," "it was down all the time," "training was inadequate and nothing like the real thing," "there was no one to go to if you had questions or concerns," "it added to my stress and workload," and the list goes on. The fact is, the system did not meet their expectations. You might not know whether those expectations were reasonable or not.

Previously we discussed the importance of clearly defining and communicating the goals and objectives of the new system. Related to goal definition is the management of user expectations. Different people may have different perspectives on what they expect from the new system; in addition, some will admit to having no expectations, and others will have joined the organization after the system was implemented and consequently are likely to have expectations derived from the people currently using the system.

Expectations come from what people see and hear about the system and the way they interpret what the system will do for them or for their organization. Expectations can be formed from a variety of sources—they may come from a comment made during a vendor presentation, a question that arises during training, a visit to another site that uses the same system, attendance at a professional conference, or a remark made by a colleague in the hallway. Furthermore, the main criterion used to evaluate the system's value or success depends on the individual's expectations and point of view. For example, the chief financial officer might measure system success in terms of the financial return on investment, the chief medical director might look at impact on physicians' time and quality of care, the nursing staff members might consider any change in their workload, public relations personnel might compare levels of patient satisfaction, and the IT staff members might evaluate the change in the number of help desk calls made since the new system was implemented. All these approaches are measures of an information system's perceived impact on the organization or individual. However, they are not all the same, and they may not have equal importance to the organization in achieving its strategic goals.

It is therefore important for the health care executive team not only to establish and communicate clearly defined goals for the new system but also to listen to needs and expectations of the various user groups and to define, meet, and manage expectations appropriately. Ways to manage expectations include making sure users understand that the first days or weeks of system use may be rocky, that the organization may need time to adjust to a new workflow, that the technology may have bugs, and that users should not expect problem-free system operation from the start. Clear and effective communication is key in this endeavor.

In managing expectations it can be enormously helpful to conduct formative assessments of the implementation process, in which the focus is on the process as well as the outcomes. Specific metrics need to be chosen and success criteria defined to determine whether or not the system is meeting expectations (Cusack & Poon, 2011). For example, if wide-scale use is a priority, collection of actual numbers of transactions or use logs may be meaningful information for the leadership team. Other categories of metrics that might be helpful are clinical outcome measures, clinical process measures, provider adoption and attitude measures, patient knowledge and attitude measures, workflow impact measures, and financial impact measures. The Agency for Healthcare Research and Quality published the *Health Information Technology Evaluation Toolkit,* which can serve as a guide for project teams involved in evaluating the system implementation process or project outcomes (Cusack & Poon, 2011).

Know Your Culture and Do Not Underestimate User Resistance

Before embarking on system implementation, it is critical to know your culture. Understanding the culture is important *before* you make the investment. For example, you might ask, How engaged and ready are the physicians and other clinicians for the new system? Are they comfortable with technology? Do you have hospitalists on staff? Or are you a community hospital in which the bulk of your medical staff members are physicians who have admitting privileges at several hospitals and make rounds only once a day? How engaged have the physicians been in the design and build of the new system? Is there strong support? If you don't have sufficient medical staff buy-in and support or hospitalists on staff who are committed to the project, you run the risk of encountering **user resistance** and system failure because of inadequate use.

During the implementation process it is also important to analyze current workflow and make appropriate changes as needed. Previously we gave an example of analyzing a patient scheduling process. Patient scheduling is a relatively straightforward process. A change in this system may not dramatically change the job responsibilities of the schedulers and may have little impact on nurses' or physicians' time. Therefore, these groups may offer little resistance to such a change. (This is not to guarantee a lack of resistance—if you mess up a practice's schedule, you can have a lot of angry people on your hands!) By contrast, changes in processes that involve the direct provision of patient care services and that do affect nurses' and physicians' time may be tougher for users to accept. The physician ordering process is a perfect example. Historically most physicians were accustomed to picking up a pen and paper and handwriting an order or calling one in to the nurses' station from their phones. With CPOE, physicians may be expected to keyboard their orders directly into the system and respond to automated reminders and decision-support alerts. A process that historically took them a few seconds to do might now take several minutes, depending on the number of prompts and reminders. Moreover, physicians are now doing things that were not asked of them before—they are checking for drug interactions, responding to reminders and alerts, evaluating whether evidence-based clinical guidelines apply to the patient, and the list goes on. All these activities take time, but in the long run they will improve the quality of patient care. Therefore, it is important for physicians to be actively involved in designing the process and in seeing its value to the patient care process.

Getting physicians, nurses, and other clinicians to accept and use clinical information systems can be challenging even when they are involved in the implementation. At times the incentives for using the system may not be aligned with their individual needs and goals. On the one hand, for example, if the physician is expected to see a certain number of patients per day and is evaluated on patient load and if writing orders used to take thirty minutes a day with the old system and now takes sixty to ninety minutes with the new CPOE system, the physician can either see fewer patients or work more hours. One should expect to see physician resistance. On the other hand, if the physician's performance and income is related to adherence to clinical practice guidelines, care coordination, and patient health outcomes, using the system may be far more enticing. A recent study among six health care organizations found that more senior physicians often feel a loss of power by having junior physicians more comfortable with computers than they are and a loss in power in the physicians' ability to shift work to others (McAlearney et al., 2015). That is, with the implementation of EHRs, the physicians were now required to use the computers and input their orders rather than delegate the tasks to junior physicians or nurses.

It perhaps goes without saying that user acceptance occurs when users see or realize the value the health care information system brings to their work and the patients they serve. This value takes different forms. Some people may realize increased efficiency, less stress, greater organization, and improved quality of information, whereas others may find that the system enables them to provide better care, avoid medical mistakes, and make better decisions. In some cases an individual may not experience the value personally yet may come to realize the value to the organization as a whole.

Allocate Sufficient Resources

Sufficient resources are needed during and after the new system has been implemented. User acceptance comes from confidence in the new system. Individuals want to know that the system works properly, is stable and secure, and that someone is available to help them when they have questions, problems, or concerns. Therefore, it is important for the organization to ensure that adequate resources are devoted to implementing and supporting the system and its users. At a minimum, adequate technical staff expertise should be available as well as sufficient IT infrastructure.

We have discussed the importance of giving the implementation team sufficient support as it carries out its charge, but what forms can this support take? Some methods of supporting the team are to make available release time, additional staff members, and development funds. Senior managers might allocate travel funds so team members can view the system in use in other facilities. They might decide that all implementation team members or super-users will receive 50 percent release time for the next six months to devote to the project. This release time will enable those involved to give up some of their normal job duties so they can focus on the project.

Providing sufficient time and resources to the implementation phase of the project is, however, only part of the overall support needed. Studies have shown that an information system's value to the organization is typically realized over time. Value is derived as more and more people use the system, offer suggestions for enhancing it, and begin to push the system to fulfill its functionality. If users are ever to fully realize the system's value, they must have access to local technical support—someone, preferably within the organization, who is readily available, is knowledgeable about the intricacies of the system, and is able to handle hardware and software problems. This individual should be able to work effectively with the vendor and others to find solutions to system problems. Even though it is ideal to have local technical support in-house, that may be difficult in small physician offices or community-based settings. In such cases the facility may need to consider such options as (1) devoting a significant portion of an employee's time to training so that he or she may assume a support role, (2) partnering with a neighboring organization that uses the same system to share technical support staff members, or (3) contracting with a local computer firm to provide the needed assistance. The vendor may be able to assist the organization in identifying and securing local technical support.

In addition to arranging for local technical support, the organization will also need to invest resources in building and maintaining a reliable, secure IT infrastructure (servers, operating systems, and networks) to support the information system, particularly if it is a mission-critical system. Many patient information systems need to be available 24 hours a day, 7 days a week, 365 days a year. Health care professionals can come to rely on having access to timely, accurate, and complete information in caring for their patents, just as they count on having electricity, water, and other basic utilities. Failing to build the IT infrastructure that will adequately support the new clinical system can be catastrophic for the organization and its IT department.

An IT infrastructure's lifetime may be relatively short. It is reasonable to expect that within three to ten years, the hardware, software, and network will likely need to be replaced as advances are made in technology, the organization's goals and needs change, and the health care environment changes. Downtime, scheduled and unscheduled, should be limited.

Provide Adequate Training

Previously we discussed the importance of training staff members on the new system prior to the go-live date. Having a training program suited to the needs of the various user groups is very important during the implementation process. People who will use the system should be relatively comfortable with it, have had ample opportunities to use it in a safe environment, and know where to turn should they have questions or need additional assistance. It is equally important to provide ongoing training months and even years after the system has been implemented. In all likelihood the system will go through a series of upgrades, changes will be made, and users will get more comfortable with the fundamental features and will be ready to push the system to the next level. Some users will explore additional functionality on their own; others will need prodding and additional training in order to learn more advanced features.

It is also critical to provide the type of training that works best for your users' needs and learning preferences. Do not be afraid to have different training methods for different user groups (Holden, 2011). Memorial Sloan-Kettering Cancer Center is a perfect example. It is one of the world's oldest private cancer centers in the world. All of its physicians are employees of the organization. When they were first implementing their CPOE, all clinical and administrative staff members underwent group training sessions (Sklarin, Granovsky, & Hagerty-Paglia, 2011). The system was not accepted by the physicians for a variety of reasons, and training was a critical issue. Once the leadership team realized this, they regrouped, changed tactics, and added three new approaches to working with the physicians: (1) they rolled out one service at a time with one hour of personalized training to each physician of that service (additional time did not seem to help); (2) support staff members were stationed at the clinical areas during the implementation period for individualized assistance; and (3) a physician champion was involved in workflow discussions and key in facilitating the placement of orders in the system and in helping ensure physician compliance (Sklarin et al., 2011). Understanding the culture and the physician training needs of the organization is vital when implementing a new system, as is a willingness to reevaluate the project. It is important to view the system as a long-term investment rather than a one-time purchase. The resources allocated or committed to the system should include not only the upfront investment in hardware and software but also the time, people, and resources needed to maintain and support it.

Manage Unintended Consequences

Management expertise and leadership are important elements to the success of any system implementation. Effective leaders help build a community of collaboration and trust. However, effective leadership also entails understanding the **unintended consequences** that can occur during complex system implementations and managing them. Unintended consequences can be positive, negative, or both, depending on one's perspective. A decade ago, Ash and colleagues (2007) conducted interviews with key individuals from 176 US hospitals that had implemented CPOE. CPOE is one of the most complex and challenging of clinical applications to implement and a key function of EHR systems. From their work, they identified eight types of unintended consequences that implementation teams should plan for and consider when implementing CPOE.

Conflicts can also occur between paper-based and electronic systems if providers who prefer paper records annotate printouts and place them in patient charts as formal documentation, in essence creating two distinct and sometimes conflicting patient records (Jones et al., 2011).

Health care executives and implementation teams should be aware of these unintended consequences, particularly those that can adversely affect the organization, and carefully plan for and manage them.

Establish Strong Working Relationships with Vendors

Developing strong working relationships with the vendor is key. The health care executive should view the vendor as a partner and an entity with which the organization will likely have a long-term relationship. This relationship often begins when the organization first selects a new information system

1. **More work or new work.** CPOEs can increase work because systems may be slow, nonstandard cases may call for more steps in ordering, training may remain an issue, some tasks may become more difficult, the computer forces the user to complete "all steps," and physicians often take on tasks that were formerly done by others.

2. **Workflow.** CPOEs can greatly alter workflow, sometimes improving workflow for some and slowing or complicating it for others.

3. **System demands.** Maintenance, training, and support efforts can be significant for an organization, not only in building the system but also in making improvements and enhancements to it.

4. **Communication.** CPOE systems affect communication within the organization; they can reduce the need to clarify orders but also lead to people failing to adequately communicate with each other in appropriate situations.

5. **Emotions.** Clinician reactions to CPOE can run the gamut from positive to negative.

6. **New kinds of errors.** Although CPOE systems are generally designed to detect and prevent errors, they can lead to new types of errors such as juxtaposition errors, in which clinicians click on the adjacent patient name or medication from a list and inadvertently enter the wrong order.

7. **Power shifts.** Shifts in power may be viewed as less of a problem than some of the other unintended consequences, but CPOE can be used to monitor physician behavior.

8. **Dependence on the system.** Clinicians become dependent on the CPOE system, so managing downtime procedures is critical. Even then, while the system is down, CPOE users view the situation as managed chaos.

Source: Adapted from Ash et al. (2007). Reproduced with permission of American Medical Informatics Association.

and continues well after the system is live and operational. The system will have upgrades, new version releases, and ongoing maintenance contracts. It behooves both parties, the health care provider organization and the vendor, to clearly define expectations, resource needs, and timelines. It is important to have open, honest, and candid conversations when problems arise or differences in expectation occur. Equally important is for both parties to demonstrate a willingness to address needs and solve problems collaboratively.

SYSTEM SUPPORT AND EVALUATION

Information systems evolve as an organization continues to grow and change. No matter how well the system was designed and tested, errors and problems will be detected and changes will need to be made. IT staff members generally assume a major role in maintaining and supporting the information systems in the health care organization. When errors or problems are detected, IT staff members correct the problem or work with the vendor to see that the problem is fixed. Moreover, the vendor may detect glitches and develop upgrades or patches that will need to be installed.

Many opportunities for enhancing and optimizing the system's performance and functionality will arise well after the go-live date. The organization will want to ensure that the system is adequately maintained, supported, and further developed over time. Selecting and implementing a health care information system is an enormous investment. This investment must be maintained, just as one would maintain one's home. In fact, health care organizations that have implemented EHR systems are now actively in the midst of optimizing use of the system in practice (Sachs & Long, 2016). Optimization can take the form of additional training, revised workflows, adding new features or functionality, or using data from the system for quality improvement initiatives, as examples. Optimizing systems and assessing their value is discussed in Chapter Seven.

As with other devices, information systems have a life cycle and eventually need to be replaced. Health care organizations typically go through a process whereby they plan, design, implement, and evaluate their health care information systems. Too often in the past the organization's work was viewed as done once the system went live. It has since been discovered how vital system maintenance and support resources are and how important it is to evaluate the extent to which the system goals are being achieved.

Evaluating or accessing the value of the health care information system is increasingly important. Acquiring and implementing systems requires large investments, and stakeholders, including boards of directors, are demanding to know the actual and future value of these projects. Evaluations must be viewed as an integral component of every major health information system project and not an afterthought. Chapter Seven is devoted to this topic.

SUMMARY

Implementing a new information system in a health care organization requires a significant amount of planning and preparation. The health care organization should begin by appointing an implementation team comprising experienced individuals, including representatives from key areas in the organization, particularly areas that will be affected by or responsible for using the new system. Key users should be involved in analyzing existing processes and procedures and making recommendations for changes. A system champion should be part of the implementation team and serve as an advocate in soliciting input, representing user views, and spearheading the project. When implementing a clinical application, it is important that the system champion be a physician or clinician, someone who is able to represent the views of the care providers.

Under the direction of a highly competent implementation team, a number of important activities should occur during the system rollout. This team should assume a leadership role in ensuring that the system is effectively incorporated into the day-to-day operations of the facility. This generally requires the organization to (1) analyze workflow and processes and perform any necessary process reengineering, (2) install and configure the system, (3) train staff members, (4) convert data, (5) adequately test the system, and (6) communicate project progress using appropriate forums at all levels throughout the organization. Attention should be given to the countless details associated with ensuring that downtime and backup procedures are in place, security plans have been developed, and the organization is ready for the go-live date.

During the days immediately following system implementation, the organization should have sufficient staff members on hand to assist users and provide individual assistance as needed. A stable and secure IT infrastructure should be in place to ensure minimal, ideally zero, downtime and adequate response time. The IT department or other appropriate unit or representative should have a formal mechanism in place for reporting and correcting errors, bugs, and glitches in the system.

Once the system has gone live, it is critical for the organization to have in place the plans and resources needed to adequately maintain and support the new system. Technical staff members and resources should be available to the users. Ongoing training should be an integral part of the organization's plans to support and further develop the new system. In addition, the leadership team should have in place a thoughtful plan for evaluating the implementation process and assessing the value of the health care information system.

Beyond taking ultimate responsibility for completion of the activities needed to implement and support and evaluate the new system, the health care executive should assume a leadership role in managing change and the organizational and human aspects of the new system. Information systems can have a profound impact on health care organizations, the people who work there, and the patients they serve. Acquiring a good product and having the right technical equipment and expertise are not enough to ensure system success. Health care executives must also be attuned to the human aspects of introducing new IT into the care delivery process.

KEY TERMS

Business owner	*System champion*
Business sponsor	*System implementation*
Implementation team	*Train the trainer*
IT manager	*Unintended consequences*
Managing change	*User resistance*
Project manager	*Workflow and process analysis*

LEARNING ACTIVITIES

1. Visit a health care organization that has recently implemented or replaced a health care information system. What process did it use to implement the system? How does that process compare with the one described in this chapter? How successful was the organization in implementing the new system? To what do staff members attribute this success?

2. Search the literature for a recent article on a system implementation project. Briefly describe the process used to implement the system and the lessons learned. How might this particular facility's experiences be useful to others? Explain.

3. Physician acceptance and use of clinical information systems are often cited as challenges. What do you think the health care leadership team can or should do to foster acceptance by physicians? Assume that a handful of physicians in your organization are actively resisting a new clinical information system. How would you approach and address their resistance and concerns?

4. Assume you are working with an implementation team in installing a new nursing documentation system for a home health agency. Historically, all its nursing documentation was recorded in paper form. The home health agency has little computerization beyond basic registration information and has no IT staff members. What recommendations might you offer to the implementation team as it begins the work of installing the new nursing documentation system?

5. Discuss the risks to a health care organization in failing to allocate sufficient support and resources to a newly implemented health care information system.

6. Assume you are the CEO of a large group practice (seventy-five physicians) that implemented an EHR system two years ago. The physicians are asking for an evaluation of the system and its impact on quality, costs, and patient satisfaction. Devise a plan for evaluating the EHR system's impact on the organization in these three areas.

7. Read the executive summary of the Institute of Medicine's (2011) report entitled *Health IT and Patient Privacy: Building Safer Systems for Better Care.* How can the introduction of health IT that is designed to enhance or improve patient quality and safety lead to patient safety concerns? Do you agree that patient safety is a partnership between the health care organization and health IT vendor when implementing health care information systems? Explain the role of each and your rationale.

REFERENCES

Ash, J. S., Anderson, N. R., & Tarczy-Hornoch, P. (2008). People and organization issues in research systems implementation. *Journal of the American Medical Informatics Association, 15,* 283–289.

Ash, J. S., Sittig, D. F., Poon, E. G., Guappone, K., Campbell, E., & Dykstra, R. (2007). The extent and importance of unintended consequences related to computerized provider order entry. *Journal of the American Medical Informatics Association, 14*(4), 415–423.

Ash, J. S., Stavri, P., Dykstra, R., & Fournier, L. (2003). Implementing computerized physician order entry: The importance of special people. *International Journal of Medical Informatics, 69*(2–3), 235–250.

Cusack, C., & Poon, E. (2011). *Health information exchange evaluation toolkit.* Agency for Healthcare Research and Quality. Retrieved February 2013 from http://healthit.ahrq.gov/portal/server.pt/community/health_it_tools_and_resources/919/health_information_exchange_(hie)_evaluation_toolkit/27870

Daly, R. (2016). The EHR evolution: New priorities and implementation changes. *Healthcare Financial Management* (Feb.), 45–50.

Elias, B., Barginere, M., Berry, P. A., & Selleck, C. S. (2015). Implementation of an electronic health records system within an interprofessional model of care. *Journal of Interprofessional Care, 29*(6), 551–554.

Holden, R. J. (2011). What stands in the way of technology-mediated patient safety improvements? A study of facilitators and barriers to physicians' use of electronic health records. *Journal of Patient Safety, 7*(4), 193–202.

Institute of Medicine (IOM). (2011). *Health IT and patient privacy: Building safer systems for better care.* Washington, DC: National Academies Press.

Jones, S. S., Koppel, R., Ridgley, M. S., Palen, T., Wu, S., & Harrison, M. I. (2011, Aug.). *Guide to reducing unintended consequences of electronic health records.* Rockville, MD: Agency for Healthcare Research and Quality.

Keen, P. (1997). *The process edge.* Boston, MA: Harvard Business School Press.

McAlearney, A. S., Hefner, J. L., Sieck, C. J., & Huerta, T. R. (2015). The journey through grief: Insights from a qualitative study of electronic health record implementation. *Health Services Research, 50*(2), 462–488.

Metzger, J., & Fortin, J. (2003). *Computerized physician order entry in community hospitals: Lessons from the field.* Oakland, CA: California HealthCare Foundation.

Miller, R. H., & Sim, I. (2004). Physicians' use of electronic medical records: Barriers and solutions. *Health Affairs, 23*(2), 116–126.

Miller, R. H., Sim, I., & Newman, J. (2003). *Electronic medical records: Lessons from small physician practices.* Oakland, CA: California HealthCare Foundation.

Sachs, P. B., & Long, G. (2016). Process for managing and optimizing radiology work flow in the electronic health record environment. *Journal of Digital Imaging, 29,* 43–46.

Sittig, D. F., & Singh, H. (2011). Defining health information technology-related errors: New developments since *To Err Is Human. Archives of Internal Medicine, 171*(14), 1281–1284.

Sklarin, N. T., Granovsky, S., & Hagerty-Paglia, J. (2011). Electronic health record implementation at an academic cancer center: Lessons learned and strategies for success. *American Society of Clinical Oncology,* pp. 411–415.

Wager, K. A., Lee, F., White, A., Ward, D., & Ornstein, S. (2000). Impact of an electronic medical record system on community-based primary care practices. *Journal of the American Board of Family Practice, 13*(5), 338–348.

Yackanicz, L., Kerr, R., & Levick, D. (2010). Physician buy-in for EMRs. *Journal of Healthcare Information Management, 24*(2), 41–44.

CHAPTER 7

Assessing and Achieving Value in Health Care Information Systems

Virtually all the discussion in this book focuses on the knowledge and management processes necessary to achieve one fundamental objective: organizational investments in IT resulting in a desired value. That value might be the furtherance of organizational strategies, improvement in the performance of core processes, or the enhancement of decision making. Achieving value requires the alignment of IT with overall strategies, thoughtful governance, solid information system selection and implementation approaches, and effective organizational change.

Failure to achieve desired value can result in significant problems for the organization. Money is wasted. Execution of strategies is hamstrung. Organizational processes can be damaged.

This chapter carries the IT value discussion further. Specifically, it covers the following topics:

- The definition of IT-enabled value
- The IT project proposal
- Ensuring the delivery of value
- Analyses of the IT value challenge

DEFINITION OF IT-ENABLED VALUE

We can make several observations about IT-enabled value:

- IT value can be tangible and intangible.
- IT value can be significant.
- IT value can be variable across organizations.
- IT value can be diverse across IT proposals.
- A single IT investment can have a diverse value proposition.
- Different IT investments have different objectives and hence different value propositions and value assessment techniques.

These observations will be discussed in more detail in the following sections.

Tangible and Intangible

Tangible value can be measured whereas intangible value is very difficult, perhaps practically impossible, to measure.

Some tangible value can be measured in terms of dollars:

- Increases in revenue
- Reductions in labor costs: for example, through staff layoffs, overtime reductions, or shifting work to less expensive staff members
- Reductions in supply costs: for example, because of improvements in purchasing
- Reductions in maintenance costs for computer systems
- Reductions in use of patient care services: for example, fewer lab tests are performed or care is conducted in less expensive settings

Some tangible value can be measured in terms of process improvements:

- Fewer errors
- Faster turnaround times for test results
- Reductions in elapsed time to get an appointment
- A quicker admissions process
- Improvement in access to data
- Improvements in the percentage of care delivery that follows medical evidence

Some tangible value can be measured in terms of strategically important operational and market outcomes:

- Growth in market share
- Reduction in turnover
- Increase in brand awareness
- Increase in patient and provider satisfaction
- Improvement in reliability of computer systems

By contrast, intangible value can be very difficult to measure. The organization is trying to measure such things as

- Improved decision making
- Improved communication
- Improved compliance
- Improved collaboration

- Increased agility
- Becoming more state of the art
- Improved organizational competencies: for example, becoming better at managing chronic disease
- Becoming more customer friendly

Significant

IT can be leveraged to achieve significant organization value. The following are some example studies:

A study that compared the quality of diabetes care between physician practices that used EHRs and practices that did not found that the EHR sites had composite standards for diabetes care that were 35.1 percent higher than paper-based sites and had 15 percent better care outcomes (Cebul, Love, Jain, & Herbert, 2011).

EMC (a company that makes data storage devices and other information technologies) reported a reduction of $200 million in health care costs over ten years through the use of data analytics, lifestyle coaches, and remote patient monitoring to help employees manage health risks and chronic diseases (Mosquera, 2011).

A cross-sectional study of hospitals in Texas (Amarasingham, Plantinga, Diener-West, Gaskin, & Powe, 2009) found that higher levels of the automation of notes and patient records were associated with a 15 percent decrease in the adjusted odds of a fatal hospitalization. Higher scores in the use of computerized provider order entry (CPOE) were associated with 9 percent and 55 percent decreases in the adjusted odds of death for myocardial infarction and coronary artery bypass graft procedures, respectively. For all cases of hospitalization, higher levels of clinical decision-support use were associated with a 16 percent decrease in the adjusted odds of complications. And higher levels of CPOE, results reporting, and clinical decision support were associated with lower costs for all hospital admissions.

A clinical decision support (CDS) module, embedded within an EHR, was used to provide early detection of situations that could result in venous thromboembolism (VTE). A study of the impact of the module showed that the VTE rate declined from 0.954 per one thousand patient days to 0.434 comparing baseline to full VTE CDS. Compared to baseline, patients benefitting from VTE CDS were 35 percent less likely to have a VTE (Amland et. al., 2015).

Variable

Even when they implement the same system, not all organizations experience the same value. Organizational factors such as change management prowess and governance have a significant impact on an organization's ability to be successful in implementing health information technology.

As an example of variability, two children's hospitals implemented the same EHR (including CPOE) in their pediatric intensive care units. One hospital experienced a significant increase in mortality (Han et al., 2005), whereas the other did not (Del Beccaro, Jeffries, Eisenberg, & Harry, 2006). The hospital that did experience an increase in mortality noted that several implementation factors contributed to the deterioration in quality; specific order sets for critical care were not created, changes in workflow were not well executed, and orders for patients arriving via critical care transportation could not be written before the patient arrived at the hospital, delaying life-saving treatments.

Even when organizations have comparable implementation skill levels, the value achieved can vary because different organizations decide to focus on different objectives. For example, some organizations may decide to improve the quality of diabetes care, and others may emphasize the reduction in care costs. Hence, if an outcome is of modest interest to an organization and it devotes few resources to achieving that outcome, it should not be surprised if the outcome does not materialize.

Diverse across Proposals

Consider three proposals (real ones from a large integrated delivery system) that might be in front of organizational leadership for review and approval: a disaster notification system, a document imaging system, and an e-procurement system. Each offers a different type of value to the organization.

The disaster notification system would enable the organization to page critical personnel, inform them that a disaster—for example, a train wreck or biotoxin outbreak—had taken place, and tell them the extent of the disaster and the steps they would need to take to help the organization respond to the disaster. The system would cost $520,000. The value would be "better preparedness for a disaster."

The document imaging system would be used to electronically store and retrieve scanned images of paper documents, such as payment reconciliations, received from insurance companies. The system would cost $2.8 million, but would save the organization $1.8 million per year ($9 million over the life of the system) through reductions in the labor required to look for paper documents and in the insurance claim write-offs that occur because a document cannot be located.

The e-procurement system would enable users to order supplies, ensure that the ordering person had the authority to purchase supplies, transmit the order to the supplier, and track the receipt of the supplies. Data from this system could be used to support the standardization of supplies, that is, to reduce the number of different supplies used. Such standardization might save $500,000 to $3 million per year. The actual savings would depend on physician willingness to standardize. The system would cost $2.5 million.

These proposals reflect a diversity of value, ranging from "better disaster response" to a clear financial return (document imaging) to a return with such a wide potential range (e-procurement) that it could be a great investment (if you really could save $3 million a year) or a terrible investment (if you could save only $500,000 a year).

Diverse in a Single Investment

Picture archiving and communication systems (PACS) are used to store radiology (and other) images, support interpretation of images, and distribute the information to the physician providing direct patient care. These systems are an example of the diversity of value that can result from one IT investment. A PACS can do the following:

- Reduce costs for radiology film and the need for film librarians.
- Improve service to the physician delivering care, through improved access to images.
- Improve productivity for the radiologists and for the physicians delivering care (both groups reduce the time they spend looking for images).
- Generate revenue, if the organization uses the PACS to offer radiology services to physician groups in the community.

This one investment has a diverse value proposition; it has the potential to deliver cost reduction, productivity gains, service improvements, and revenue gains.

Different Analyses for Different Objectives

The Committee to Study the Impact of Information Technology on the Performance of Service Activities (1994), organized by the National Research

Council (NRC), has identified six categories of IT investments in service industries, reflecting different objectives. The techniques used to assess IT investment value should vary by the type of objective that the IT investment intends to support. One technique does not fit all IT investments.

Infrastructure

IT investments may be for infrastructure that enables other investments or applications to be implemented and deliver desired capabilities. Examples of infrastructure are data communication networks, workstations, and clinical data repositories. A delivery system–wide network enables a large organization to implement applications to consolidate clinical laboratories, implement organization-wide collaboration tools, and share patient health data between providers.

It is difficult to quantitatively assess the impact or value of infrastructure investments because of the following:

- They enable applications. Without those applications, infrastructure has no value. Hence, infrastructure value is indirect and depends on application value.

- The allocation of infrastructure value across applications is complex. When millions of dollars are invested in a data communication network, it may be difficult or impossible to determine how much of that investment should be allocated to the ability to create delivery system–wide EHRs.

- A good IT infrastructure is often determined by its agility, potency, and ability to facilitate integration of applications. It is very difficult to assign return on investment (ROI) numbers or any meaningful numerical value to most of these characteristics. What, for instance, is the value of being agile enough to speed up the time it takes to develop and enhance applications?

Information system infrastructure is as hard to evaluate as other organizational infrastructure, such as having talented, educated staff members. As with other infrastructure,

- Evaluation is often instinctive and experientially based.

- In general, underinvesting can severely limit the organization.

- Investment decisions involve choosing between alternatives that are assessed for their ability to achieve agreed-on goals. For example,

Four Types of IT Investment

Complementing the NRC study, Jeanne Ross and Cynthia Beath (2002) studied the IT investment approaches of thirty companies from a wide range of industries. They identified four classes of investment:

- **Transformation.** These IT investments had an impact that would affect the entire organization or a large number of business units. The intent of the investment was to effect a significant improvement in overall performance or change the nature of the organization.
- **Renewal.** Renewal investments were intended to upgrade core IT infrastructure and applications or reduce the costs or improve the quality of IT services. Examples of these investments include application replacements, upgrades of the network, or expansion of data storage.
- **Process improvement.** These IT investments sought to improve the operations of a specific business entity—for example, to reduce costs and improve service.
- **Experiments.** Experiments were designed to evaluate new information technologies and test new types of applications. Given the results of the experiments, the organization would decide whether broad adoption was desirable.

Different organizations will allocate their IT budgets differently across these classes. An office products company had an investment mix of experiments (15 percent), process improvement (40 percent), renewal (25 percent), and transformation (20 percent). An insurance firm had an investment mix of experiments (3 percent), process improvement (25 percent), renewal (18 percent), and transformation (53 percent).

The investment allocation is often an after-the-fact consideration—the allocation is not planned, it just "happens." However, ideally, the organization decides its desired allocation structure and does so before the budget discussions. An organization with an ambitious and perhaps radical strategy may allocate a very large portion of its IT investment to the transformation class, whereas an organization with a conservative, stay-the-course strategy may have a large process improvement portion to its IT investments.

Source: Ross and Beath (2002, p. 54).

if an organization wishes to improve security, it might ask whether it should invest in network monitoring tools or enhanced virus protection. Which of these investments would enable it to make the most progress toward its goal?

Mandated

Information system investment may be necessary because of mandated initiatives. Mandated initiatives might involve reporting quality data to accrediting organizations, making required changes in billing formats, or improving disaster notification systems. Assessing these initiatives is generally approached by identifying the least expensive and the quickest to implement alternative that will achieve the needed level of compliance.

Cost Reduction

Information system investments directed to cost reduction are generally highly amenable to ROI and other quantifiable dollar-impact analyses. The ability to conduct a quantifiable ROI analysis is rarely the question. The ability of management to effect the predicted cost reduction or cost avoidance is often a far more germane question.

Specific New Products and Services

IT can be critical to the development of new products and services. At times the information system delivers the new service, and at other times it is itself the product. Examples of information system–based new services include bank cash-management programs and programs that award airline mileage for credit card purchases. A new service offered by some health care providers is a personal health record that enables a patient to communicate with his or her physician and to access care guidelines and consumer-oriented medical textbooks.

The value of some of these new products and services can be quantifiably assessed in terms of a monetary return. These assessments include analyses of potential new revenue, either directly from the service or from service-induced use of other products and services. An ROI analysis will need to be supplemented by techniques such as sensitivity analyses of consumer response. Despite these analyses, the value of this IT investment usually has a speculative component. This component involves consumer utilization, competitor response, and impact on related businesses.

Quality Improvement

Information system investments are often directed to improving the quality of service or medical care. These investments may be intended to reduce waiting times, improve the ability of physicians to locate information, improve treatment outcomes, or reduce errors in treatment. Evaluation of these initiatives, although quantifiable, is generally done in terms of service parameters that are known or believed to be important determinants of organizational success. These parameters might be measures of aspects of organizational processes that customers encounter and then use to judge the organization, for example, waiting times in the physician's office. A quantifiable dollar outcome for the service of care quality improvement can be very difficult to predict. Service quality is often necessary to protect current business, and the effect of a failure to continuously improve service or medical care can be difficult to project.

Major Strategic Initiative

Strategic initiatives in information technology are intended to significantly change the competitive position of the organization or redefine the core nature of the enterprise. In health care it is unusual that information systems are the centerpiece of a redefinition of the organization, although as we discussed in Chapter Four IT is a critical foundation for provider efforts to manage population health. However, several other industries have attempted IT-centric transformations.

Amazon is an effort to transform retailing. Venmo (which enables micropayments between individuals) is an effort to disrupt aspects of the branch bank. There can be a ROI core or component to analyses of such initiatives, because they often involve major reshaping or reengineering of fundamental organizational processes. However, assessing the ROIs of these initiatives and their related information systems with a high degree of accuracy can be very difficult. Several factors contribute to this difficulty:

- These major strategic initiatives usually recast the organization's markets and its roles. The outcome of the recasting, although visionary, can be difficult to see with clarity and certainty.
- The recasting is evolutionary; the organization learns and alters itself as it progresses over what are often lengthy periods of time. It is difficult to be prescriptive about this evolutionary process. Most accountable care organizations are confronting this phenomenon.
- Market and competitor responses can be difficult to predict.

IT value is diverse and complex. This diversity indicates the power of IT and the diversity of its use. Nonetheless, the complexity of the value proposition means that it is difficult to make choices between IT investments and also difficult to assess whether the investment ultimately chosen delivered the desired value or not.

THE IT PROJECT PROPOSAL

The **IT project proposal** is a cornerstone in examining value. Clearly, ensuring that all proposals are well crafted does not ensure value. To achieve value, alignment with organizational strategies must occur, factors for sustained IT excellence must be managed, budget processes for making choices between investments must exist, and projects must be well managed. However, the proposal (as will be discussed in Chapter Thirteen) does describe the intended outcome of the IT investment. The proposal requests money and an organizational commitment to devote management attention and staff effort to implementing an information system. The proposal describes why this investment of time, effort, and money is worth it—that is, the proposal describes the value that will result. In this section we discuss the value portion of the proposal and some common problems encountered with it.

Sources of Value Information

As project proponents develop their case for an IT investment, they may be unsure of the full gamut of potential value or of the degree to which a desired value can be truly realized. The organization may not have had experience with the proposed application and may have insufficient analyst resources to perform its own assessment. It may not be able to answer such questions as, What types of gains have organizations seen as a result of implementing a population health system? To what degree will IT be a major contributor to our efforts to improve patient access through telehealth?

Information about potential value can be obtained from several sources (discussed in Appendix A). Conferences often feature presentations that describe the efforts of specific individuals or organizations in accomplishing initiatives of interest to many others. Industry publications may offer relevant articles and analyses. Several industry research organizations—for example, Gartner and the Advisory Board—can offer advice. Consultants can be retained who have worked with clients who are facing or have addressed similar questions. Vendors of applications can describe the outcomes experienced by their customers. And colleagues can be contacted to determine the experiences of their organizations.

Garnering an understanding of the results of others is useful but insufficient. It is worth knowing that Organization Y adopted computerized provider order entry (CPOE) and reduced unnecessary testing by *x* percent. However, one must also understand the CPOE features that were critical in achieving that result and the management steps taken and the process changes made in concert with the CPOE implementation.

Formal Financial Analysis

Most proposals should be subjected to formal financial analyses regardless of their value proposition. Several types of financial measures are used by organizations. An organization's finance department will work with leadership to determine which measures will be used and how these measures will be compiled.

Two common financial measures are **net present value** and **internal rate of return:**

1. *Net present value* is calculated by subtracting the initial investment from the future cash flows that result from the investment. The cash can be generated by new revenue or cost savings. The future cash is discounted, or reduced, by a standard rate to reflect the fact that a dollar earned one or more years from now is worth less than a dollar one has today (the rate depends on the time period considered). If the cash generated exceeds the initial investment by a certain amount or percentage, the organization may conclude that the IT investment is a good one.

2. *Internal rate of return* is the discount rate at which the present value of an investment's future cash flow equals the cost of the investment. Another way to look at this is to ask, Given the amount of the investment and its promised cash, what rate of return am I getting on my investment? On the one hand, a return of 1 percent is not a good return (just as one would not think that a 1 percent return on one's savings was good). On the other hand, a 30 percent return is very good.

Table 7.1 shows the typical form of a financial analysis for an IT application.

Table 7.1 Financial analysis of a patient accounting document imaging system

	Current Year	Year 1	Year 2	Year 3	Year 4	Year 5	Year 6	Year 7
COSTS								
One-time capital expense	$1,497,466	$1,302,534						
System operations								
System maintenance	—	288,000	$288,000	$288,000	$288,000	$288,000	$288,000	$288,000
System maintenance	—	152,256	152,256	152,256	152,256	152,256	152,256	152,256
TOTAL COSTS	1,497,466	1,742,790	440,256	440,256	440,256	440,256	440,256	440,256
BENEFITS								
Revenue gains								
Rebilling of small secondary balances	—	651,000	868,000	868,000	868,000	868,000	868,000	868,000
Medicaid billing documentation	—	225,000	300,000	300,000	300,000	300,000	300,000	300,000
Disallowed Medicare bad debt audit	—	—	—	—	100,000	100,000	100,000	100,000
Staff savings								
Projected staff savings	—	36,508	136,040	156,504	169,065	169,065	169,065	171,096
Operating savings								
Projected operating savings	—	64,382	77,015	218,231	222,550	226,436	226,543	229,935
TOTAL BENEFITS	—	976,891	1,381,055	1,542,735	1,659,615	1,663,502	1,663,608	1,669,031
CASH FLOW	(1,497,466)	(765,899)	940,799	1,102,479	1,219,359	1,223,246	1,223,352	1,228,775
CUMULATIVE CASH FLOW	(1,497,466)	(2,263,365)	(1,322,566)	(220,087)	999,272	2,222,517	3,445,869	4,674,644
NPV (12% discount)	1,998,068							
IRR	33%							

Comparing Different Types of Value

Given the diversity of value, it is very challenging to compare IT proposals that have different value propositions. How does one compare a proposal that promises to increase revenue and improve collaboration to one that offers improved compliance, faster turnaround times, and reduced supply costs?

At the end of the day, judgment is used to choose one proposal over another. Health care executives review the various proposals and associated value statements and make choices based on their sense of organizational priorities, available monies, and the likelihood that the proposed value will be seen. These judgments can be aided by developing a scoring approach that enables leaders to apply a common metric across proposals. For example, the organization might decide to score each proposal according to how much value it promises to deliver in each of the following areas:

- Revenue impact
- Cost reduction
- Patient or customer satisfaction
- Quality of work life
- Quality of care
- Regulatory compliance
- Potential learning value

In this approach, each of these areas in each proposal is assigned a score, ranging from 5 (significant contribution to the area) to 1 (minimal or no contribution). The scores are then totaled for each proposal, and, in theory, one picks those proposals with the highest aggregate scores. In practice, IT investment decisions are rarely that purely algorithmic. However, such scoring can be very helpful in sorting through complex and diverse value propositions:

- Scoring forces the leadership team to discuss why different members of the team assigned different scores—why, for example, did one person assign a score of 2 for the revenue impact of a particular proposal and another person assign a 4? These discussions can clarify people's understandings of proposal objectives and help the team arrive at a consensus on each project.
- Scoring means that the leadership team will have to defend any decision not to fund a project with a high score or to fund one with a low score. In the latter case, team members will have to discuss why they are all in favor of a project when it has such a low score.

PERSPECTIVE
Prerequisites for Effective IT Project Prioritization

Jeanne Ross and Emmett Johnson (2009) identified four prerequisites to effective IT project prioritization.

Explicit operating vision of the business. An operating vision is more than the sum of the operations of individual departments. Rather, it is a solid understanding of how the organization wants to operate as a whole. For example, how will the organization manage patients with a chronic disease? What processes must be in place to ensure a superior patient experience?

Operating visions lead to enterprise-wide requirements for integration and standardization. IT projects should support this vision and conform to these requirements.

Business process owners. Process owners are those senior leaders who are responsible for the performance of core organization processes, such as patient access. These owners must sponsor IT initiatives and be held accountable for their successful completion and value delivery. These owners are in a good position to understand the IT priorities of their processes.

Transparent IT operating costs. Organizational leadership must understand IT costs and the drivers of those costs. This understanding prepares them to thoughtfully assess the risks and benefits of proposed new systems and to identify alternative approaches to achieving desired process gains.

Rigorous project governance. Excellent IT governance must exist for the overall IT agenda (to be discussed in Chapter Twelve) and for individual projects (to be discussed in Chapter Thirteen).

Source: Ross and Johnson (2009).

The organization can decide which proposal areas to score and which not to score. Some organizations give different areas different weights—for example, reducing costs might be considered twice as important as improving organizational learning. The resulting scores are not binding, but they can be helpful in arriving at a decision about which projects will be approved and what value is being sought.

Tactics for Reducing the Budget

Proposals for IT initiatives may originate from a wide variety of sources in an organization. The IT group will submit proposals, as will department directors and physicians. Many of these proposals will not be directly related to an overall strategy but may nevertheless be good ideas that if implemented would lead to improved organizational performance. So it is common for an organization to have more proposals than it can fund. For example, during the IT budget discussion, the leadership team may decide that although it is looking at $2.2 million in requests, the organization can afford to spend only $1.7 million, so $500,000 worth of requests must be denied. Table 7.2 presents a sample list of requests.

Table 7.2 Requests for new information system projects

Community General Hospital

Project Name	Operating Cost
TOTAL	$2,222,704
Clinical portfolio development	38,716
Enterprise monitoring	70,133
HIPAA security initiative	36,950
Accounting of disclosure—HIPAA	35,126
Ambulatory Center patient tracking	62,841
Bar-coding infrastructure	64,670
Capacity management	155,922
Chart tracking	34,876
Clinical data repository	139,902
CRP research facility	7,026
Emergency Department data warehouse	261,584
Emergency Department order entry	182,412
Medication administration system	315,323
Order communications	377,228
Transfusion services replacement system	89,772
Wireless infrastructure	44,886
Next-generation order entry	3,403
Graduate medical education duty hours	163,763

Reducing the budget in situations such as this requires a value discussion. The leadership is declaring some initiatives to have more value than others. Scoring initiatives according to criteria is one approach to addressing this challenge.

In addition to such scoring, other assessment tactics can be employed, prior to the scoring, to assist leaders in making reduction decisions.

- Some requests are mandatory. They may be mandatory because of a regulation requirement (such as a new Medicare rule) or because a current system is so obsolete that it is in danger of crashing—permanently—and it must be replaced soon. These requests must be funded.

- Some projects can be delayed. They are worthwhile, but a decision on them can be put off until next year. The requester will get by in the meantime.

- Key groups within IT, such as the staff members who manage clinical information systems, may already have so much on their plate that they cannot possibly take on another project. Although the organization wants to do the project, it would be ill-advised to do so now, and so the project can be deferred to next year.

- The user department proposing the application may not have strong management or may be experiencing some upheaval; hence, implementing a new system at this time would be risky. The project could be denied or delayed until the management issues have been resolved.

- The value proposition or the resource estimates or both are shaky. The leadership team does not trust the proposal, so it could be denied or sent back for further analysis. Further analysis means that the proposal will be examined again next year.

- Less expensive ways of addressing the problems cited in the proposal may exist, such as a less expensive application or a non-IT approach. The proposal could be sent back for further analysis.

- The proposal is valuable, and the leadership team would like to move it forward. However, the team may reduce the budget, enabling progress to occur but at a slower pace. This delays realizing the value but ensures that resources are devoted to making progress.

These tactics are routinely employed during budget discussions aimed at trying to get as much value as possible given finite resources.

Common Proposal Problems

During the review of IT investment proposals, organizational leadership might encounter several problems related to the estimates of value and the estimates of the resources needed to obtain the value. If undetected, these problems might lead to a significant overstatement of potential return or understatement of costs. An overstatement or understatement, obviously, may result in significant organizational unhappiness when the value that people thought they would see never materializes and never could have materialized.

Fractions of Effort

Proposal analyses might indicate that the new IT initiative will save fractions of staff time, for example, that each nurse will spend fifteen minutes less per shift on clerical tasks. To suggest a total value, the proposal might multiply as follows (this example is highly simplified): 200 nurses $\times$ 15 minutes saved per 8-hour shift $\times$ 250 shifts worked per year = 12,500 hours saved. The math might be correct, and the conclusion that 12,500 hours will become available for doing other work such as direct patient care might also be correct. But the analysis will be incorrect if it then concludes that the organization would thus "save" the salary dollars of six nurses (assuming 2,000 hours worked per year per nurse).

Saving fractions of staff effort does not always lead to salary savings, even when there are large numbers of staff members, because there may be no practical way to realize the savings—to, for example, lay off six nurses. If, for example, there are six nurses working each eight-hour shift in a particular nursing unit, the fifteen minutes saved per nurse would lead to a total savings of 1.5 hours per shift. But if one were then to lay off one nurse on a shift, it would reduce the nursing capacity on that shift by eight hours, damaging the unit's ability to deliver care. Saving fractions of staff member effort does not lead to salary savings when staff members are geographically highly fragmented or when they work in small units or teams. It leads to possible salary savings only when staff members work in very large groups and some work of the reduced staff members can be redistributed to others.

Reliance on Complex Behavior

Proposals may project with great certainty that people will use systems in specific ways. For example, several organizations expect that consumers will use Internet-based quality report cards to choose their physicians and hospitals. However, few consumers appear to actually rely on such sites. Organizations may expect that nurses will readily adopt systems that help them discharge patients faster. However, nurses often delay entering discharge transactions so that they can grab a moment of peace in an otherwise overwhelmingly busy day.

System use is often not what was anticipated. This is particularly true when the organization has no experience with the relevant class of users or with the introduction of IT into certain types of tasks. The original value projection can be thrown off by the complex behaviors of system users. People do not always behave as we expect or want them to. If user behavior is uncertain, the organization would be wise to pilot an application and learn from this demonstration.

Unwarranted Optimism

Project proponents are often guilty of optimism that reflects a departure from reality. Proponents may be guilty of any of four mistakes:

- They assume that nothing will go wrong with the project.
- They assume that they are in full control of all variables that might affect the project—even, for example, quality of vendor products and organizational politics.
- They believe that they know exactly what changes in work processes will be needed and what system features must be present, when what they really have, at best, are close approximations of what must happen.
- They believe that everyone can give full time to the project and forget that people get sick or have babies and that distracting problems unrelated to the project will occur, such as a sudden deterioration in the organization's fiscal performance, and demand attention.

Decisions based on such optimism eventually result in overruns in project budgets and timetables and compromises in system goals. Overruns and compromises change the value proposition.

Shaky Extrapolations

Projects often achieve gains in the first year of their implementation, and proponents are quick to project that such gains will continue during the remaining life of the project. For example, an organization may see 10 percent of its physicians move from using dictation when developing a progress note to using structured, computer-based templates. The organization may then erroneously extrapolate that each year will see an additional 10 percent shift. In fact, the first year might be the only year in which such a gain will occur. The organization has merely convinced the more computer-facile physicians to change, and the rest of the physicians have no interest in ever changing.

Underestimating the Effort

Project proposals might count the IT staff member effort in the estimates of project costs but not count the time that users and managers will have to devote to the project. A patient care system proposal, for instance, may not include the time that will be spent by dozens of nurses working on system design, developing workflow changes, and attending training. These efforts are real costs. They often lead to the need to hire temporary nurses to provide coverage on the inpatient care units, or they might lead to a reduced patient census because there are fewer nursing hours available for patient care. Such miscounting of effort understates the cost of the project.

Fairy-Tale Savings

IT project proposals may note that the project can reduce the expenses of a department or function, including costs for staff members, supplies, and effort devoted to correcting mistakes that occur with paper-based processes. Department managers will swear in project approval forums that such savings are real. However, when asked if they will reduce their budgets to reflect the savings that will occur, these same managers may become significantly less convinced that the savings will result. They may comment that the freed-up staff member effort or supplies budgets can be redeployed to other tasks or expenses. The managers may be right that the expenses should be redeployed, and all managers are nervous when asked to reduce their budgets and still do the same amount of work. However, the savings expected have now disappeared.

Failure to Account for Post-Implementation Costs

After a system goes live, the costs of the system do not go away. System maintenance contracts are necessary. Hardware upgrades will be required. Staff members may be needed to provide enhancements to the application. These support costs may not be as large as the costs of implementation, but they are costs that will be incurred every year, and over the course of several years they can add up to some big numbers. Proposals often fail to adequately account for support costs.

ENSURING THE DELIVERY OF VALUE

Achieving value from IT investments requires management effort. There is no computer genie that descends on the organization once the system is live and waves its wand and—shazzam!—value has occurred. Achieving value is hard work but doable work. Management can take several steps to ensure the delivery of value (Dragoon, 2003; Glaser, 2003a, 2003b). These steps are discussed in the sections that follow.

Make Sure the Homework Was Done

IT investment decisions are often based on proposals that are not resting on solid ground. The proposer has not done the necessary homework, and this elevates the risk of a suboptimal return.

Clearly, the track record of the investment proposer will have a significant influence on the investment decision and on leaders' thinking about whether or not the investment will deliver value. However, regardless of the proposer's track record, an IT proposal should enable the leadership team to respond with a strong yes to each of the following questions:

- Is it clear how the plan advances the organization's strategy?
- Is it clear how care will improve, costs will be reduced, or service will be improved? Are the measures of current performance and expected improvement well researched and realistic? Have the related changes in operations, workflow, and organizational processes been defined?
- Are the senior leaders whose areas are the focus of the IT plan clearly supportive? Could they give the project proposal presentation?
- Are the resource requirements well understood and convincingly presented? Have these requirements been compared to those experienced by other organizations undertaking similar initiatives?
- Have the investment risks been identified, and is there an approach to addressing these risks?
- Do we have the right people assigned to the project, have we freed up their time, and are they well organized?

Answering with a no, a maybe, or an equivocal yes to any of these questions should lead one to believe that the discussion is perhaps focusing on an expense rather than an investment.

Require Formal Project Proposals

It is a fact of organizational life that projects are approved as a result of hallway conversations or discussions on the golf course. Organizational life is a political life. While recognizing this reality, the organization should require that every IT project be written up in the format of a proposal and that each proposal should be reviewed and subjected to scrutiny before the organization will commit to supporting it. However, an organization may also decide that small projects—for example, those that involve less than $25,000 in costs and less than 120 person-hours—can be handled more informally.

Increase Accountability for Investment Results

Few meaningful organizational initiatives are accomplished without establishing appropriate accountability for results. Accountability for IT investment results can be improved by taking three major steps.

First, the business owner of the IT investment should defend the investment—for example, the director of clinical laboratories should defend the request for a new laboratory system and the director of nursing should defend the need for a new nursing system. The IT staff members will need to work with the business owner to define IT costs, establish likely implementation time frames, and sort through application alternatives. But the IT staff members should never defend an application investment.

Second, as will be discussed in Chapter Thirteen, project sponsors and business owners must be defined, and they must understand the accountability that they now have for the successful completion of the project.

Third, the presentation of these projects should occur in a forum that routinely reviews such requests. Seeing many proposals, and their results, over the course of time will enable the forum participants to develop a seasoned understanding of good versus not-so-good proposals. Forum members are also able to compare and contrast proposals as they decide which ones should be approved. A manager might wonder (and it's a good question), "If I approve this proposal, does that mean that we won't have resources for another project that I might like even better?" Examining as many proposals together as possible enables the organization to take a portfolio view of its potential investments.

Figure 7.1 IT investment portfolio

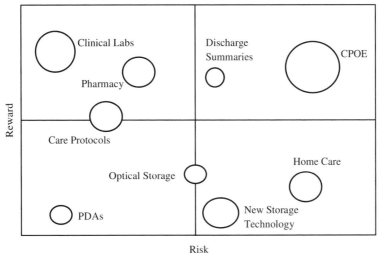

Source: Adapted from Arlotto and Oakes (2003). Copyright 2003 Healthcare Information and Management Systems Society (HIMSS) Used with permission.

Figure 7.1 displays an example of a project investment portfolio represented graphically. The size of each bubble reflects the magnitude of a particular IT investment. The axes are labeled "reward" (the size of the expected value) and "risk" (the relative risk that the project will not deliver the value). Other axes may be used. One commonly used set of axes consists of "support of operations" and "support of strategic initiatives."

Diagrams such as the one in Figure 7.1 serve several functions:

- They summarize IT activity on one piece of paper, enabling leaders to consider a new request in the context of prior commitments.
- They help to ensure a balanced portfolio, promptly revealing imbalances such as a clustering of projects in the high-risk quadrant.
- They help to ensure that the approved projects cover an appropriate spectrum of organizational needs: for example, that projects are directed to revenue cycle improvement, to operational improvement, and to patient safety.

Manage the Project Well

One guaranteed way to reduce value is to mangle the management of the implementation project. Implementation failures or significant budget

PERSPECTIVE
Types of Portfolio Investments

Peter Weill and Sinan Aral (2006) note that organizations should manage their IT investments as a portfolio. Specifically, they describe four types of IT investments in a portfolio.

Infrastructure. Infrastructure refers to the core information technology that serves as the foundation for all applications. Examples of infrastructure include networks, servers, operating systems, and mobile devices.

Transactional. Transactional systems are those applications that support the core operations processes. Examples of transactional systems include CPOE, scheduling, clinical laboratory automation, and clinician documentation.

Informational. Informational IT assets are those that support decision making such as clinical decision support, quality measurement and analyses, market assessment, and budget performance.

Strategic. Strategic investments are IT systems that are critical to the furthering of an organization's strategy. These investments could be infrastructure, transactional, and informational, but they differ in that they are clearly directed to furthering a strategic initiative as distinct from being helpful to support ongoing operations.

Weill and Aral note that different industries have different allocations of IT investments across these categories. Financial services emphasize infrastructure in an effort to ensure high reliability and low costs. However, retail has emphasized informational as they seek to understand customer buying patterns.

Source: Weill and Aral (2006).

and timetable overruns or really unhappy users—any of these can dilute value.

Among the many factors that can lead to mangled project management are the following:

- The project's scope is poorly defined.
- The accountability is unclear.

- The project participants are marginally skilled.
- The magnitude of the task is underestimated.
- Users feel like victims rather than participants.
- All the world has a vote and can vote at any time.

Many of these factors were discussed in Chapters Five and Six.

Manage Outcomes

Value is not an automatic result of implementing an information system. Value must be managed into existence. Figure 7.2 depicts a reduction in days in accounts receivable (AR) at a physician practice. During the interval depicted, a new practice management system was implemented. The practice did not see a precipitous decline in days in AR (a sign of improved revenue performance) in the time immediately following the implementation in the second quarter of 2015. The practice did see a progressive improvement in days in AR because someone was managing that improvement using the new capabilities that came with the new system.

If the gain in revenue performance had been an "automatic" result of the information system implementation, the practice would have seen a quick, sharp drop in days in AR. Instead it saw a gradual improvement over time. This gradual change reflects the following:

- The gain occurred through day-in, day-out changes in operational processes, fine-tuning of system capabilities, and follow-ups in staff training.

Figure 7.2 Days in accounts receivable

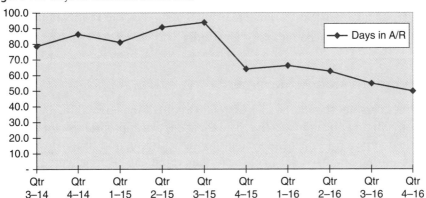

- A person had to be in charge of obtaining this improvement. Someone had to identify and make operational changes, manage changes in system capabilities, and ensure that needed training occurred.

Conduct Post-Implementation Audits

Rarely do organizations revisit their IT investments to determine if the promised value was actually achieved. They tend to believe that once the implementation is over and the change settles in, value will have been automatically achieved. This is unlikely.

Post-implementation audits can be conducted to identify value achievement progress and the steps still needed to achieve maximum gain. An organization might decide to audit two to four systems each year, selecting systems that have been live for at least six months. During the course of the audit meeting, these five questions can be asked:

1. What goals were expected at the time the project investment was approved?
2. How close have we come to achieving those original goals?
3. What do we need to do to close the goal gap?
4. How much have we invested in system implementation, and how does that compare to our original budget?
5. If we had to implement this system again, what would we do differently?

Post-implementation audits assist value achievement by the following:

- Signaling leadership interest in ensuring the delivery of results
- Identifying steps that still need to be taken to ensure value
- Supporting organizational learning about IT **value realization**
- Reinforcing accountability for results

Celebrate Value Achievement

Business value should be celebrated. Organizations usually hold parties shortly after applications go live. These parties are appropriate; a lot of people worked very hard to get the system up and running and used. However, up and running and used does not mean that value has been delivered. In addition to go-live parties, organizations should consider business value parties, celebrations conducted once the value has been achieved—for example, a party that celebrates the achievement of service improvement goals. Go-live parties alone risk sending the inappropriate signal that implementation is the end point of the IT initiative. Value delivery is the end point.

Leverage Organizational Governance

The creation of an IT committee of the board of directors can enhance organizational efforts to achieve value from IT investments. At times the leadership team of an organization is uncomfortable with some or all of the IT conversation. Board members may not understand why infrastructure is so expensive or why large implementations can take so long and cost so much. They may feel uncomfortable with the complexity of determining the likely value to be obtained from IT investments. The creation of a subcommittee made up of the board members most experienced with such discussions can help to ensure that hard questions are being asked and that the answers are sound.

Shorten the Deliverables Cycle

When possible, projects should have short deliverable cycles. In other words, rather than asking the organization to wait twelve or eighteen months to see the first fruits of its application implementation labors, make an effort to deliver a sequence of smaller implementations. For example, one might conduct pilots of an application in a subset of the organization, followed by a staged rollout. Or one might plan for serial implementation of the first 25 percent of the application features.

Pilots, staged rollouts, and serial implementations are not always doable. When they are possible, however, they enable the organization to achieve some value earlier rather than later, support organizational learning about which system capabilities are really important and which were only thought to be important, facilitate the development of reengineered operational processes, and create the appearance (whose importance is not to be underestimated) of more value delivery.

Benchmark Value

Organizations should benchmark their performance in achieving value against the performance of their peers. These benchmarks might focus on process performance—for example, days in accounts receivable or average time to get an appointment. An important aspect of value benchmarking is the identification of the critical IT application capabilities and related operational changes that enabled the achievement of superior results. This understanding of how other organizations achieved superior IT-enabled performance can guide an organization's efforts to continuously achieve as much value as possible from its IT investments.

Communicate Value

Once a year the IT department should develop a communication plan for the twelve months ahead. This plan should indicate which presentations will be made in which forums and how often IT-centric columns will appear in organizational newsletters. The plan should list three or so major themes—for example, specific regional integration strategies or efforts to improve IT service—that will be the focus of these communications. Communication plans try to remedy the fact that even when value is being delivered, most people in the organization may not be fully aware of it.

ANALYSES OF THE IT VALUE CHALLENGE

The IT investment and value challenge plagues all industries. It is not a problem peculiar to health care. The challenge has been with us for fifty years, ever since organizations began to spend money on big mainframes. This challenge is complex and persistent, and we should not believe we can fully solve it. We should believe we can be better at dealing with it. This section highlights the conclusions of several studies and articles that have examined this challenge.

Factors That Hinder Value Return

The Committee to Study the Impact of Information Technology on the Performance of Service Activities (1994) found these major contributors to failures to achieve a solid return on IT investments:

- The organization's overall strategy is wrong, or its assessment of its competitive environment is inadequate.
- The strategy is fine, but the necessary IT applications and infrastructure are not defined appropriately. The information system, if it is solving a problem, is solving the wrong problem.
- The organization fails to identify and draw together well all the investments and initiatives necessary to carry out its plans. The IT

investment then falters because other changes, such as reorganization or reengineering, fail to occur.

- The organization fails to execute the IT plan well. Poor planning or less than stellar management can diminish the return from any investment.

Value may also be diluted by factors outside the organization's control. Weill and Broadbent (1998) noted that the more strategic the IT investment, the more its value can be diluted. An IT investment directed to increasing market share may have its value diluted by non-IT decisions and events—for example, pricing decisions, competitors' actions, and customers' reactions. IT investments that are less strategic but have business value—for example, improving nursing productivity—may be diluted by outside factors—for example, shortages of nursing staff members. And the value of an IT investment directed toward improving infrastructure characteristics may be diluted by outside factors—for example, unanticipated technology immaturity or business difficulties confronting a vendor.

The Investment-Performance Relationship

A study by Strassmann (1990) examined the relationship between IT expenditures and organizational effectiveness. Data from an *Information Week* survey of the top one hundred users of IT were used to correlate IT expenditures per employee with profits per employee. Strassmann concluded that there is no overall obvious direct relationship between expenditure and organizational performance. This finding has been observed in several other studies (for example, Keen, 1997). It leads to several conclusions:

- Spending more on IT is no guarantee that the organization will be better off. There has never been a direct correlation between spending and outcomes. Paying more for care does not give one correspondingly better care. Clearly, one can spend so little that nothing effective can be done. And one can spend so much that waste is guaranteed. But moving IT expenditures from 4 percent of the operating budget to 6 percent of the operating budget does not inherently lead to a 50 percent increase in desirable outcomes.

- Factors other than the appropriateness of the tool to the task also influence the relationship between IT investment and organizational performance. These factors include the nature of the work (for example, IT is likely to have a greater impact on bank performance than on consulting firm performance), the basis of competition in an industry (for example, cost per unit of manufactured output versus prowess in marketing), and an organization's relative competitive position in the market.

The Value of the Overall Investment

Many analyses and academic studies have been directed to answering this broad question: How can an organization assess the value of its overall investments in IT? Assessing the value of the aggregate IT investment is different from assessing the value of a single initiative or other specific investment. And it is also different from assessing the caliber of the IT department.

Developing a definitive, accurate, and well-accepted way to answer this question has so far eluded all industries and may continue to be elusive. Nonetheless there are some basic questions that can be asked in pursuit of answering the larger question. Interpreting the answers to these basic questions is a subjective exercise, making it difficult to derive numerical scores. Bresnahan (1998) suggests five questions:

1. How does IT influence the customer experience?
2. Do patients and physicians, for example, find that organizational processes are more efficient, less error prone, and more convenient?
3. Does IT enable or retard growth? Can the IT organization support effectively the demands of a merger? Can IT support the creation of clinical product lines—for example, cardiology—across the integrated delivery system?
4. Does IT favorably affect productivity?
5. Does IT advance organizational innovation and learning?

Progressive Realization of IT Value

Brown and Hagel (2003) made three observations about IT value.

First, IT value requires innovation in business practices. If an organization merely computerizes existing processes without rectifying (or at times eliminating) process problems, it may have merely made process problems occur faster. In addition, those processes are now more expensive because there is a computer system to support. Providing appointment scheduling systems may not make waiting times any shorter or enhance patients' ability to get an appointment when they need one.

All IT initiatives should be accompanied by efforts to materially improve the processes that the system is designed to support. IT often enables the organization to think differently about a process or expand its options for improving a process. If the process thinking is narrow or unimaginative, the value that could have been achieved will have been lost, with the organization settling for an expensive way to achieve minimal gain.

For example, if Amazon had thought that the Internet enabled it to simply replace the catalogue and telephone as a way of ordering something, it would have missed ideas such as presenting products to the customer based on data about prior orders or enabling customers to leave their own ratings of books and music.

Second, the economic value of IT comes from incremental innovations rather than "big bang" initiatives. Organizations will often introduce very large computer systems and process change all at once. Two examples of such big bangs are the replacement of all systems related to the revenue cycle and the introduction of a new EHR over the course of a few weeks.

Big bang implementations are very tricky and highly risky. They may be haunted by series of technical problems. Moreover, these systems introduce an enormous number of process changes affecting many people. It is exceptionally difficult to understand the ramifications of such change during the analysis and design stages that precede implementation. A full understanding is impossible. As a result, the implementing organization risks material damage. This damage destroys value. It may set the organization back, and even if the organization grinds its way through the disruption, the resulting trauma may make the organization unwilling to engage in future ambitious IT initiatives.

By contrast, IT implementations (and related process changes) that are more incremental and iterative reduce the risk of organizational damage and permit the organization to learn. The organization has time to understand the value impact of phase n and then can alter its course before it embarks upon phase $n + 1$. Moreover, incremental change leads the organization's members to understand that change, and realizing value, are never-ending aspects of organizational life rather than things to be endured every couple of years.

Third, the strategic impact of IT investments comes from the cumulative effect of sustained initiatives to innovate business practices. If economic value is derived from a series of thoughtful, incremental steps, then the aggregate effect of those steps should be a competitive advantage. Most of the time, organizations that wind up dominating an industry do so through incremental movement over the course of several years (Collins, 2001).

Persistent innovation by a talented team, over the course of years, will result in significant strategic gains. The organization has learned how to improve itself, year in and year out. Strategic value is a marathon. It is a long race that is run and won one mile at a time.

Companies with Digital Maturity

CapGemini (2012) examined digital innovations at four hundred large companies. The study examined the **digital maturity** of these companies and compared this maturity with the performance of the companies. Digital maturity is defined according to two variables:

- Digital intensity, or the extent to which the company had invested in technology-enabled initiatives to change how the company operates. Example investments included advanced analytics, social media, digital design of products, and real-time monitoring of operations.
- Transformation management intensity, or the extent of the leadership capabilities necessary to drive digital transformation throughout the company. Example capabilities included vision, governance, and ability to change culture.

The study examined the degree to which digital intensity and transformation-management intensity separated those that performed well from those that did not. (See Figure 7.3.)

The study found that companies that had low scores on both intensity dimensions fared the poorest (24 percent less profitable than their competitors), whereas companies that had high scores on both intensity dimensions performed the best (26 percent more profitable than their competitors).

However, the study found that transformation-management intensity was more important than digital intensity. Companies that had high transformation-management intensity but low digital intensity performed 9 percent better than their competitors. And companies that had high digital intensity but low transformation intensity were 11 percent less profitable than competitors.

Transformation ability was more important than investment in IT although IT investments enabled transformation skills to achieve more value.

SUMMARY

IT value is complex, multifaceted, and diverse across and within proposed initiatives. The techniques used to analyze value must vary with the nature of the value.

Figure 7.3 Digital intensity versus transformation intensity

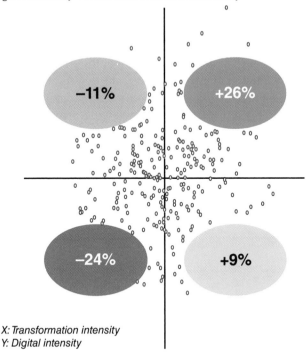

X: Transformation intensity
Y: Digital intensity

Source: CapGemini (2012). CapGemini Consulting and the MIT Center for Digital Business, "The Digital Advantage: How digital leaders outperform their peers in every industry," Nov. 5, 2012. Used with permission.

The project proposal is the core means for assessing the potential value of an IT initiative. IT proposals have a commonly accepted structure. And approaches exist for comparing proposals with different types of value propositions. Project proposals often present problems in the way they estimate value—for example, they may unrealistically combine fractions of effort saved, fail to appreciate the complex behavior of system users, or underestimate the full costs of the project.

Many factors can dilute the value realized from an IT investment. Poor linkage between the IT agenda and the organizational strategy, the failure to set goals, and the failure to manage the realization of value all contribute to dilution.

There are steps that can be taken to improve the achievement of IT value. Leadership can ensure that project proponents have done their homework, that accountability for results has been established, that formal proposals are used, and that post-implementation audits are conducted. Even though there are many approaches and factors that can enhance the realization of IT-enabled value, the challenges of achieving this value will remain a management issue for the foreseeable future.

Health care organization leaders often feel ill-equipped to address the IT investment and value challenge. However, no new management techniques are required to evaluate IT plans, proposals, and progress. Leadership teams are often asked to make decisions that involve strategic hunches (such as a belief that developing a continuum of care would be of value) about areas where they may have limited domain knowledge (new surgical modalities) and where the value is fuzzy (improved morale). Organizational leaders should treat IT investments just as they would treat other types of investments; if they don't understand, believe, or trust the proposal or its proponent, they should not approve it.

KEY TERMS

Digital maturity

Internal rate of return

IT project proposal

IT value

Net present value

Value realization

LEARNING ACTIVITIES

1. Interview the CIO of a local health care provider or payer. Discuss how his or her organization assesses the value of IT investments and ensures that the value is delivered.

2. Select two articles from a health care IT trade journal that describe the value an organization received from its IT investments. Critique and compare the articles.

3. Select two examples of intangible value. Propose one or more approaches that an organization might use to measure each of those values.

4. Prepare a defense of the value of a significant investment in an electronic health record system.

REFERENCES

Amarasingham, R., Plantinga, L., Diener-West, M., Gaskin, D. J., & Powe, N. R. (2009). Clinical information technologies and inpatient outcomes. *Archives of Internal Medicine, 169*(2), 108–114.

Amland, R., Dean, B., Yu, H., Ryan, H., Orsund, T., Hackman, J., & Roberts, S. (2015). Computerized clinical decision support to prevent venous thrombo-embolism among hospitalized patients: Proximal outcomes from a multi-year quality improvement project. *Journal for Healthcare Quality, 37*(4), 221–231.

Arlotto, P., & Oakes, J. (2003). *Return on investment: Maximizing the value of healthcare information technology.* Chicago, IL: Healthcare Information and Management Systems Society.

Bresnahan, J. (1998, July 15). What good is technology? *CIO Enterprise,* pp. 25–26, 28, 30.

Brown, J., & Hagel, J. (2003). Does IT matter? *Harvard Business Review, 81,* 109–112.

CapGemini. (2012). *The digital advantage: How digital leaders outperform their peers in every industry.* Paris, France: CapGemini.

Cebul, R. D., Love, T. E., Jain, A. K., & Herbert, C. J. (2011). Electronic health records and the quality of diabetes care. *New England Journal of Medicine, 365,* 825–833.

Collins, J. (2001). *Good to great.* New York, NY: HarperCollins.

Committee to Study the Impact of Information Technology on the Performance of Service Activities. (1994). *Information technology in the service society.* Washington, DC: National Academies Press.

Del Beccaro, M. A., Jeffries, H. E., Eisenberg, M. A., & Harry, E. D. (2006). Computerized provider order entry implementation: No association with increased mortality rates in an intensive care unit. *Pediatrics, 118*(1), 290–295.

Dragoon, A. (2003, Aug. 15). Deciding factors. *CIO,* pp. 49–59.

Glaser, J. (2003a, March). Analyzing information technology value. *Healthcare Financial Management,* pp. 98–104.

Glaser, J. (2003b, Sept.). When IT excellence goes the distance. *Healthcare Financial Management,* pp. 102–106.

Han, Y. Y., Carcillo, J. A., Venkataraman, S. T., Clark, R.S.B., Watson, R. S., Nguyen, T. C., Bayir, H., & Orr, R. A. (2005). Unexpected increased mortality after implementation of a commercially sold computerized physician order entry system. *Pediatrics, 116*(6), 1506–1512.

Keen, P. (1997). *The process edge.* Boston, MA: Harvard Business School Press.

Mosquera, M. (2011). *How PHRs boosted shareholder value at EMC.* Government Health IT. Retrieved August 2011 from http://govhealthit.com/news/some-employers-say-phrs-cut-healthcare-costs

Ross, J., & Beath, C. (2002). Beyond the business case: New approaches to IT investment. *MIT Sloan Management Review, 43*(2), 51–59.

Ross, J. W., & Johnson, E. (2009). Prioritizing IT investments. *Research Briefing, IX*(3). Cambridge, MA: MIT Center for Information Systems Research.

Strassmann, P. (1990). *The business value of computers.* New Canaan, CT: Information Economics Press.

Weill, P., & Aral, S. (2006). Generating premium returns on your IT investments. *MIT Sloan Management Review, 47*(2), 54–60.

Weill, P., & Broadbent, M. (1998). *Leveraging the new infrastructure.* Boston, MA: Harvard Business School Press.

CHAPTER 8

Organizing Information Technology Services

LEARNING OBJECTIVES

- To be able to describe the roles, responsibilities, and major functions of the IT department or organization.

- To be able to discuss the role and responsibility of the chief information officer (CIO), chief medical informatics officer (CMIO), chief security officer (CSO), chief technology officer (CTO), and other key IT staff members.

- To be able to describe the different ways IT services might be organized and governed within a health care organization.

- To be able to identify key attributes of highly effective IT organizations.

- To be able to describe the role and function of the data analytics department or unit.

- To be able to develop a plan for evaluating the effectiveness of the IT function within an organization.

By now you should have an understanding of health care data, the various clinical and administrative applications that are used to manage those health care data, and the processes of selecting, acquiring, and implementing health care information systems. You should also have a basic understanding of the core technologies that are common to many health care applications, and you can appreciate some of what it takes to ensure that information systems are reliable and secure.

In many health care organizations, an information technology (IT) function requires staff members who are involved in these and other IT-related activities—everything from customizing a software application to setting up and maintaining a wireless network to performing system backups. In a solo physician practice, this responsibility may lie with the office manager or lead physician. In a large hospital setting, this responsibility may lie with the IT department in conjunction with the medical staff, the administration, and the major departmental units—for example, admissions, finance, radiology, and nursing.

Some health care organizations outsource a portion or all of their IT services; however, they are still responsible for ensuring that those services are of high quality and support the IT needs of the organization. This responsibility cannot be delegated entirely to an outside vendor or IT firm. Health care executives must manage IT resources just as they do human, financial, and other facility resources.

This chapter provides an overview of the various functions and responsibilities that one would typically find in the IT department of a large health care organization. We describe the different groups or units that are typically seen in an IT department. We review a typical organizational structure for IT and discuss the variations that are often seen in that structure and the reasons for them. This chapter also presents an overview of the senior IT management roles and the roles with which health care executives will often work in the course of projects and IT initiatives. IT outsourcing, in which the health care organization asks an outside vendor to run IT, is reviewed. Finally, we examine approaches to evaluating the efficiency and effectiveness of the IT department.

INFORMATION TECHNOLOGY FUNCTIONS

The IT department has been an integral part of most hospitals or health care systems since the early days of mainframe computing. If the health care facility was relatively large and complex and used a fair amount of information technology, one would find IT staff members behind the scenes developing or enhancing applications, building system interfaces, maintaining databases, managing networks, performing system backups, and carrying out a host of other IT support activities. Today the IT department is becoming increasingly important, not only in hospitals but also in all health care organizations that use IT to manage clinical and administrative data and processes.

Throughout this chapter we refer to the IT department usually found in an integrated health care system. We chose this setting because it is typically the most complex and IT intensive. Moreover, many of the principles that apply to managing IT resources in this setting also apply in other types of health care facilities, such as an ambulatory care clinic or rural community health center. The breadth and scope of the services provided may differ considerably, however, depending on the extent to which IT is used in the organization.

IT Department Responsibilities

The IT department has several responsibilities:

- Ensuring that an IT plan and strategy have been developed for the organization and that the plan and strategy are kept current as the organization evolves; these activities are discussed in Chapter Twelve

- Working with the organization to acquire or develop and implement needed new applications; these processes were discussed in Chapters Five and Six

- Providing day-to-day support for users: for example, fixing broken workstations, responding to questions about application use, training new users, and applying vendor-supplied upgrades to existing applications

- Managing the IT infrastructure: for example, performing backups of databases, installing network connections for new organizational locations, monitoring system performance, and securing the infrastructure from denial of service attacks

- Examining the role and relevance of emerging information technologies

Core Functions

To fulfill their responsibilities, all IT departments have four core functions. Depending on the size of the IT group and the diversity of applications and responsibilities, a function may require several subsidiary departments or subgroups.

Operations and Technical Support

The **operations and technical support** function manages the IT infrastructure—for example, the servers, networks, operating systems, database management systems, and workstations. This function installs new technology, applies upgrades, troubleshoots and repairs the infrastructure, performs "housekeeping" tasks such as backups, and responds to user problems, such as a printer that is not working.

This function may have several IT subgroups:

- Data center management: manages the equipment in the organization's computer center
- Network engineers: manage the organization's network technologies
- Server engineers: oversee the installation of new servers and perform such tasks as managing server space utilization
- Database managers: add new databases, support database query tools, and respond to database problems such as file corruptions
- Security: ensure that virus and intrusion detection software is current, physical access to the computer room is constrained, disaster recovery plans are current, and processes are in place to manage application and system passwords
- Help desk: provide support to users who call in with problems such as broken office equipment, trouble operating an application, a forgotten password, or uncertainty about how to perform a specific task on the computer
- Deployments: install new workstations and printers, move workstations when groups move to new buildings, and the like
- Training: train organization staff members on new applications and office software, such as presentation development applications

Applications Management

The applications management group manages the processes of acquiring new application systems, developing new application systems, implementing these new systems, providing ongoing enhancement of applications, troubleshooting application problems, and working with application suppliers to resolve these problems.

This function may have several IT groups:

- Groups that focus on major classes of applications: for example, a financial systems group and a clinical systems group

- Groups dedicated to specific applications (this is most likely in large organizations): for example, a group to support the applications in the clinical laboratory or in radiology
- An applications development group (this is found in organizations that perform a significant amount of internal development)
- Groups that focus on specific types of internal development: for example, a web or mobile device development group

Specialized Groups

Health care organizations may develop groups that have very specialized functions, depending on the type of organization or the organization's approach to IT. For example:

- Groups that support the needs of the research community in academic medical centers
- Process redesign groups in organizations that engage in a significant degree of process reengineering during application implementation
- Decision-support groups that help users and management perform analyses and create reports from corporate databases—for example, quality-of-care reports or financial performance reports

In addition, the **chief information officer (CIO),** who is the most senior IT executive, is often responsible for managing the organization's telecommunications function—the staff members who manage the phone system, overhead paging system, and nurse call systems. Depending on the organization's structure and the skill and interests of the CIO, one occasionally finds these other organizational functions reporting to the CIO. These additional functions are often added because of the executive skills of the CIO and not strictly because they are IT-related:

- The health information management or medical records department
- The function that handles the organization's overall strategic plan development
- The marketing department

IT Administration

Depending on the size of the IT department, one may find groups that focus on supporting IT administrative activities. These groups may perform such tasks as these:

- Overseeing the development of the IT strategic plan
- Managing contracts with vendors
- Developing and monitoring the IT budget
- Providing human resource support for the IT staff members
- Providing support for the management of IT projects: for example, developing project status reports or providing project management training
- Managing the space occupied by an IT department or group

A typical organizational structure for an IT department in a large health system is shown in Figure 8.1.

Figure 8.1 shows the enterprise-wide CIO, a deputy CIO, and CIOs for each of the major divisions, for example, an academic medical center and the physician network of the health system. The division CIOs must ensure that the IT needs of each division are met and that the division needs are considered during the development and execution of enterprise-level initiatives such as the implementation of a common revenue cycle system.

Figure 8.1 also shows roles for specialized functions: telehealth, genomics IT, research, medical imaging, and medical informatics. The figure shows the operations and technical support groups (technical services and operations and network services and communications), **application management** groups (clinical systems and finance and administrative systems), the IT administration group (IS administration), and health information management.

Finally, the figure shows the presence of a CTO (chief technology officer) and CISO (chief information security officer), which will be discussed in the following section on IT senior leadership roles.

IT Senior Leadership Roles

Within the overall IT group, several positions and roles are typically present ranging from senior leadership—for example, the chief information officer—to staff members who do the day-in, day-out work of implementing application systems—for example, systems analysts. In the following sections we will describe several senior-level IT positions:

- Chief information officer (CIO)
- Chief technology officer (CTO)
- Chief information security officer (CISO)
- Chief clinical informatics officer (CCIO), specifically the chief medical information officer (CMIO)

Figure 8.1 IT organizational chart: Large health system

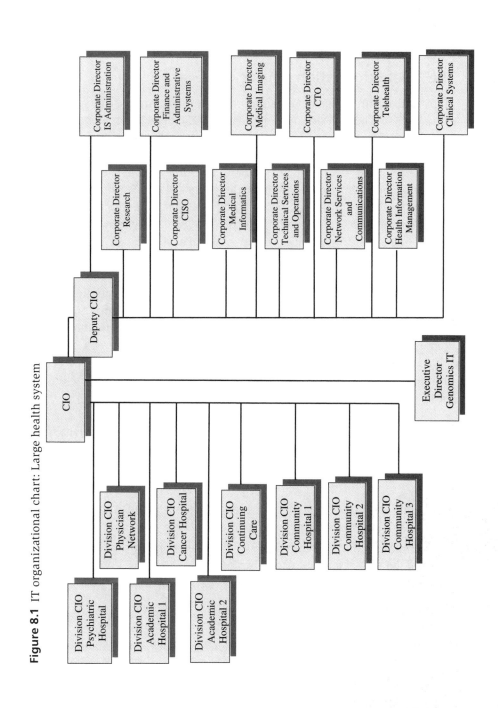

This is not an exhaustive list of all possible senior-level positions, but the discussion provides an overview of typical roles and functions.

The Chief Information Officer

Many midsize and large health care organizations employ a chief information officer (CIO). The CIO not only manages the IT department but also is seen as the executive who can successfully lead the organization in its efforts to apply IT to advance its strategies.

The role of the CIO in health care and other industries has been the subject of research and debate over the years (Glaser & Kirby, 2009; Glaser & Williams, 2007). Studies conducted by College of Healthcare Information Management Executives (CHIME) (1998, 2008) have chronicled the evolution of the health care CIO. This evolution has involved debates on CIO reporting relationships, salaries, and titles and the role of the CIO in an organization's strategic planning. Through extensive research, CHIME has identified seven key attributes, or competencies, exhibited by high-performing CIOs (CHIME, 2008). CHIME provides intensive "boot camp" training sessions for its CIO members to aid in their professional development of these competencies.

Earlier work by Earl and Feeney (1995) found that CIOs from a wide range of industries who added value to their respective organizations had many of these same characteristics:

- Obsessively and continuously emphasize business imperatives so that they focus the IT direction correctly
- Have a track record of delivery that causes IT performance problems to drop off management's agenda
- Interpret for the rest of the leadership team the meaning and nature of the IT success stories of other organizations
- Establish and maintain good working relationships with the members of the organization's leadership
- Establish and communicate the IT performance record.
- Concentrate the IT development efforts on those areas of the organization where the most leverage is to be gained
- Work with the organization's leadership to develop a shared vision of the roles and contributions of IT
- Make important general contributions to business thinking and operations

PERSPECTIVE
Seven Key Attributes of a High-Performing CIO

1. **Sets vision and strategy.** Collaborates well with senior leaders to set organization vision and strategy and to determine how technology can best serve the organization.

2. **Integrates information technology for business success.** Applies knowledge of the organization's systems, structures, and functions to determine how best to advance the performance of the business with technology.

3. **Makes change happen.** Is able to lead the organization in making the process changes necessary to fully capitalize on IT investments.

4. **Builds technological confidence.** Helps the business assess the value of IT investments and the steps needed to achieve that value.

5. **Partners with customers.** Interacts with internal and external customers to ensure continuous customer satisfaction.

6. **Ensures information technology talent.** Creates a work environment and community that draws, develops, and retains top IT talent.

7. **Builds networks and community.** Develops and maintains professional networks with internal and external sources and effectively leverages those networks to further the effective use of IT.

Source: CHIME (2008).

Earl and Feeney (1995) also found that the value-added CIO, as a person, has integrity, is goal directed, is experienced with IT, and is a good consultant and communicator. Those organizations that have such a CIO tend to describe IT as critical to the organization, find that IT thinking is embedded in business thinking, note that IT initiatives are well focused, and speak highly of IT performance.

Organizational excellence in IT doesn't just happen. It is managed and led. If the health care organization decides that the effective application of IT is a major element of its strategies and plans, it will need a very good CIO. Failure to hire and retain such talent will severely hinder the organization's aspirations.

Whom the CIO should report to has been a topic of industry debate and an issue inside organizations as well. CIOs will often argue that they should report to the chief executive officer (CEO). This argument is not wrong nor is it necessarily right. The CIO does need access to the CEO and clearly should be a member of the executive committee and actively involved in strategy discussions. However, the CIO needs a boss who is a good mentor, provides appropriate political support, and is genuinely interested in the application of IT. Chief financial officers (CFOs) and chief operating officers (COOs) can be terrific in these regards. In general about one-third of all health care provider CIOs report to the CEO, one-third report to the CFO, and one-third report to the COO.

The Chief Technology Officer

The **chief technology officer (CTO)** has several responsibilities. The CTO must guide the definition and implementation of the organization's technical architecture. This role includes defining technology standards (for example, defining the operating systems and network technologies the organization will support), ensuring that the technical infrastructure is current (for example, that major vendor releases and upgrades have been applied), and ensuring that all the technologies fit. The CTO's role in ensuring fit is similar to an architect's role in ensuring that the materials used to construct a house come together in a way that results in the desired house.

The CTO is also responsible for tracking emerging technologies, identifying the ones that might provide value to the organization, assessing them, and when appropriate, working with the rest of the IT department and the organization to implement these technologies. For example, the CTO may be asked to investigate the possible usefulness of the Internet of Things. The CTO role is not often found in smaller organizations but is increasingly common in larger ones. In smaller organizations, the CIO also wears the CTO hat.

The Chief Information Security Officer

As will be discussed in Chapter Nine, the **chief information security officer (CISO)** is a relatively new position that has emerged as a result of the growing threats to information security and the health care organization's need to comply with federal and state security regulations. The primary role and functions of the CISO are to ensure that the health care organization has an effective information security plan, appropriate technical and administrative procedures are in place to ensure that information systems are secure and safe from tampering or misuse, and appropriate disaster recovery procedures exist.

The Chief Clinical Informatics Officer

There are several roles that fall under the broad umbrella of the chief clinical informatics officer (AMIA Task Force Report on CCIO Knowledge, Education and Skillset Requirements, 2016). These roles include the chief nursing informatics officer (CNIO) and the chief pharmacy informatics officer. Of these roles the **chief medical information officer (CMIO)** is the most common (approximately 30 percent of CIOs employ a CMIO (AMIA Task Force Report on CCIO Knowledge, Education and Skillset Requirements, 2016) although still a relatively new position. The CMIO position emerged as a result of the growing interest in adopting clinical information systems and leveraging those systems to improve care. The CMIO is usually a physician, and this role may be filled through a part-time commitment by a member of the organization's medical staff.

Murphy (2011) identified the skills of the CCIO (including the CMIO and CNIO):

- Guide an EHR selection process
- Define a clinical information systems governance process
- Engage senior executives in an EHR culture and practice changes
- Advise on implementation methodologies and the sequencing of EHR modules
- Identify the value proposition and key performance indicator metrics of EHR use
- Determine an EHR enhancement request system and prioritization process
- Staff ongoing clinical process improvement initiatives
- Educate about health technology and the interactions between people and process changes
- Develop strong relationships with key stakeholders in the organization

The CIO, CTO, CISO, and CMIO all play important roles in helping to ensure that information systems acquired and implemented are consistent with the strategic goals of the health care organization, are well accepted and effectively used, and are adequately maintained and secured. Sample job descriptions for the CIO and the CMIO positions are given in Appendix B.

IT Staff Roles

The IT leadership team cannot carry out the organization's IT agenda unilaterally. The department's work relies heavily on highly trained, qualified professional and technical staff members to perform a host of IT-related functions. In this section are brief descriptions of some key professionals who work in IT:

- The project leader
- The systems analyst
- The programmer
- The database administrator
- The network administrator

The Project Leader

The *project leader* manages IT projects such as the implementation of a new revenue cycle application, deployment of infrastructure in a new medical office building, or determination of the need for a new system. At times project leaders are staff members from user departments, though in general they are members of the IT department. This role was discussed in more depth in Chapter Six.

The Systems Analyst

The role of the **systems analyst** will vary considerably depending on the analyst's background and the needs of the organization. Some analysts have a strong computer programming background, whereas others have a business orientation or come from clinical disciplines, such as nursing, pharmacy, or the laboratory. In fact, because of the increased interest in the adoption of clinical information systems, systems analysts with clinical backgrounds in nursing, pharmacy, medical technology, and the like (often referred to as *clinical systems analysts*) are in high demand. Most systems analysts work closely with managers and end users in identifying information system needs and problems, evaluating workflow, and determining strategies for optimizing the use and effectiveness of particular systems.

When an organization decides to develop a new information system, systems analysts are often called on to determine what computer hardware and software will be needed. They prepare specifications, flowcharts, and process diagrams for computer programmers to follow.

They work with programmers and vendor staff members to test new systems and system upgrades, recommend solutions, and determine whether program requirements have been met. They may also prepare cost-benefit and return-on-investment analyses to help management decide whether implementing a proposed system will deliver the desired value.

The Programmer

Programmers write, test, and maintain the programs that computers must follow to perform their functions. They also conceive, design, and test logical structures for solving problems with computers. Many technical innovations in programming—advanced computing technologies and sophisticated new languages and programming tools—have redefined the role of programmers and elevated much of the programming work done today.

Programmers are often grouped into two broad types—applications programmers and systems programmers. Applications programmers write programs to handle specific user tasks, such as a program to track inventory within an organization. They may also revise existing packaged software or customize generic applications such as integration technologies. Systems programmers write programs to maintain and control infrastructure software, such as operating systems, networked systems, and database systems. They are able to change the sets of instructions that determine how the network, workstations, and central processing units within a system handle the various jobs they have been given and how they communicate with peripheral equipment such as other workstations, printers, and disk drives.

The Database Administrator

Database administrators work with database management systems software and determine ways to organize and store data. They identify user requirements, set up computer databases, and test and coordinate modifications to these systems. An organization's database administrator ensures the performance of the database systems, understands the platform on which the databases run, and adds new users to the systems. Because they may also design and implement system security, database administrators often plan and coordinate security measures. With the volume of sensitive data growing rapidly, data integrity, backup systems, and database security have become increasingly important aspects of the job for database administrators.

The advent of payment reform is placing increasing pressure on providers to improve the efficiency and quality of clinical, operational, and financial performance. Moreover, the arrival of population health requires that providers define their populations and manage the health and care received by that population. These pressures result in the need for a group that provides superior analytics support to the organization.

Most providers have had an analytics group for some time. Providers have used analytics to measure referral patterns, DRG performance, payer mix, and expected reimbursement and patient volumes. However, these pressures have elevated the importance of this group and often expanded their staff and the scope of their work.

This group can be a department within the IT organization but increasingly the group reports up through a non-IT function, usually the function responsible for clinical quality or finance.

Wadsworth (2016) defines a proposed structure and role for a typical provider analytics group. A content and analytics team, composed of data architects and outcomes analysts, mines the data contained in an enterprise data warehouse (which is the aggregation, across the organization, of the clinical, financial, operational, and market data deemed most important to the organization). The team works with a senior leadership committee to identify potential areas of organizational improvement. The committee prioritizes the areas and assigned workgroups to engage in process improvement.

Workgroups are teams that identify steps that should be taken to improve clinical, operational, and financial performance of a particular area (e.g., pharmacy) or process (e.g., total joint replacement). This work usually defines a current state and outlines a desired future state. The core

The Network Administrator

It is essential that the organization has an adequate network or network infrastructure to support all its clinical and administrative applications and also its general applications (such as e-mail, intranets, and videoconferencing). Networks come in many variations, so **network administrators** are needed to design, test, and evaluate systems such as local area networks of the workgroup typically consists of a physician lead, an operations lead, and a nurse who understands the patient workflow.

Members of the workgroup typically fulfill these functions:

- **Data architect:** Builds a solid architecture to capture and provide data from disparate source systems into an integrated platform

- **Application administrator:** Ensures source-system applications function to capture needed data elements

- **Outcomes analyst:** Mines data to identify statistically valid trends and variability that may exist

- **Knowledge manager:** Acts as a liaison between the technical and clinical teams; usually staffed by a nurse, this critical role helps the technical team understand and interpret clinical data as he or she seeks to build algorithms that mimic clinical workflow

- **Clinical implementation team (CIT):** Consists of practicing clinicians who own a clinical process within an organization, will champion adoption of the improvements, and guide the rollout of the improvement process

- **Guidance team:** Provides governance over all the workgroups and CITs under a clinical program—for example, a guidance team for the women and children's clinical program may oversee three separate workgroups focusing on gynecology, pregnancy, or normal newborn; takes into account resources, organizational readiness, and political climate to determine which workgroups receive priority; reports to the senior leadership committee

Source: Wadsworth (2016).

(LANs), wireless networks, the Internet, intranets, and other data communications systems. Networks can range from a connection between two offices in the same building to globally distributed connectivity to voice mail and e-mail systems across a host of different health care organizations. Network administrators perform network modeling, analysis, and planning; they may also research related products and make hardware and software recommendations.

Staff Positions in High Demand

As the technology evolves (for example, advances in analytics) and the focus of organizations shifts (for example, shifts to population health) various IT staff roles will become in high demand. The core positions will always be needed but new roles and refinements of existing roles emerge constantly. In 2016 high-demand positions (across industries) include these functions (Florentine, 2015):

- User interface designers
- Web infrastructure developers
- Network engineers
- Security and cyber security professionals
- Mobile application developers
- Systems analysts
- Industry knowledgeable project managers
- Cloud application architects
- Data scientists

When positions are in high demand organizations may face significant challenges hiring the staff members they need; salaries may be very high, availability will be limited, and organization's will need to sell themselves to prospective recruits. A CHIME (2012) survey of CIOs found 67 percent were experiencing IT staff shortages. The positions in greatest demand were clinical information systems project managers and systems analysts.

Staff Attributes

In addition to ensuring that it has the appropriate IT functions and IT roles (and that the individuals filling these roles are competent), the health care organization must ensure that the IT staff members have certain attributes. These attributes are unlikely to arise spontaneously; they must often be managed into existence. An assessment of the IT function (as discussed further on in this chapter) can highlight problems in this area and then lead to management steps designed to improve staff member attributes.

High-performing IT staff members have several general characteristics:

- **They execute well.** They deliver applications, infrastructure, and services that reflect a sound understanding of organizational needs.

These deliverables occur on time and on budget so that those involved in a project give the project team high marks for professional comportment.

- **They are good consultants.** They advise organizational members on the best approach to the application of IT given the problem or opportunity. They advise when IT may be inappropriate or the least important component of the solution. This advice ranges from help desk support to systems analyses to new technology recommendations to advice on the suitability of IT for furthering an aspect of organizational strategy.

- **They provide world-class support.** Information systems require daily care and feeding and problem identification and correction. This support needs to be exceptionally efficient and effective.

- **They stay current in their field of expertise.** They keep up to date on new techniques and technologies that may improve the ability of the organization to apply IT effectively.

ORGANIZING IT STAFF MEMBERS AND SERVICES

Now that we have introduced the various roles and functions found in the health care IT arena, we will examine how these roles and functions can be organized. Essentially, three factors influence the structure of the IT department:

- Degree of **IT centralization or decentralization**
- Core IT competencies
- Departmental attributes

Degree of IT Centralization or Decentralization

A critical factor in determining the structure for the IT department is the degree of centralization of organizational decision making. A health care organization might be a highly structured hierarchy in which decisions are made by a few senior leaders. Conversely, an organization might delegate authority to make many decisions to the department level or to the hospital level in an integrated delivery system, resulting in decentralized decision making. Referring to Figure 8.1, in a highly centralized organization, division CIOs may not be necessary because virtually all decisions are made at the enterprise level. Conversely, in a highly decentralized organization, the central role of corporate director, clinical systems shown in Figure 8.1 may not be necessary because all EHR decisions are made at the local level.

The following describes some of the advantages to centralizing IT services (Oz, 2006):

- **Enforcement of hardware and software standards.** In a centralized structure, the organization typically develops software and hardware standards, which can lead to cost savings, facilitate the exchange of data among systems, make installations easier, and promote sharing of applications.
- **Efficient administration of resources.** Centralizing the administration of contracts and licenses and inventories of hardware and software can lead to greater efficiency.
- **Better staffing.** Because it results in a pool of IT staff members from which to choose, the centralized approach may be able to identify and assign the most appropriate individuals to a particular project.
- **Easier training.** In a centralized department, staff members can specialize in certain areas (hardware, software, networks) and do not need to be jacks of all trades.
- **Effective planning of shared systems.** A centralized IT services unit typically sees the big picture and can facilitate the deployment of systems that are to be used by all units of a health care system or across organizational boundaries.
- **Easier strategic IT planning.** A strategic IT plan should be well aligned with the overall strategic plan of the organization. This alignment may be easier when IT management is centralized.
- **Tighter control by senior management.** A centralized approach to managing IT services permits senior management to maintain tighter control of the IT budget and resources.

The following describes some of the advantages to a decentralized structure (Oz, 2006):

- **Better fit of IT to business needs.** The individual IT units are familiar with their business unit's or department's needs and can develop or select systems that fit those needs more closely.
- **Quick response time.** The individual IT units are typically better equipped to respond promptly to requests or can arrange IT projects to fit the priorities of their business unit or department.

- **Encouragement of end user development of applications.** In a decentralized IT services structure, end users are often encouraged to develop their own small applications to increase productivity.

- **Innovative use of information systems.** Given that IT staff members are closer in proximity to users and know their needs, the decentralized structure may have a better chance of implementing innovative systems.

Most IT services in a health care organization are not fully centralized or decentralized but a combination of the two. For example, training and support for applications may be decentralized, with other IT functions such as application development, network support, and database management being managed centrally. The size, complexity, and culture of the health care organization might also determine the degree to which IT services should be managed centrally.

For example, in an ambulatory care clinic with three sites that are fairly autonomous, it may be appropriate to divide IT services into three functional units, each dedicated to a specific clinic. In a larger, more complex organization, such as an integrated delivery network (with multiple hospitals, outpatient clinics, and physician practices), it may be appropriate to form a centralized IT services unit that is responsible for specific IT areas such as systems planning and integration, network administration, and telecommunications, with all other functions being managed at the individual facility level.

There is no right level of centralization. Centralized organizations can be as effective as decentralized organizations. Ideally, the management and structure of IT will parallel that of the executive team's management philosophy; centralized management tends to want centralized control over IT, whereas decentralized management is more likely to be comfortable with IT that can be locally responsive.

Core IT Competencies

Organizations should identify a small number of areas that constitute core IT capabilities and competencies. These are areas where getting an A+ from the "customers" matters. For example, an organization focused on transforming its care processes would want to ensure A+ competency in this area and would perhaps settle for B− competency in its supply chain operations. An organization dedicated to being very efficient would want A+ competency in areas such as supplier management and productivity improvement and would perhaps settle for a B− in delivering superb customer service.

This definition of core competencies has a bearing on the form of the IT organization. If A+ competency is desired in care transformation, the IT department should be organized into functions that specialize in supporting care transformation—for example, a clinical information systems implementation group and a care reengineering group.

Partners HealthCare, for example, defined three areas of core capabilities: base support and services, care improvement, and technical infrastructure.

Base Support and Services

The category of core capabilities at Partners HealthCare included two subcategories:

- Frontline support: for example, mobile device problem resolution
- Project management skills

The choice of these areas of emphasis resulted in many management actions and steps—for example, the selection of criteria to be used during annual performance reviews. The emphasis on frontline support also led to the creation of an IT function responsible for all frontline support activities, including the help desk, workstation deployments, training, and user account management. The emphasis on project management led to the creation of a project management office to assist in monitoring the status of all projects and a project center of excellence to offer training on project management and established project management standards.

Care Improvement

Central to the Partners agenda was the application of IT to improve the process of care. One consequence was to establish, as a core IT capability, the set of skills and people necessary to innovatively apply IT to medical care improvement. An applied medical informatics function was established to oversee a research and development agenda. Staff members skilled in clinical information systems application development were hired. A group of experienced clinical information system implementers was established.

An IT unit of health services researchers was formed to analyze deficiencies in care processes, identify IT solutions that would reduce or eliminate these deficiencies, and assess the impact of clinical information systems on care improvement. Organizational units possessing unique technical and clinical knowledge in radiology imaging systems and telemedicine were also created.

Technical Infrastructure

Because Partners HealthCare recognized the critical role of a well-conceived, well-executed, and well-supported technical architecture, infrastructure architecture and design continued to serve as a core competency. A technology strategy function was created, and the role of chief technology officer was created. Significant attention was paid to ensuring that extremely talented architectural and engineering staff members were hired along with staff members with terrific support skills.

Departmental Attributes

IT departments, similar to people, have characteristics or attributes. They may be agile or ossified. They may be risk tolerant or risk averse. These characteristics can be stated, and strategies to achieve desired characteristics can be defined and implemented. To illustrate, this section will discuss briefly two characteristics—agility and innovativeness—and discuss how they might affect the organization of IT functions. These two characteristics are representative and are generally viewed as desirable.

There are many steps that an organization can take to increase its overall agility and also that of the IT department (Glaser, 2008a). For example, it is likely to try to chunk its initiatives so that there are multiple points at which a project can be reasonably stopped and yet still deliver value. Thus, the rollout of an EHR might call for implementation at ten clinics per year but could be stopped temporarily at four clinics and still deliver value to those four. Chunking allows an organization and its departments to quickly shift emphasis from one project to another.

An agile IT department will have the ability to form and disband teams quickly (perhaps every three months) as staff members move from project to project. This requires that organizational structures and reporting relationships be flexible so staff members can move rapidly between projects. It also means that during a project, the project manager is (temporarily anyway) the boss of the project team members. The team members might report to someone else according to the organizational chart, but their real boss at this time is the project manager. Because team members might move rapidly from project to project, they might have several bosses during the course of a year. And a person might be the boss on one project and the subordinate on another project. (Many consulting firms operate with this model.) Agile organizations and departments are organized less around functions and more around projects. The IT structure must accommodate continuous project team formation, and project managers must have significant authority.

An organization or department that wants to be innovative might take steps such as implementing reward systems that encourage new ideas and successful implementation of innovative applications and also punishment systems that are loath to discipline those involved in experiments that failed (Glaser, 2008b). The innovative IT department might create dedicated research and development groups. It might form teams composed of IT and vendor staff members in an effort to cross-fertilize each group with the ideas of the other. It might also permit staff members to take sabbaticals or accept internships with other departments in the organization in an effort to expand IT members' awareness of organizational operations, cultures, and issues.

IN-HOUSE VERSUS OUTSOURCED IT

For many years, health care organizations have generally provided IT services in-house. By in-house we mean that the organization hired its own IT staff members and formed its own IT department. In recent years, however, health care organizations have shown a growing interest in outsourcing part or all of their IT services. **Outsourced IT** means that an organization asks a third party to provide the IT staff members and be responsible for the management of IT.

The reasons for outsourcing IT functions are varied. Some health care organizations may simply not have staff members with the skills, time, or resources needed to take on new IT projects or provide sufficient IT service. Others may choose to outsource certain IT functions, such as help desk services or website development, so that internal IT staff members can focus their time on implementing or supporting applications central to the organization's strategic goals.

Outsourcing IT may enable organizations to better control costs. Because a contract is typically established for a defined scope of work to be done over a specific period of time, the IT function becomes a line item that can be more effectively budgeted over time. This does not mean, however, that outsourcing IT services is necessarily more cost-effective than providing IT services in-house.

At times, new organizational leadership finds an IT function that is in disastrous condition. After years of mismanagement, applications may function poorly, the infrastructure may be unstable, and the IT staff members may be demoralized. An outsourcing company may be brought in as a form of rescue mission.

A number of factors come into play and should be considered when evaluating whether outsourcing part or all of IT services is in the best interest of the organization. The following questions should be asked:

- Does our organization have IT staff members with the knowledge and skills needed to provide necessary services? Effectively manage projects? Adequately support current applications and infrastructure?

- How easy or difficult is it to recruit and retain qualified IT staff members?

- What are our organization's major IT priorities? How equipped is our organization to address these priorities? Do we have the right mix of skills, time, and resources?

- What benefits might be realized from outsourcing this IT function? What are the risks? Do the benefits outweigh the risks?

- What parts, if any, of the IT department does it make the most sense to outsource?

- If we opt to outsource IT services, with whom do we want to do business? How will we monitor and evaluate IT performance and service? What provisions will we make in the contract with the outsourcing company to ensure timeliness and quality of service? How will the terms of the contract be monitored?

It is important to evaluate the cost and effectiveness of the IT function and services, whether they are performed by in-house staff members or outsourced. There are pros and cons to each approach, and the organization must make its decision based on its strategy goals and priorities. There is no silver bullet or one solution for all.

Related to decisions to outsource all or a portion of the organization's IT staff are decisions to have a third-party supplier run the organization's applications in the third party's data center. Cloud computing growth has been explosive recently. Gartner (2013) estimates that by the time this book is published the majority of business computing will involve a cloud. The cloud approach can be full (all of an organization's applications are run on a third-party cloud) or hybrid (the third party runs some applications and the organization runs the remaining applications in its data centers).

Cloud computing can be less expensive, easier to scale, and more able to adopt newer technologies. Keeping some applications internally enables the organization to maintain control over sensitive or critical applications and data.

PERSPECTIVE
Future Demands on the IT Function

Broaden the knowledge base. For the IT staff members steeped in inpatient care, knowledge of hospital operations must expand to include knowledge of the operations and needs of long-term care facilities, patient support communities, and small physician practices. Understanding of the intricacies of fee-for-service must expand to include payments based on bundles and capitation.

Skills in managing complex implementations will still be necessary, but those skills must broaden to include redesigning processes that traverse care settings, turning clinical decision-support logic to achieve chronic care outcomes, and assisting clinicians and managers in developing the analytics capabilities necessitated by new payment arrangements.

Address IT innovation and management. The IT staff members must grapple with IT innovation that continues at a remarkable pace. Social media use continues to grow and become more sophisticated and capable. Mobile personal devices have become the device of choice for personal and professional activities. Big data has exceptional potential, although it is cloaked in a dense fog of hype.

In addition, the organization's dependence on IT for it to function heightens the importance of a well-managed and secure IT infrastructure and application base.

A shift in strategic emphasis. With the EHR core in place (courtesy of Meaningful Use), the IT function must shift from focusing on the large-scale implementation of EHRs to extending that investment to support care management, enabling the management of a population's health, introducing extensive evidence-based decision support, developing superior analytics capabilities, creating and redesigning processes, and improving the efficiency of clinical and administrative processes.

Step up leadership skills. Leadership skills and attributes include emotional intelligence, communication skills, integrity, business understanding, and the ability to hire, grow, and manage a world-class team. As the pressures on operations and clinical practice increase, there will be a growing premium placed on having superlative leadership skills.

Source: Glaser (2016).

EVALUATING IT EFFECTIVENESS

Whether IT services are provided by in-house staff or are outsourced, it is important to evaluate IT performance. Is the function efficient? Does it deliver good service? Is it on top of new developments in its field? Does the function have a strong management team?

At times, health care executives become worried about the performance of an IT function. Other organizations have IT functions that seem to accomplish more or spend less. Management and physicians frequently express dissatisfaction with IT: nothing is getting done, it costs too much, or it takes too long to get a new application implemented. Many factors may result in user dissatisfaction: poor expectation setting, unclear priorities, limited funding, or inadequate IT leadership. An assessment of IT services can help management understand the nature of the problems and identify opportunities for improvement.

One desirable approach to assessing IT services is to use outside consultants. Consultants can bring a level of objectivity to the assessment process that is difficult to achieve internally. They can also share their experiences, having worked with a variety of different health care organizations and having observed different ways of handling some of the same issues or problems.

Whether the assessment is done by internal staff members or by consultants, several key areas should be addressed:

- Governance
- Budget development and resource allocation
- System acquisition
- System implementation
- IT service levels

Governance

How effective is the **governance** structure? To what degree are IT strategies well aligned with the organization's overall strategic goals? Is the CIO actively involved in strategy discussions? Does senior leadership discuss IT agenda items on a regular basis? We will discuss governance in Chapter Thirteen.

Budget Development and Resource Allocation

The IT budget is often compared to the IT budgets of comparable health care organizations. The question behind a budget benchmark is, Are we spending too much or too little on IT? Budget benchmarks are expressed in terms of the IT operating budget as a percentage of the overall organization's operating budget and the IT capital budget as a percentage of the organization's total capital budget.

These budget benchmarks are useful and in some sense required because most boards of directors expect to see them. Management has to be careful in interpreting the results, however. These percentages do not necessarily reflect the quality of IT services or the extent and size of the organization's application base or infrastructure. Hence, one can find a poorly performing IT group that has implemented little having the same percentage of the organization's budgetary resources as a world-class IT group that has implemented a stunning array of applications.

Spending a high percentage of the operating budget does not per se mean that the organization is spending too much and should reduce its IT budget. The organization may have decided to ramp up its IT investments in order to achieve certain strategic objectives. A low percentage—for example, 1 percent—does not necessarily mean that underinvestment is occurring and the IT budget should be significantly increased. The organization may be very efficient, or it may have decided that given its strategies its investments should be made elsewhere.

We will discuss the IT budget and resource allocation in Chapter Thirteen.

System Acquisition

How effective are system acquisitions? How long did they take? What process was used to select the systems? We discussed system acquisition in Chapter Five.

System Implementation

Are new applications delivered on time, within budget, and according to specification? Do the participants in the implementation speak fondly of the professionalism of the IT staff members or do they view IT staff members as forms of demonic creatures? We discussed system implementation in Chapter Six.

IT Service Levels

IT staff members deliver service every day—for example, they manage system performance, respond to help desk calls, and manage projects. The quality of these services can be measured. An assessment of the IT function invariably reviews these measures and the management processes in place to monitor and improve IT services. IT users in the organization are interested in measures such as these:

- **Infrastructure.** Are the information systems reliable, that is, do they rarely "go down"? Are response times fast?
- **Day-to-day support.** Does the help desk quickly, patiently, and effectively resolve my problems? If I ask for a new workstation, does it arrive in a reasonable period of time?
- **Consultation.** Are the IT folks good at helping me think through my IT needs? Are they realistic in helping me to understand what the technology will and will not do?

An organization faces a challenge in defining what level of IT service it would like and also how much it is willing to pay for IT services. All of us would love to have systems analysts with world-class consulting skills, but we may not be able to afford their salaries. Similarly, all of us would love to have systems that never go down and are as fast as greased lightning, but we might not be willing to pay the cost of engineering very, very high reliability and blazing speed. The IT service conversation attempts to establish formal and measurable levels of service and the cost of providing that service. The organization seeks an informed conversation about the desirability and the cost of improving the service or the possibility of degrading the service in an effort to reduce costs.

In general, it can be very difficult to measure quality and consequences of consultative services. This makes it difficult to understand whether it is worth investing to improve the service other than at the service extremes. For example, it can be clear that you need to fire a very ineffective systems analyst and that you need to treat your all-star analyst very well. But it may not be clear whether paying $10,000 extra for an IT staff member is worth it or not.

Formal, measurable service levels can be established for many infrastructure attributes and day-to-day support. Moreover, industry benchmarks exist for these measures. Common infrastructure metrics are as follows:

- **Reliability:** for example, the percentage of time that systems have unscheduled downtime
- **Response time:** for example, how quickly an application moves from one screen to the next
- **Resiliency:** for example, how quickly a system can recover after it goes down

Glaser (2006) proposes a series of questions that can be used to assess the IT function. These questions cover the areas of infrastructure and application performance, execution, and strategic alignment.

Infrastructure and Application Performance

External and internal auditors' reports on IT controls and management. Do these reports note material problems with significant downtime, failure to perform adequate management of the data center, and adequacy of security controls?

IT infrastructure management processes. Does IT track downtime and what steps have been taken to reduce it? Are they current with vendor releases? How does IT manage virus protection? When the infrastructure has problems, what are the procedures for responding?

Execution

Achieving desired application outcomes. Picking three recent implementations, what were the objectives? To what degree were the objectives achieved? If the organization fell short in achieving objectives, why did this happen?

User engagement. Do implemented systems improve the operation of key departments? Was the training good? Were the IT group and the vendor responsive to issues and problems?

- **Software bugs:** for example, the number of bugs detected in an application per line of program code or hour of use

Common day-to-day support metrics are as follows:

- The percentage of help desk calls that are resolved within twenty-four hours
- The percentage of help desk calls that are not resolved after five days
- The percentage of help desk calls that are repeat calls, that is, the problem was not resolved the first time
- The time that elapses between ordering a workstation and its installation

PERSPECTIVE
Assessing the IT Function

Managing the implementation. Were clear project charters developed? Are sound project management techniques used? Do most projects get done on time and on budget?

Frontline support. Does the IT organization measure its service? Has the IT organization established service goals? Was the organization's management involved in setting those goals?

Departmental IT liaisons. Who are the IT liaisons to major user departments? Do they do a good job? Do the liaisons keep the department up-to-date on IT plans? Are liaisons considered to be members of the department's team?

Alignment of the IT Agenda with the Organization's Agenda

IT linkage to organizational strategy. Can the major elements of the organization's strategy be mapped to the IT initiatives needed to support the strategic plan? Is there a regular senior leadership discussion of the IT agenda, and does the leadership take responsibility for making decisions about which IT initiatives to fund?

Governance. What processes and committees are used to set priorities? Is the process for setting the IT budget well understood, efficient, sufficiently rigorous, and perceived as fair? Is there a well-accepted approach for acquiring new applications?

Source: Glaser (2006).

It is important that the management team define the desired level of IT service. For example, is the goal to achieve an uptime of 99.99 percent, or does the organization want to have 90 percent of help desk calls closed within twenty-four hours? If the service levels are deemed to be inadequate, a discussion can be held with IT managers to identify the costs of achieving a higher level of service. Additional staff members may be needed at the help desk, or the organization may need to develop a redundant network to improve resiliency. Conversely, if the organization needs to reduce IT costs, the management team may need to examine the service consequences of reducing the number of help desk staff members.

The assessment of the IT function requires examining areas that range from strategy development to service levels. And the assessment can use a

PERSPECTIVE
Managing Core IT Processes

Agarwal and Sambamurthy (2002) have identified eight core IT processes that must be managed well for an IT department to be effective:

1. **Human capital management** involves the development of IT staff skills and the attraction and retention of IT talent.

2. **Platform management** is a series of activities that designs the IT architecture and constructs and manages the resulting infrastructure.

3. **Relationship management** centers on developing and maintaining relationships between the IT function and the rest of the organization and on partnerships with IT vendors.

4. **Strategic planning** links the IT agenda and plans to the organization's strategy and plans.

5. **Financial management** encompasses a wide range of management processes—developing the IT budget, defining the business case for IT investments, and benchmarking IT costs.

6. **Value innovation** involves identifying new ways for IT to improve business operations and ensuring that IT investments deliver value.

7. **Solutions delivery** includes the selection, development, and implementation of applications and infrastructure.

8. **Services provisioning** centers on the day-to-day support of applications and infrastructure—for example, the help desk, workstation deployments, and user training.

Source: Agarwal and Sambamurthy (2002).

variety of data collection techniques. Appendix B contains a sample survey used by an IT services department to assess user satisfaction.

Answers to these questions provide an indication, clearly rough, of how well the IT function is being run and, to a degree, of whether the aggregate IT investment is providing value. All these questions come from commonsense management beliefs about what is involved in running an organization well and tests of IT domain knowledge.

SUMMARY

It is critical that health care organizations have access to appropriate IT staff members and resources to support their health care information systems and system users. IT staff members perform several common functions and have several common roles. In large organizations, the IT department often has a management team comprising the chief information officer, chief technology officer, chief information security officer, and chief medical information officer, who provide leadership to ensure that the organization fulfills its IT strategies and goals. Having a CIO with strong leadership skills, vision, and experience is critical to the organization achieving its strategic IT goals. Working with the CIO and IT management team, one will often find a team of professional and technical staff members including systems analysts, computer programmers, network administrators, database administrators, web designers, and support personnel. Each brings a unique set of knowledge and skills to support the IT operations of the health care organization.

The organizational structure of the IT department is influenced by several factors: level of centralization, core IT competencies, and desired attributes of the IT department.

IT services may be provided by in-house staff members or outsourced to an outside vendor or company. Many factors come into play in deciding if and when to outsource all or part of the IT services. Availability of staff members, time constraints, financial resources, and the executive management team's view of IT may determine the appropriateness of outsourcing.

Whether IT services are provided in-house or outsourced, it is important for the management team to assess the efficiency and effectiveness of IT services. The governance structure, how the IT resources are allocated, the track record of system acquisitions and system implementations, and user satisfaction with current IT service levels are some of the key elements that should be examined in any assessment. Consultants may be employed to conduct the assessment and offer the organization an outsider's objective view.

KEY TERMS

Application management

Chief information officer (CIO)

Chief information security officer
   (CISO)

Chief medical information officer
   (CMIO)

Chief technology officer (CTO)

Database administrators

Governance

IT centralization and decentralization

Network administrators

Operations and technical support

Outsourced IT

Programmers

Systems analyst

LEARNING ACTIVITIES

1. Visit an IT department in a health care facility in your community and interview the CIO or department director. Examine the IT department's organizational structure. What functions or services does the IT department provide? How centralized are IT services within the organization? Does the organization employ a CMIO, CISO, or CTO? If so, what are each person's job qualifications and responsibilities?

2. Find an article in the literature that outlines either the advantages or disadvantages or both of outsourcing IT. Discuss the findings with your classmates. What have others learned about outsourcing that may be important to your organization?

3. Plan and organize a panel discussion with CIOs from local health care facilities. Find out what some of their greatest challenges are and what a typical day is like for them. To what degree are their organizations facing workforce shortages? In what areas, if any? What strategies do they employ to recruit and retain top-notch staff members?

4. Investigate any one of the following roles and interview someone working in this type of position. Find out the individual's roles, responsibilities, qualifications, background, experience, and challenges.

   o Chief medical information officer

   o Chief information security officer

   o Chief technology officer

   o Clinical systems analyst

   o Mobile application developer

REFERENCES

Agarwal, R., & Sambamurthy, V. (2002). *Organizing the IT function for business innovation leadership.* Chicago, IL: Society for Information Management.

AMIA Task Force Report on CCIO Knowledge, Education and Skillset Requirements (2016). *The chief clinical informatics officer (CCIO).* Washington, DC: American Medical Informatics Association.

College of Healthcare Information Management Executives (CHIME). (1998). *The healthcare CIO: A decade of growth.* Ann Arbor, MI: Author.

College of Healthcare Information Management Executives (CHIME). (2008). *The seven CIO success factors.* Retrieved April 2008 from http://www.cio-chime.org/events/ciobootcamp/measure.asp

College of Healthcare Information Management Executives (CHIME). (2012). *Demand persists for experienced health IT staff.* Retrieved in April 2016 from http://www.hhnmag.com/ext/resources/inc-hhn/pdfs/resources/CHIME_Work-force-_survey_report-2012.pdf

Earl, M., & Feeney, D. (1995). Is your CIO adding value? *McKinsey Quarterly, 2,* 144–161.

Florentine, S. (2015). *10 hot IT skills for 2016.* Retrieved April 2016 from http://www.cio.com/article/3014161/careers-staffing/10-hot-it-job-skills-for-2016.html#slide1

Gartner. (2013). *Gartner says cloud computing will become the bulk of new IT spend by 2016.* Retrieved April 2016 from http://www.gartner.com/newsroom/id/2613015

Glaser, J. (2006, Jan.). Assessing the IT function in less than one day. *Healthcare Financial Management,* pp. 104–108.

Glaser, J. (2008a, April). Creating IT agility. *Healthcare Financial Management,* pp. 36–39.

Glaser, J. (2008b, Feb. 6). The four cornerstones of innovation. *Most Wired Online.*

Glaser, J. (2016, Feb. 8). The evolution of the health care chief information officer. *H&HN Daily.*

Glaser, J., & Kirby, J. (2009). Evolution of the healthcare CIO. *Healthcare Financial Management, 63*(11), 38–41.

Glaser, J., & Williams, R. (2007). The definitive evolution of the role of the CIO. *Journal of Healthcare Information Management, 21*(1), 9–11.

Murphy, J. (2011). The nursing informatics workforce: Who are they and what do they do? *Nursing Economics, 42*(11), 20–23.

Oz, E. (2006). *Management information systems: Instructor edition* (4th ed.). Boston, MA: Course Technology.

Wadsworth, J. (2016). *The best organizational structure for healthcare analytics.* Health Catalyst. Retrieved May 31, 2016, from https://www.healthcatalyst.com/best-organizational-structure-healthcare-analytics

PART THREE

Laws, Regulations, and Standards That Affect Health Care Information Systems

CHAPTER 9

Privacy and Security

LEARNING OBJECTIVES

- To be able to distinguish among privacy, confidentiality, and security as they relate to health information.

- To be able to identify the purpose of the Privacy Act of 1974 and 42 C.F.R. (Code of Federal Regulations) Part 2, Confidentiality of Substance Abuse Patient Records.

- To be able to describe and discuss the impact of the HIPAA Privacy, Security, and Breach Notification rules.

- To be able to identify threats to health care information and information systems caused by humans (intentional and unintentional), natural causes, and the environment.

- To be able to understand the purpose and key components of the health care organization security program and the need to mitigate security risks.

- To be able to discuss the increased need for and identify resources to improve cybersecurity in health care organizations.

Privacy is an individual's constitutional right to be left alone, to be free from unwarranted publicity, and to conduct his or her life without its being made public. In the health care environment, privacy is an individual's right to limit access to his or her health care information. In spite of this constitutional protection and other legislated protections discussed in this chapter, approximately 112 million Americans (a third of the United States population) were affected by breaches of **protected health information (PHI)** in 2015 (Koch, 2016). Three large insurance-related corporations accounted for nearly one hundred million records being exposed (Koch, 2016). In one well-publicized security breach at Banner Health, where hackers gained entrance through food and beverage computers, approximately 3.7 million individuals' information was accessed, much of it health information (Goedert, 2016).

Health information privacy and security are key topics for health care administrators. In today's ever-increasing electronic world, where the Internet of Things is on the horizon and nearly every health care organization employee and visitor has a smart mobile device that is connected to at least one network, new and more virulent **threats** are an everyday concern. In this chapter we will examine and define the concepts of privacy, confidentiality, and security as they apply to health information. Major legislative efforts, historic and current, to protect health care information are outlined, with a focus on the **Health Insurance Portability and Accountability Act (HIPAA)** Privacy, Security, and Breach Notification rules. Different types of threats, intentional and unintentional, to health information will be discussed. Basic requirements for a strong health care organization security program will be outlined, and the chapter will conclude with the **cybersecurity** challenges in today's environment of mobile and cloud-based devices, wearable fitness trackers, social media, and remote access to health information.

PRIVACY, CONFIDENTIALITY, AND SECURITY DEFINED

As stated, **privacy** is an individual's right to be left alone and to limit access to his or her health care information. **Confidentiality** is related to privacy but specifically addresses the expectation that information shared with a health care provider during the course of treatment will be used only for its intended purpose and not disclosed otherwise. Confidentiality relies on trust. **Security** refers to the systems that are in place to protect health information and the systems within which it resides. Health care organizations must protect their health information and health information systems from a range of potential threats. Certainly, security systems must protect against unauthorized access and disclosure of patient information, but they must also be designed to protect the organization's IT assets—such as the networks, hardware, software, and applications that make up the organization's health care information systems—from harm.

LEGAL PROTECTION OF HEALTH INFORMATION

There are many sources for the legal and ethical requirements that health care professionals maintain the confidentiality of patient information and protect patient privacy. Ethical and professional standards, such as those published by the American Medical Association and other organizations, address professional conduct and the need to hold patient information in confidence. Accrediting bodies, such as the Joint Commission, state facility licensure rules, and the government through Centers for Medicare and Medicaid, dictate that health care organizations follow standard practice and state and federal laws to ensure the confidentiality and security of patient information.

Today, legal protection specially addressing the unauthorized disclosure of an individual's health information generally comes from one of three sources (Koch, 2016):

- Federal HIPAA Privacy, Security, and Breach Notification rules
- State privacy laws. These laws typically apply more stringent protections for information related to specific health conditions (HIV/AIDS, mental or reproductive health, for example).
- **Federal Trade Commission (FTC) Act** consumer protection, which protects against unfair or deceptive practices. The FTC issued the Health Breach Notification Rule in 2010 to require certain businesses not covered by HIPAA, including PHR vendors, PHR-related entities, or third-party providers for PHR vendors or PHR-related entities to notify individuals of a security breach.

However, there are two other major federal laws governing patient privacy that, although they have been essentially superseded by HIPAA, remain important, particularly from a historical perspective.

- The Privacy Act of 1974 (5 U.S.C. §552a; 45 C.F.R. Part 5b; OMB Circular No. A-108 [1975])
- Confidentiality of Substance Abuse Patient Records (42 U.S.C. §290dd-2, 42 C.F.R. Part 2)

The Privacy Act of 1974

In 1966, the Freedom of Information Act (FOIA) was passed. This legislation provides the American public with the right to obtain information from federal agencies. The act covers all records created by the federal government, with nine exceptions. The sixth exception is for personnel and medical information, "the disclosure of which would constitute a clearly unwarranted invasion of personal privacy." There was, however, concern that this exception to the FOIA was not strong enough to protect federally created patient records and other health information. Consequently, Congress enacted the **Privacy Act of 1974.** This act was written specifically to protect patient confidentiality only in *federally operated* health care facilities, such as Veterans Administration hospitals, Indian Health Service facilities, and military health care organizations. Because the protection was limited to those facilities operated by the federal government, most general hospitals and other nongovernment health care organizations did not have to comply. Nevertheless, the Privacy Act of 1974 was an important piece of legislation, not only because it addressed the FOIA exception for patient information but also because it explicitly stated that patients had a right to access and amend their medical records. It also required facilities to maintain documentation of all disclosures. Neither of these things was standard practice at the time.

Confidentiality of Substance Abuse Patient Records

During the 1970s, people became increasingly aware of the extra-sensitive nature of drug and alcohol treatment records. This led to the regulations currently found in **42 C.F.R. (Code of Federal Regulations) Part 2, Confidentiality of Substance Abuse Patient Records.** These regulations have been amended twice, with the latest version published in 1999. They offer specific guidance to federally assisted health care organizations that provide referral, diagnosis, and treatment services to patients with alcohol or drug problems. Not surprisingly, they set stringent release of information standards, designed to protect the confidentiality of patients seeking alcohol or drug treatment.

HIPAA

HIPAA is the first comprehensive federal regulation to offer specific protection to private health information. Prior to the enactment of HIPAA there was no single federal regulation governing the privacy and security of patient-specific information, only the limited legislative protections previously discussed. These laws were not comprehensive and protected only specific groups of individuals.

The Health Insurance Portability and Accountability Act of 1996 consists of two main parts:

- **Title I** addresses health care access, portability, and renewability, offering protection for individuals who change jobs or health insurance policies. (Although Title I is an important piece of legislation, it does not address health care information specifically and will therefore not be addressed in this chapter.)
- **Title II** includes a section titled, "Administrative Simplification."

The requirements establishing privacy and security regulations for protecting individually identifiable health information are found in Title II of HIPAA. The **HIPAA Privacy Rule** was required beginning April 2003 and the **HIPAA Security Rule** beginning April 2005. Both rules were subsequently amended and the Breach Notification Rule was added as a part of the HITECH Act in 2009.

The information protected under the HIPAA Privacy Rule is specifically defined as PHI, which is information that

- Relates to a person's physical or mental health, the provision of health care, or the payment for health care
- Identifies the person who is the subject of the information
- Is created or *received* by a covered entity
- Is transmitted or maintained in *any* form (paper, electronic, or oral)

Unlike the Privacy Rule, the Security Rule addressed only PHI transmitted or maintained in electronic form. Within the Security Rule this information is identified as ePHI.

The HIPAA rules also define covered entities (CEs), those organizations to which the rules apply:

- Health plans, which pay or provide for the cost of medical care
- Health care clearinghouses, which process health information (for example, billing services)
- Health care providers who conduct certain financial and administrative transactions electronically (These transactions are defined broadly so that the reality of HIPAA is that it governs nearly all health care providers who receive any type of third-party reimbursement.)

If any CE shares information with others, it must establish contracts to protect the shared information. The HITECH Act amended HIPAA and added "Business Associates" as a category of CE. It further clarified that certain entities, such as health information exchange organizations, regional health information organizations, e-prescribing gateways, or a vendor that contracts with a CE to allow the CE to offer a personal health record as a part of its EHR, are business associates if they require access to PHI on a routine basis (Coppersmith, Gordon, Schermer, & Brokelman, PLC, 2012).

HIPAA Privacy Rule

Although the HIPAA Privacy Rule is a comprehensive set of federal standards, it permits the enforcement of existing state laws that are more protective of individual privacy, and states are also free to pass more stringent laws. Therefore, health care organizations must still be familiar with their own state laws and regulations related to privacy and confidentiality.

The major components to the HIPAA Privacy Rule in its original form include the following:

- **Boundaries.** PHI may be disclosed for health purposes only, with very limited exceptions.
- **Security.** PHI should not be distributed without patient authorization unless there is a clear basis for doing so, and the individuals who receive the information must safeguard it.
- **Consumer control.** Individuals are entitled to access and control their health records and are to be informed of the purposes for which information is being disclosed and used.
- **Accountability.** Entities that improperly handle PHI can be charged under criminal law and punished and are subject to civil recourse as well.
- **Public responsibility.** Individual interests must not override national priorities in public health, medical research, preventing health care fraud, and law enforcement in general.

With HITECH, the Privacy Rule was expanded to include creation of new privacy requirements for HIPAA-covered entities and business associates. In addition, the rights of individuals to request and obtain their PHI are strengthened, as is the right of the individual to prevent a health care organization from disclosing PHI to a health plan, if the individual paid in full out of pocket for the related services. There were also some new provisions for accounting of disclosures made through an EHR for treatment, payment, and operations (Coppersmith et al., 2012).

The HIPAA Privacy Rule attempts to sort out the *routine and nonroutine use of health information* by distinguishing between patient consent *to use* PHI and patient authorization *to release* PHI. Health care providers and others must obtain a patient's written consent prior to disclosure of health information for routine uses of treatment, payment, and health care operations. This consent is fairly general in nature and is obtained prior to patient treatment. There are some exceptions to this in emergency situations, and the patient has a right to request restrictions on the disclosure. However, health care providers can deny treatment if they feel that limiting the disclosure would be detrimental. Health care providers and others must obtain the patient's specific written authorization for all nonroutine uses or disclosures of PHI, such as releasing health records to a school or a relative.

Exhibit 9.1 is a sample release of information form used by a hospital, showing the following elements that should be present on a valid release form:

- Patient identification (name and date of birth)
- Name of the person or entity to whom the information is being released
- Description of the specific health information authorized for disclosure
- Statement of the reason for or purpose of the disclosure
- Date, event, or condition on which the authorization will expire, unless it is revoked earlier
- Statement that the authorization is subject to revocation by the patient or the patient's legal representative
- Patient's or legal representative's signature
- Signature date, which must be after the date of the encounter that produced the information to be released

Health care organizations need clear policies and procedures for releasing PHI. A central point of control should exist through which all nonroutine requests for information pass, and all disclosures should be well documented.

In some instances, PHI can be released without the patient's authorization. For example, some state laws require disclosing certain health information. It is always good practice to obtain a patient authorization prior to releasing information when feasible, but in state-mandated cases it is not required. Some examples of situations in which information might need to be disclosed to authorized recipients without the patient's consent are the

Exhibit 9.1 Sample release of information form

MUSC Health

AUTHRELSE

AUTHORIZATION TO DISCLOSE PROTECTED HEALTH INFORMATION
Page 1 of 1
Form Origination Date: 1/2000

Version: 9   Version Date: 12/15

Patient Name:_____

Date of Birth:_____

Last 4 digits of SSN:_____

Phone #:_____

MRN (internal only):_____

This form must be completed in its entirety in order to be considered valid.

Check ONE box **Release Records To:** ☐ (*Where* do you want the information sent? *Who* may have the information?) **OR** **Obtain Records From:** ☐ (*Who* has the information you want released?) Please list the specific Hospital and /or clinic.	NAME/ ORGANIZATION:_____ Attention to: _____ Address _____ City:_____ State _____ Zip code: _____ Day Phone Number: _____ Fax Number _____
Release Instructions: (*How* do you want the information?)	Release Method/Format requested: (check one) ☐ *Mail* ☐ *DVD/CD* ☐ *My Chart/Epic* ☐ *Fax* (To healthcare provider ONLY)☐ *Other*_____
Purpose of Release: (*Why* is it needed?)	☐ Continuing Care ☐ Legal ☐ Patient Request ☐ Military ☐ Insurance ☐ Disability ☐ School ☐ Other _____ I understand that fees for copies of medical records /Images and postage fees may be charged as provided by S.C. Law.
Treatment Date(s): (*When* were you seen?)	☐ Treatment dates from_____ to_____(Please be specific) OR ☐ All Treatment Dates
Information to be Released: (*What* do you want sent or released? Check the appropriate box.)	☐ ENTIRE RECORD ☐ Images/DVD ☐ Immunization records ☐ Medication list ☐ Physician progress/ visit notes	☐ Abstract Information History & Physical, consults, lab & radiology reports, discharge summary, operative/procedure reports, Emergency Department reports, and Occupational/Physical Therapy reports. ☐ Psychotherapy ☐ Other:_____

I understand this information may include reference to psychiatric / psychological care, sexual assault, drug abuse, results of tests for all infectious diseases including HIV / AIDS and / or alcohol abuse.

I understand that I have a right to cancel / revoke this authorization at any time. I understand that if I cancel / revoke this authorization I must do so in writing and present my written cancellation / revocation to the Health Information Services Department (Medical Records). I understand that the cancellation / revocation will not apply to information that has already been released in response to this authorization, as stated in the Notice of Privacy Practice. Unless otherwise canceled / revoked, this authorization will expire / end one year from this date or_____.

I understand that authorizing the disclosure of protected health information is voluntary. I can refuse to sign this authorization. I do not need to sign this form to receive treatment. I understand I may review and / or copy the information to be disclosed, as provided in 45 CFR §164.524. I understand that any disclosure of information carries with it the possibility of unauthorized disclosure by the person / organization receiving the information. I understand I will be given a copy of this authorization.

A copy of my identification will be made and attached to this authorization. (NOTE: STATE LAW ALLOWS 45 DAYS for Processing.)

_____
Printed Name of Patient or Legal Guardian / Representative

_____
Date

X_____
Signature of Patient or Legal Guardian/Representative

_____
Relationship to Patient, if signed by Legal Guardian

_____
Witness Signature

Document(s) of patient representative's authority must be attached if patient is not signing.
To contact Health Information Services (Medical Records) in writing, the address is: 169 Ashley Avenue / MSC 349 /Suite 200/ Attn: Release of Information / Charleston, South Carolina 29425; the phone number is (843) 792-3881. Fax number is (843) 876-8080 or (843) 876-8055.

Original to Health Information Services (medical records department)   **Copy to patient**

all_all_consent_authorelease   OTE 700078 Rev. 12/15

Source:

presence of a communicable disease, such as AIDS and sexually transmitted diseases, which must be reported to the state or county department of health; suspected child abuse or adult abuse that must be reported to designated authorities; situations in which there is a legal duty to warn another person of a clear and imminent danger from a patient; bona fide medical emergencies; and the existence of a valid court order.

The HIPAA Security Rule

The HIPAA Security Rule is closely connected to the HIPAA Privacy Rule. The Security Rule governs only ePHI, which is defined as protected health information maintained or transmitted in electronic form. It is important to note that the Security Rule does not distinguish between electronic forms of information or between transmission mechanisms. ePHI may be stored in any type of electronic media, such as magnetic tapes and disks, optical disks, servers, and personal computers. Transmission may take place over the Internet or on local area networks (LANs), for example.

The standards in the final rule are defined in general terms, focusing on what should be done rather than on how it should be done. According to the Centers for Medicare and Medicaid Services (CMS, 2004), the final rule specifies "a series of administrative, technical, and physical security procedures for covered entities to use to assure the confidentiality of **electronic protected health information (ePHI).** The standards are delineated into either *required* or *addressable* implementation specifications." A required specification *must* be implemented by a CE for that organization to be in compliance. However, the CE is in compliance with an addressable specification if it does any one of the following:

- Implements the specification as stated
- Implements an alternative security measure to accomplish the purposes of the standard or specification
- Chooses not to implement anything, provided it can demonstrate that the standard or specification is not reasonable and appropriate and that the purpose of the standard can still be met; because the Security Rule is designed to be technology neutral, this flexibility was granted for organizations that employ nonstandard technologies or have legitimate reasons not to need the stated specification (AHIMA, 2003)

The standards contained in the HIPAA Security Rule are divided into sections, or categories, the specifics of which we outline here. You will notice overlap among the sections. For example, contingency plans are covered under both administrative and physical safeguards, and access controls are addressed in several standards and specifications.

The HIPAA Security Rule

The **HIPAA Security Administrative Safeguards** section of the Final Rule contains nine standards:

1. **Security management functions.** This standard requires the CE to implement policies and procedures to prevent, detect, contain, and correct security violations. There are four implementation specifications for this standard:
   - *Risk analysis* (required). The CE must conduct an accurate and thorough assessment of the potential risks to and **vulnerabilities** of the confidentiality, integrity, and availability of ePHI.
   - *Risk management* (required). The CE must implement security measures that reduce risks and vulnerabilities to a reasonable and appropriate level.
   - *Sanction policy* (required). The CE must apply appropriate sanctions against workforce members who fail to comply with the CE's security policies and procedures.
   - *Information system activity review* (required). The CE must implement procedures to regularly review records of information system activity, such as audit logs, access reports, and security incident tracking reports.

2. **Assigned security responsibility.** This standard does not have any implementation specifications. It requires the CE to identify the individual responsible for overseeing development of the organization's security policies and procedures.

3. **Workforce security.** This standard requires the CE to implement policies and procedures to ensure that all members of its workforce have appropriate access to ePHI and to prevent those workforce members who do not have access from obtaining access. There are three implementation specifications for this standard:
   - *Authorization and/or supervision* (addressable). The CE must have a process for ensuring that the workforce working with ePHI has adequate authorization and supervision.

- *Workforce clearance procedure* (addressable). There must be a process to determine what access is appropriate for each workforce member.
- *Termination procedures* (addressable). There must be a process for terminating access to ePHI when a workforce member is no longer employed or his or her responsibilities change.

4. **Information access management.** This standard requires the CE to implement policies and procedures for authorizing access to ePHI. There are three implementation specifications within this standard. The first (not shown here) applies to health care clearinghouses, and the other two apply to health care organizations:

- *Access authorization* (addressable). The CE must have a process for granting access to ePHI through a workstation, transaction, program, or other process.
- *Access establishment and modification* (addressable). The CE must have a process (based on the access authorization) to establish, document, review, and modify a user's right to access a workstation, transaction, program, or process.

5. **Security awareness and training.** This standard requires the CE to implement awareness and training programs for all members of its workforce. This training should include periodic security reminders and address protection from malicious software, log-in monitoring, and password management. (These items to be addressed in training are all listed as addressable implementation specifications.)

6. **Security incident reporting.** This standard requires the CE to implement policies and procedures to address security incidents.

7. **Contingency plan.** This standard has five implementation specifications:

- Data backup plan (required)
- Disaster recovery plan (required)
- Emergency mode operation plan (required)
- Testing and revision procedures (addressable); the CE should periodically test and modify all contingency plans
- Applications and data criticality analysis (addressable); the CE should assess the relative criticality of specific applications and data in support of its contingency plan

8. **Evaluation.** This standard requires the CE to periodically perform technical and nontechnical evaluations in response to changes that may affect the security of ePHI.

9. **Business associate contracts and other arrangements.** This standard outlines the conditions under which a CE must have a formal agreement with business associates in order to exchange ePHI.

The **HIPAA Security Physical Safeguards** section contains four standards:

1. **Facility access controls.** This standard requires the CE to implement policies and procedures to limit physical access to its electronic information systems and the facilities in which they are housed to authorized users. There are four implementation specifications with this standard:
   - *Contingency operations* (addressable). The CE should have a process for allowing facility access to support the restoration of lost data under the disaster recovery plan and emergency mode operation plan.
   - *Facility security plan* (addressable). The CE must have a process to safeguard the facility and its equipment from unauthorized access, tampering, and theft.
   - *Access control and validation* (addressable). The CE should have a process to control and validate access to facilities based on users' roles or functions.
   - *Maintenance records* (addressable). The CE should have a process to document repairs and modifications to the physical components of a facility as they relate to security.
2. **Workstation use.** This standard requires the CE to implement policies and procedures that specify the proper functions to be performed and the manner in which those functions are to be performed on a specific workstation or class of workstation that can be used to access ePHI and that also specify the physical attributes of the surroundings of such workstations.
3. **Workstation security.** This standard requires the CE to implement physical safeguards for all workstations that are used to access ePHI and to restrict access to authorized users.
4. **Device and media controls.** This standard requires the CE to implement policies and procedures for the movement of hardware and electronic media that contain ePHI into and out of a facility and within a facility. There are four implementation specifications with this standard:
   - *Disposal* (required). The CE must have a process for the final disposition of ePHI and of the hardware and electronic media on which it is stored.

- *Media reuse* (required). The CE must have a process for removal of ePHI from electronic media before the media can be reused.
- *Accountability* (addressable). The CE must maintain a record of movements of hardware and electronic media and any person responsible for these items.
- *Data backup and storage* (addressable). The CE must create a retrievable, exact copy of ePHI, when needed, before movement of equipment.

The **HIPAA Security Technical Safeguards** section has five standards:

1. **Access control.** This standard requires the CE to implement technical policies and procedures for electronic information systems that maintain ePHI in order to allow access only to those persons or software programs that have been granted access rights as specified in the administrative safeguards. There are four implementation specifications within this standard:
   - *Unique user identification* (required). The CE must assign a unique name or number for identifying and tracking each user's identity.
   - *Emergency access procedure* (required). The CE must establish procedures for obtaining necessary ePHI in an emergency.
   - *Automatic log-off* (addressable). The CE must implement electronic processes that terminate an electronic session after a predetermined time of inactivity.
   - *Encryption and decryption* (addressable). The CE should implement a mechanism to encrypt and decrypt ePHI as needed.
2. **Audit controls.** This standard requires the CE to implement hardware, software, and procedures that record and examine activity in the information systems that contain ePHI.
3. **Integrity.** This standard requires the CE to implement policies and procedures to protect ePHI from improper alteration or destruction.
4. **Person or entity authentication.** This standard requires the CE to implement procedures to verify that a person or entity seeking access to ePHI is in fact the person or entity claimed.
5. **Transmission security.** This standard requires the CE to implement technical measures to guard against unauthorized access to ePHI

being transmitted across a network. There are two implementation specifications with this standard:

- *Integrity controls* (addressable). The CE must implement security measures to ensure that electronically transmitted ePHI is not improperly modified without detection.
- *Encryption* (addressable). The CE should encrypt ePHI whenever it is deemed appropriate.

The Policies, Procedures, and Documentation section has two standards:

1. **Policies and procedures.** This standard requires the CE to establish and implement policies and procedures to comply with the standards, implementation specifications, and other requirements.
2. **Documentation.** This standard requires the CE to maintain the policies and procedures implemented to comply with the Security Rule in written form. There are three implementation specifications:

- *Time limit* (required). The CE must retain the documentation for six years from the date of its creation or the date when it was last in effect, whichever is later.
- *Availability* (required). The CE must make the documentation available to those persons responsible for implementing the policies and procedures.
- *Updates* (required). The CE must review the documentation periodically and update it as needed.

HIPAA Breach Notification Rule

The **HIPAA Breach Notification Rule** requires CEs and their business associates to provide notification following a breach of *unsecured* protected health information. "'Unsecured' PHI is PHI that has not been rendered unusable, unreadable, or indecipherable to unauthorized persons through the use of a technology or methodology specified by the Secretary in guidance" (US Department of Health and Human Services, n.d.c). To meet the requirement of "secured" PHI, it must have been encrypted using a valid encryption process, or the media on which the PHI is stored have been destroyed. Paper or other hard copy media, such as film, must be shredded or otherwise destroyed so that it cannot be read or reconstructed. Electronic media must be "sanitized" according to accepted standards so that PHI cannot be retrieved (US Department of Health and Human Services, n.d.c).

The notification requirements include, depending on the circumstances, notification to these sources:

- Individuals affected
- The Health and Human Services Secretary (via the Office for Civil Rights [OCR])
- Major media outlets

All individuals affected by breaches of unsecured PHI must be notified within a reasonable length of time—less than sixty days—after the breach is discovered. If the CE does not have sufficient information to contact ten or more individuals directly, the notification must be made on the home page of its website for at least ninety days or by a major media outlet. A CE that experiences a breach involving five hundred or more individuals must, in addition to sending individual notices, provide notice to a major media outlet serving the area. This notification must also be made within sixty days. All breaches must also be reported to the secretary of HHS; the breaches involving more than five hundred individuals must be reported within sixty days; all others may be reported on an annual basis (US Department of Health and Human Services, n.d.b).

HIPAA Enforcement and Violation Penalties

The Department of Health and Human Services (HHS) **Office for Civil Rights (OCR)** is responsible for enforcing HIPAA Privacy and Security rules. In addition, HITECH gave state attorneys general the authority to bring civil actions on behalf of the residents of their states for HIPAA violations. From April 2003 until May 2016, OCR has received over 134,000 HIPAA complaints and has initiated 879 compliance reviews. The resolution of the complaints and reviews is as follows (US Department of Health and Human Services, 2016):

- Settled thirty-five cases resulting in $36,639,200 in penalties
- Resolved 24,241 cases by requiring a change in privacy practices and corrective actions by, or providing technical assistance to, CEs or business associates
- Identified 11,018 cases as no violation and 79,865 cases as non-eligible

HIPAA criminal and civil penalties for noncompliance are applied using a tiered schedule that ranges from $100 for a single violation, when the individual did not know he or she was not in compliance, to $1,500,000 for multiple violations because of willful neglect. It is important to note that

Table 9.1 HIPAA violation categories

Violation Category	Category Fine*
Category 1: A violation that the CE was unaware of, and could not have realistically avoided, had a reasonable amount of care been taken to abide by HIPAA rules	Minimum fine of $100 per violation up to $50,000
Category 2: A violation that the CE should have been aware of but could not have avoided even with a reasonable amount of care (but falling short of willful neglect of HIPAA rules)	Minimum fine of $1,000 per violation up to $50,000
Category 3: A violation suffered as a direct result of "willful neglect" of HIPAA rules, in cases in which an attempt has been made to correct the violation	Minimum fine of $10,000 per violation up to $50,000
Category 4: A violation of HIPAA rules constituting willful neglect, and no attempt has been made to correct the violation	Minimum fine of $50,000 per violation

*The fines are issued per violation category, per year that the violation was allowed to persist. The maximum fine per violation category, per year, is $1,500,000.

Source: What are the penalties for HIPAA violations? (2015).

civil penalties cannot be levied in situations when the violation is corrected within a specified period of time.

The structure for HIPAA violations reflect four categories of violations and associated penalties. Table 9.1 outlines the categories and penalties.

In addition to these civil penalties, a HIPAA violation may result in criminal charges. The criminal penalties are divided into the following three tiers (What are the penalties for HIPAA violations, 2015):

- Tier 1: Reasonable cause or no knowledge of violation—Up to one year in jail
- Tier 2: Obtaining PHI under false pretenses—Up to five years in jail
- Tier 3: Obtaining PHI for personal gain or with malicious intent—Up to ten years in jail

As stated, most HIPAA violations are resolved with corrective action. In 2015 six financial penalties were issued. However, a serious violation can cost a health care organization a significant about of money. One such case resulting in a substantial financial settlement is outlined in the Perspective. The top ten largest fines levied for HIPAA violations as of August 2016 are listed in Table 9.2.

Table 9.2 Top ten largest fines levied for HIPAA violations as of August 2016

Organization	Individuals Affected	Fine Awarded ($ million)	Data Awarded
Advocate Health Care: Lacked appropriate safeguards, including an unencrypted laptop was left in a vehicle overnight	4 million	5.55	August 2016
New York Presbyterian Hospital and Columbia University: PHI accessible on Google and other search engines	6,800	4.8	May 2014
Cignet Health: Did not allow patients access to medical records and refused to cooperate with OCR	41	4.3	February 2011
Feinstein Institute for Medical Research: Lacked appropriate safeguards leading to theft	Unknown	3.9	March 2016
Triple-S Management Corp (Blue Cross/ Blue Shield licensee in Puerto Rico): Did not deactivate user IDs and passwords, allowing previous employees to access PHI	398,000	3.5	November 2015
University of Mississippi Medical Center: Did not manage risks appropriately, although aware of risks and vulnerabilities	10,000	2.75	July 2016
Oregon Health & Science University: Lacked safeguards with regards to stolen laptop and used cloud storage without a business associate agreement in place	7,000	2.7	July 2016
CVS Pharmacy: Improperly disposed of PHI such as prescription labels	Unknown	2.25	January 2009
New York Presbyterian Hospital: Allowed filming of two patients for a TV series creating the potential for PHI to be compromise. (*Note:* Hospital continues to maintain it was not a violation.)	Unknown	2.2	April 2016
Concentra Health Services: Failed to remediate an identified lack of encryption after an unencrypted laptop was stolen	870	1.73	April 2014

Source: Bazzoli (2016).

PERSPECTIVE
$750,000 HIPAA Settlement Underscores
the Need for Organization-Wide Risk Analysis

The University of Washington Medicine (UWM) has agreed to settle charges that it potentially violated the Health Insurance Portability and Accountability Act of 1996 (HIPAA) Security Rule by failing to implement policies and procedures to prevent, detect, contain, and correct security violations. UWM is an affiliated covered entity, which includes designated health care components and other entities under the control of the University of Washington, including University of Washington Medical Center, the primary teaching hospital of the University of Washington School of Medicine. Affiliated covered entities must have in place appropriate policies and processes to assure HIPAA compliance with respect to each of the entities that are part of the affiliated group. The settlement includes a monetary payment of $750,000, a corrective action plan, and annual reports on the organization's compliance efforts.

The US Department of Health and Human Services Office for Civil Rights (OCR) initiated its investigation of the UWM following receipt of a breach report on November 27, 2013, which indicated that the electronic protected health information (e-PHI) of approximately 90,000 individuals was accessed after an employee downloaded an email attachment that contained malicious malware. The malware compromised the organization's IT system, affecting the data of two different groups of patients: (1) approximately 76,000 patients involving a combination of patient names, medical record numbers, dates of service, and/or charges or bill balances; and (2) approximately 15,000 patients involving names, medical record numbers, other demographics such as address and phone number, dates of birth, charges or bill balances, Social Security numbers, insurance identification or Medicare numbers.

OCR's investigation indicated UWM's security policies required its affiliated entities to have up-to-date, documented system-level risk assessments and to implement safeguards in compliance with the Security Rule. However, UWM did not ensure that all of its affiliated entities were properly conducting risk assessments and appropriately responding to the potential risks and vulnerabilities in their respective environments.

Source: HHS.gov (2015). Used with permission.

THREATS TO HEALTH CARE INFORMATION

What are the threats to health care information systems? In general, threats to health care information systems fall into one of these three categories:

- Human tampering threats
- Natural and environmental threats, such as floods and fire
- Environmental factors and technology malfunctions, such as a drive that fails and has no backup or a power outage

Threats to health care information systems from human beings can be intentional or unintentional. They can be *internal,* caused by employees, or *external,* caused by individuals outside the organization.

Intentional threats include knowingly disclosing patient information without authorization, theft, intentional alteration of data, and intentional destruction of data. The culprit could be a computer **hacker,** a disgruntled employee, or a prankster. Cybercrime directed at health information systems has increased significantly in recent years. In the 2014–2015 two-year period, more than 90 percent of health care organizations reported a health information security breach, and of these reports, nearly half were because of criminal activity (Koch, 2016). Intentional destruction or disruption of health care information is generally caused by some form of **malware,** a general term for software that is written to "infect" and subsequently harm a host computer system. The best-known form of malware is the computer virus, but there are others, including the particularly virulent ransomware, attacks from which are on the rise in health care.

The following list includes common forms of malware with a brief description of each (Comodo, 2014):

- **Viruses** are generally spread when software is shared among computers. It is a "contagious" piece of software code that infects the host system and spreads itself.
- **Trojans** (or Trojan Horses) are a type of virus specifically designed to look like a safe program. They can be programmed to steal personal information or to take over the resources of the host computer making it unavailable for its intended use.
- **Spyware** tracks Internet activities assisting the hacker in gathering information without consent. Spyware is generally hidden and can be difficult to detect.

- **Worms** are software code that replicates itself and destroys files that are on the host computer, including the operating system.
- **Ransomware** is an advanced form of malware that hackers use to cripple the organization's computer systems through malicious code, generally launched via an e-mail that is opened unwittingly by an employee, a method known as *phishing*. The malicious code then encrypts and locks folders and operating systems. The hacker demands money, generally in the form of bitcoins, a type of digital currency, to provide the decryption key to unlock the organization's systems (Conn, 2016).

Some of the causes of unintentional health information breaches are lack of training in proper use of the health information system or human error. Users may unintentionally share patient information without proper authorization. Other examples include users sharing **passwords** or downloading information from nonsecure Internet sites, creating the potential for a breach in security. Some of the more common forms of internal breaches of security across all industries are the installation or use of unauthorized software, use of the organization's computing resources for illegal or illicit communications or activities (porn surfing, e-mail harassment, and so forth), and the use of the organization's computing resources for personal profit. Losing or improperly disposing of electronic devices, including computers and portable electronic devices, also constitute serious forms of unintentional health information exposure. In 2015, the OCR portal, which lists breach incidents potentially affecting five hundred or more individuals, reported more than seventy-five thousand individuals' data were breached either because of loss or improper disposal of a device containing PHI (OCR, n.d.).

Threats from natural causes, such as fire or flood, are less common than human threats, but they must also be addressed in any comprehensive health care information security program. Loss of information because of environmental factors and technical malfunctions must be secured against by using appropriate safeguards.

THE HEALTH CARE ORGANIZATION'S SECURITY PROGRAM

The realization of any of the threats discussed in the previous section can cause significant damage to the organization. Resorting to manual operations if the computers are down for days, for example, can lead to organizational chaos. Theft or loss of organizational data can lead to litigation by the individuals harmed by the disclosure of the data and HIPAA violations. Malware can corrupt databases, corruption from which there may be no recovery. The function of the health care organization's security program is to identify potential threats and implement processes to remove these threats or mitigate their ability to cause damage. The primary challenge of developing an effective security program in a health care organization is balancing the need for security with the cost of security. An organization does not know how to calculate the likelihood that a hacker will cause serious damage or a backhoe will cut through network cables under the street. The organization may not fully understand the consequences of being without its network for four hours or four days. Hence, it may not be sure how much to spend to remove or reduce the risk.

Another challenge is maintaining a satisfactory balance between health care information system security and health care data and information availability. As we saw in Chapter Two, the major purpose of maintaining health information and health records is to facilitate high-quality care for patients. On the one hand, if an organization's security measures are so stringent that they prevent appropriate access to the health information needed to care for patients, this important purpose is undermined. On the other hand, if the organization allows unrestricted access to all patient-identifiable information to all its employees, the patients' rights to privacy and confidentiality would certainly be violated and the organization's IT assets would be at considerable risk.

The ONC (2015) publication *Guide to Privacy and Security of Electronic Health Information* for health care providers includes a chapter describing a seven-step approach for implementing a security management process. The guidance is directed at physician practices or other small health care organizations, and it does not include specific technical solutions. Specific solutions for security protection will be driven by the organization's overall plan and will be managed by the organizations IT team. Larger organizations must also develop comprehensive security programs and will follow the same basic steps, but it will likely have more internal resources for security than smaller practices.

Each step in the ONC security management process for health care providers is listed in the following section.

Step 1: Lead Your Culture, Select Your Team, and Learn

This step includes six actions:

1. Designate a security officer, who will be responsible for developing and implementing the security practices to meet HIPAA requirements and ensure the security of PHI.

2. Discuss HIPAA security requirements with your EHR developer to ensure that your system can be implemented to meet the security requirements of HIPAA and Meaningful Use.

3. Consider using a qualified professional to assist with your security risk analysis. The security risk analysis is the opportunity to discover as much as possible about risks and vulnerabilities to health information within the organization.

4. Use tools to preview your security risk analysis. Examples of available tools are listed within Step 3.

5. Refresh your knowledge base of the HIPAA rules.

6. Promote a culture of protecting patient privacy and securing patient information. Make sure to communicate that all members of the organization are responsible for protecting patient information.

Step 2: Document Your Process, Findings, and Actions

Documenting the processes for risk analysis and implementation of safeguards is very important, not to mention a requirement of HIPAA. The following are some examples cited by the ONC of records to retain:

- Policies and procedures
- Completed security checklists (ESET, n.d.)
- Training materials presented to staff members and volunteers and any associated certificates of completion
- Updated business associate (BA) agreements
- Security risk analysis report
- EHR audit logs that show utilization of security features and efforts to monitor users' actions
- Risk management action plan or other documentation that shows appropriate safeguards are in place throughout your organization, implementation timetables, and implementation notes
- Security incident and breach information

Step 3: Review Existing Security of ePHI (Perform Security Risk Analysis)

Risk analysis assesses potential threats and vulnerabilities to the "confidentiality, integrity and availability" (ONC, 2015, p. 41) of PHI. Several excellent

Table 9.3 Resources for conducting a comprehensive risk analysis

OCR's Guidance on Risk Analysis Requirements under the HIPAA Rule	http://www.hhs.gov/hipaa/for-professionals/security/guidance/final-guidance-risk-analysis/index.html
OCR Security Rule Frequently Asked Questions (FAQs)	http://www.hhs.gov/hipaa/for-professionals/faq
ONC SRA (Security Risk Assessment) Tool for small practices	https://www.healthit.gov/providers-professionals/security-risk-assessment
National Institute of Standards and Technology (NIST) HIPAA Security Rule Toolkit	https://scap.nist.gov/hipaa/

government-sponsored guides and toolsets available for conducting a comprehensive risk analysis are listed in Table 9.3 with a corresponding web address.

The three basic actions recommended for the organization's first comprehensive security risk analysis are as follows:

1. Identify where ePHI exists.
2. Identify potential threats and vulnerabilities to ePHI.
3. Identify risks and their associated levels.

Step 4: Develop an Action Plan

As discussed, the HIPAA Security Plan provides flexibility in how to achieve compliance, which allows an organization to take into account its specific needs. The action plan should include five components. Once in place, the plan should be reviewed regularly by the security team, led by the security officer.

1. Administrative safeguards
2. Physical safeguards
3. Technical safeguards
4. Organizational standards
5. Policies and procedures

Table 9.4 lists common examples of vulnerabilities and mitigation strategies that could be employed.

Table 9.4 Common examples of vulnerabilities and mitigation strategies

Security Component	Examples of Vulnerabilities	Examples of Security Mitigation Strategies
Administrative safeguards	No security officer is designated. Workforce is not trained or is unaware of privacy and security issues.	Security officer is designated and publicized. Workforce training begins at hire and is conducted on a regular and frequent basis. Security risk analysis is performed periodically and when a change occurs in the practice or the technology.
Physical safeguards	Facility has insufficient locks and other barriers to patient data access. Computer equipment is easily accessible by the public. Portable devices are not tracked or not locked up when not in use.	Building alarm systems are installed. Offices are locked. Screens are shielded from secondary viewers.
Technical safeguards	Poor controls enable inappropriate access to EHR. Audit logs are not used enough to monitor users and other HER activities. No measures are in place to keep electronic patient data from improper changes. No contingency plan exists. Electronic exchanges of patient information are not encrypted or otherwise secured.	Secure user IDs, passwords, and appropriate role-based access are used. Routine audits of access and changes to EHR are conducted. Anti-hacking and anti-malware software is installed. Contingency plans and data backup plans are in place. Data are encrypted.
Organizational standards	No breach notification and associated policies exist. BA agreements have not been updated in several years.	Regular reviews of agreements are conducted and updates made accordingly.

Security Component	Examples of Vulnerabilities	Examples of Security Mitigation Strategies
Policies and procedures	Generic written policies and procedures to ensure HIPAA security compliance were purchased but not followed. The manager performs ad hoc security measures.	Written policies and procedures are implemented and staff members are trained. Security team conducts monthly review of user activities. Routine updates are made to document security measures.

Source: ONC (2015).

Step 5: Manage and Mitigate Risks

The security plan will reduce risk only if it is followed by all employees in the organization. This step has four actions associated with it.

1. Implement your plan.
2. Prevent breaches by educating and training your workforce.
3. Communicate with patients.
4. Update your BA contracts.

Step 6: Attest for Meaningful Use Security Related Objective

Organizations can attest to the EHR Incentive Program security-related objective *after* the security risk analysis and correction of any identified deficiencies.

Step 7: Monitor, Audit, and Update Security on an Ongoing Basis

The security officer, IT administrator, and EHR developer should work together to ensure that the organization's monitoring and auditing functions are active and configured appropriately. Auditing and monitoring are necessary to determine the adequacy and effectiveness of the security plan and infrastructure, as well as the "who, what, when, where and how" (ONC, 2015, p. 54) patients' ePHI is accessed.

BEYOND HIPAA: CYBERSECURITY FOR TODAY'S WIRED ENVIRONMENT

Clearly, HIPAA is an important legislative act aimed at protecting health data and information. However, in today's increasingly wired environment, health care organizations face threats that were not present when HIPAA was enacted. In June 2016, 41 percent of all data breaches were because of cyber-crime—hacking. In July of the same year a single hacker was responsible for 30 percent of the health care data breached (Sullivan, 2016). Experts argue that health care organizations are easy targets for **cybercriminals** because they are inadequately prepared. The average health care provider spends less than 6 percent of its total IT budget on security, compared to the government, which spends 16 percent, and the banking industry, which spends between 12 and 15 percent. By one estimate the increase in cybercrime against health care organizations is because of, at least in part, PHI's value on the black market, estimating that PHI is fifty times more valuable than financial infor-mation (Koch, 2016; Siwicki, 2016).

The reality of today's environment is that there are more entry points into health care information networks and computers than ever before. Mobile devices, cloud use, the use of smart consumer products, health care devices with Internet connectivity, along with more employees connecting to health care networks from remote locations create an increased need for cyberse-curity in health care organizations. One recent survey found that among medical students and physicians 93.7 percent owned smartphones and 82.9 percent had used them in a clinical setting. Perhaps the most surprising aspect of the survey was that none of respondents *believed* using the devices increased risk of breaching patient information (Buchholz, Perry, Weiss, & Cooley, 2016).

So-called *mHealth technologies,* which include entities that support per-sonal health records and cloud-based or mobile applications that collect patient information directly from patients or allow uploading of health-related data from wearable devices, are also on the rise, as is the use of health-related social media sites. These technologies were not addressed in HIPAA and, therefore, do not meet the criteria as a CE (DeSalvo & Samuels, 2016).

To provide assistance to health care organizations to combat cyber attacks and improve cybersecurity, the ONC (n.d.) published the *Top 10 Tips for Cybersecurity in Health Care.* The first tip reminds health care organiza-tions to establish a security culture, the same initial tip in their guidance for developing a security plan, clearly emphasizing the importance of this aspect of any security program. The other tips in the publication contain some more specific ways to mitigate the threat from cyber attacks. These tips are listed with specific checkpoints to ensure security (ONC, n.d.). The full version of the top-ten document is available at HealthIT.gov.

Protect Mobile Devices

- Ensure your mobile devices are equipped with strong authentication and access controls.
- Ensure laptops have password protection.
- Enable password protection on handheld devices (if available). Take extra physical control precautions over the device if password protection is not provided.
- Protect wireless transmissions from intrusion.
- Do not transmit unencrypted PHI across public networks (e.g., Internet, Wi-Fi).
- When it is absolutely necessary to commit PHI to a mobile device or remove a device from a secure area, encrypt the data.
- Do not use mobile devices that cannot support encryption.
- Develop and enforce policies specifying the circumstances under which devices may be removed from the facility.
- Take extra care to prevent unauthorized viewing of the PHI displayed on a mobile device.

Maintain Good Computer Habits

- Uninstall any software application that is not essential to running the practice (e.g., games, instant message clients, photo-sharing tools).
- Do not simply accept defaults or "standard" configurations when installing software.
- Find out whether the EHR developer maintains an open connection to the installed software (a "back door") in order to provide updates and support.
- Disable remote file sharing and remote printing within the operating system (e.g., Windows Operating System).
- Automate software updates to occur weekly (e.g., use Microsoft Windows Automatic Update).
- Monitor for critical and urgent patches and updates that require immediate attention and act on them as soon as possible.

- Disable user accounts for former employees quickly and appropriately.
- If an employee is to be involuntarily terminated, close access to the account before the notice of termination is served.
- Prior to disposal, sanitize computers and any other devices that have had data stored on them.
- Archive old data files for storage if needed or clean them off the system if not needed, subject to applicable data retention requirements.
- Fully uninstall software that is no longer needed (including trial software and old versions of current software).
- Work with your IT team or other resources to perform malware, vulnerability, configuration, and other security audits on a regular basis.

Use a Firewall

- Unless your **electronic health record (EHR)** and other systems are totally disconnected from the Internet, you must install a **firewall** to protect against intrusions and threats from outside sources.
- Larger health care organizations that use a local area network (LAN) should consider a hardware firewall.

Install and Maintain Antivirus Software

- Use an antivirus product that provides continuously updated protection against viruses, malware, and other code that can attack your computers through web downloads, CDs, e-mail, and flash drives.
- Keep **antivirus software** up-to-date.
- Most antivirus software automatically generates reminders about these updates, and many are configurable to allow for automated updating.

Plan for the Unexpected

- Create data **backups** regularly and reliably.
- Begin backing up data from day one of a new system.
- Ensure the data are being captured correctly.

- Ensure the data can be quickly and accurately restored.
- Use an automated backup system, if possible.
- Consider storing the backup far away from the main system.
- Protect backup media with the same type of access controls described in the next section.
- Test backup media regularly for their ability to restore data properly, especially as the backups age.
- Have a sound recovery plan. Know the following:
  - o What data was backed up (e.g., databases, pdfs, tiffs, docs)
  - o When the backups were done (time frame and frequency)
  - o Where the backups are stored
  - o What types of equipment are needed to restore them
- Keep the recovery plan securely at a remote location where someone has responsibility for producing it in the event of an emergency.

Control Access to PHI

- Configure your EHR system to grant PHI access *only to people with a "need to know."*
  - o This access control system might be part of an operating system (e.g., Windows), built into a particular application (e.g., an e-prescribing module), or both.
- Manually set file access permissions using an **access control** list.
  - o This can only be done by someone with authorized rights to the system.
  - o Prior to setting these permissions, identify which files should be accessible to which staff members.
- Configure role-based access control as needed.
  - o In role-based access, a staff member's role within the organization (e.g., physician, nurse, billing specialist, etc.) determines what information may be accessed.
- Assign staff members to the correct roles and then set the access permissions for each role correctly on a need-to-know basis.

The following case on access control provides additional examples of access control.

CASE STUDY

Access Control

Mary Smith is the director of the health information management department in a hospital. Under a user-based access control scheme, Mary would be allowed read-only access to the hospital's laboratory information system because of her personal identity—that is, because she is Mary Smith and uses the proper log-in and password(s) to get into the system. Under a role-based control scheme, Mary would be allowed read-only access to the hospital's lab system because she is part of the health information management department and all department employees have been granted read-only privileges for this system. If the hospital were to adopt a context-based control scheme, Mary might be allowed access to the lab system only from her own workstation or another workstation in the health information services department, provided she used her proper log-in and password. If she attempted to log in from the emergency department or another administrative office, she might be denied access. The context control could also involve time of day. Because Mary is a daytime employee, she might be denied access if she attempted to log in at night.

Use Strong Passwords

- Choose a password that is not easily guessed. Following are some examples of strong password characteristics:
  - At least eight characters in length (the longer the better)
  - A combination of uppercase and lowercase letters, one number, and at least one special character, such as a punctuation mark
- Strong passwords should *not include* personal information:
  - Birth date
  - Names of self, family members, or pets
  - Social Security number
  - Anything that is on your social networking sites or could otherwise be discovered easily by others
- Use multifactor authentication for more security. Multifactor authentication combines multiple authentication methods, such as a password plus a fingerprint scan; this results in stronger security

protections. If you e-prescribe controlled substances, you must use multifactor authentication for your accounts.

- Configure your systems so that passwords must be changed on a regular basis.

- To discourage staff members from writing down their passwords, develop a password reset process to provide quick assistance in case of forgotten passwords.

Limit Network Access

- Prohibit staff members from installing software without prior approval.

- When a wireless router is used, set it up to operate only in encrypted mode.

- Prohibit casual network access by visitors.

- Check to make sure file sharing, instant messaging, and other peer-to-peer applications have not been installed without explicit review and approval.

Control Physical Access

- Limit the chances that devices (e.g., laptops, handhelds, desktops, servers, thumb drives, CDs, backup tapes) may be tampered with, lost, or stolen.

- Document and enforce policies limiting physical access to devices and information:

  o Keep machines in locked rooms.

  o Manage keys to facilities.

  o Restrict removal of devices from a secure area.

National Institute of Standards and Technology (NIST) Cybersecurity Framework

Recognizing the severity of the rise in cybercrime, President Obama issued an executive order in February 2013 to "enhance the security and resilience of the Nation's critical infrastructure" (Executive Order 13636). As a result the **National Institute of Standards and Technology (NIST)** was directed to develop, with help of stakeholder organizations, a voluntary cybersecurity

Exhibit 9.2 Cybersecurity framework core

Function	Category	Subcategory
Identify	Asset Management	**ID.BE-1:** The organization's role in the supply chain is identified and communicated.
	Business Environment	
	Governance	
	Risk Assessment	**ID. BE-2:** The organization's place in critical infrastructure and its industry sector is identified and communicated.
	Risk Management Strategy	
Protect	Access Control	
	Awareness and Training	
	Data Security	
	Information Protection Processes and Procedures	**ID.BE-3:** Priorities for organizational mission, objectives, and activities are established and communicated.
	Maintenance	
	Protective Technology	
Detect	Anomalies and Events	
	Security Continuous Monitoring	
	Detection Processes	**ID.BE-4:** Dependencies and critical functions for delivery of critical services are established.
Respond	Response Planning	
	Communications	
	Analysis	
	Mitigation	**ID.BE-5:** Resilience requirements to support delivery of critical services are established.
	Improvements	
Recover	Recovery Planning	
	Improvements	
	Communications	

Source: NIST (2016).

framework to reduce cyber-attack risks. The resulting **NIST cybersecurity framework** consists of three components (NIST, n.d.):

1. The **Framework Core** consists of "five concurrent and continuous Functions—Identify, Protect, Detect, Respond, Recover." The functions provide "the highest level, strategic view of an organization's management of cybersecurity risk" (NIST, n.d., p. 4). The functions are divided into categories and subcategories as shown in Exhibit 9.2.

2. The **Framework Implementation Tiers** characterize an organization's actual cybersecurity practices compared to the framework, using a range of tiers from partial (Tier 1) to adaptive (Tier 4).

3. The **Framework Profile** documents outcomes obtained by reviewing all of the categories and subcategories and comparing them to the organization's business needs. Profiles can be identified as "current," documenting where the organization is now, or as "target," where the organization would like to be in the future.

Since its initial publication in 2014, the HHS, OCR, and the ONC have cited the framework as an important tool for health care organizations to consider when developing a comprehensive security program. In 2016, OCR published a crosswalk that maps the HIPAA Security Rule to the NIST framework, which can be found at HHS.gov/hipaa (US Department of Health and Human Services, n.d.a).

SUMMARY

In this chapter we gained insight into why health information privacy and security are key topics for health care administrators. In today's ever-increasing electronic world with new and more virulent threats, the security of health information is an ongoing concern. In this chapter we examined and defined the concepts of privacy, confidentiality, and security and explored major legislative efforts, historical and current, to protect health care information, with a focus on the HIPAA Privacy, Security, and Breach Notification rules. Different types of threats, human, natural and environmental, intentional and unintentional, were identified, with a focus on the increase in cybercrime. Basic requirements for a strong health care organization security program were outlined and the chapter ended with a discussion of the cybersecurity challenges within the current health care environment.

KEY TERMS

*42 C.F.R. (Code of Federal
  Regulations) Part 2, Confidentiality
  of Substance Abuse Patient Records*
Access control
Antivirus software
Backups
Business associate contracts
Confidentiality
Cybercriminals
Cybersecurity
Electronic health record (EHR)
*Electronic protected health
  information (ePHI)*
Federal Trade Commission (FTC) Act
Firewall
Hacker
*Health Insurance Portability and
  Accountability Act (HIPAA)*
HIPAA Breach Notification Rule
HIPAA Privacy Rule
*HIPAA Security Administrative
  Safeguards*

HIPAA Security Physical Safeguards
HIPAA Security Rule
HIPAA Security Technical Safeguards
Malware
*National Institute of Standards and
  Technology (NIST)*
NIST Cybersecurity Framework
Office for Civil Rights (OCR)
Passwords
Privacy
Privacy Act of 1974
Protected health information (PHI)
Ransomware
Security
Security management
Spyware
Threats
Trojan
Viruses
Vulnerabilities
Worms

LEARNING ACTIVITIES

1. Do an Internet search for a recent article discussing a significant breach under the HIPAA Privacy and Security rules. Write a summary of the article. Discuss how the organization cited in the article could have prevented or mitigated the risk of the breach.

2. Contact a health care provider to talk with the person responsible for maintaining the legal health record. Ask about the organization's release of information, retention, and destruction policies. Do they comply with the requirements of HIPAA? Explain why or why not.

3. Contact a physician's office or clinic and ask if the organization has a security plan. Discuss the process that staff members undertook to complete the plan, or develop an outline of a plan for them.

4. Visit the Office for Civil Rights Enforcement Activities and Results website. Read at least five case examples involving HIPAA security violations. What do these cases have in common? What are their

differences? Do all of the Security Rule violations you read also involve Privacy Rule violations? What were your impressions of the types of cases you read and their resolutions?

REFERENCES

American Health Information Management Association (AHIMA). (2003). *Final Rule for HIPAA security standards.* Chicago, IL: Author.

Bazzoli, F. (2016, Aug. 9). 12 largest fines levied for HIPAA violations. *Health Data Management.* Retrieved August 9, 2016, from http://www.healthdatamanagement .com/list/12-largest-fines-levied-for-hipaa-violations

Buchholz, A., Perry, B., Weiss, L. B., & Cooley, D. (2016). Smartphone use and perceptions among medical students and practicing physicians. *Journal of Mobile Technology in Medicine, 5*(1), 27–32. doi:10.7309/jmtm.5.1.5

Centers for Medicare and Medicaid Services (CMS). (2004). *HIPAA administrative simplification: Security—Final Rule.* Retrieved November 2004 from http:// www.cms.hhs.gov/hipaa/hipaa2/regulations/security

Comodo. (2014, Aug. 4). *Malware versus viruses: What's the difference?* Retrieved August 10, 2016, from https://antivirus.comodo.com/blog/computer-safety/ malware-vs-viruses-whats-difference/

Conn, J. (2016, Feb. 18). *Hospital pays hackers $17,000 to unlock EHRs frozen in "ransomware" attack.* Retrieved November 11, 2016, from http://www .modernhealthcare.com/article/20160217/NEWS/160219920

Coppersmith, Gordon, Schermer, & Brockelman, PLC. (2012). *HITECH Act expands HIPAA privacy and security rules.* Retrieved March 2012 from http://www .azhha.org/member_and_media_resources/documents/HITECHAct.pdf

DeSalvo, K. B., & Samuels, J. (2016, July 19). Examining oversight of the privacy & security of health data collected by entities not regulated by HIPAA. *Health IT Buzz.* Retrieved August 10, 2016, from https://www.healthit.gov/buzz-blog/ privacy-and-security-of-ehrs/examining-oversight-privacy-security-health-data-collected-entities-not-regulated-hipaa/

Goedert, J. (2016, Aug. 8). *Hack of Banner systems highlights the need for more firewalls.* Retrieved August 10, 2016, from http://www.healthdatamanagement .com/news/hack-of-banner-systems-highlights-the-need-for-more-firewalls?utm_ medium=email

HHS.gov. (2015). *$750,000 HIPAA settlement underscores the need for organization-wide risk analysis.* Retrieved from http://www.hhs.gov/about/news/2015/12/14/ 750000-hipaa-settlement-underscores-need-for-organization-wide-risk-analysis.html

ESET. (n.d.). *HIPAA security checklist* [Brochure]. Retrieved August 8, 2016, from https://www.healthit.gov/sites/default/files/comments_upload/hipaa-security-checklist.pdf

Koch, D. D. (2016, Spring). Is HIPAA Security Rule enough to protect electronic personal health information (PHI) in the cyber age? *Journal of Health Care Finance.* Retrieved August 8, 2016, from http://www.healthfinancejournal.com/index.php/johcf/article/view/67

National Institute of Standards and Technology (NIST). (2016). *Framework for improving critical infrastructure cybersecurity.* Retrieved from http://www.nist.gov/cyberframework/upload/CSF-for-law-policy-symposium.pdf

National Institute of Standards and Technology (NIST). (n.d.). *Cybersecurity framework.* Retrieved August 10, 2016, from http://www.nist.gov/cyberframework/

ONC. (2015). *Guide to privacy and security of electronic health information.* Retrieved from https://www.healthit.gov/sites/default/files/pdf/privacy/privacy-and-security-guide.pdf

ONC. (n.d.). *Top 10 tips for cybersecurity in health care* [Brochure]. Retrieved August 8, 2016, from https://www.healthit.gov/sites/default/files/Top_10_Tips_for_Cybersecurity.pdf

Siwicki, B. (2016, May 17). Cybersecurity special report: Ransomware will get worse, hackers targeting whales, medical devices and IoT trigger new vulnerabilities. *Healthcare IT News.* Retrieved August 10, 2016, from http://www.healthcareitnews.com/node/525131

Sullivan, T. (2016, Aug. 9). "DarkOverLord" ransomware accounts for nearly 30 percent of health data breaches in July. *Healthcare IT News.* Retrieved August 10, 2016, from http://www.healthcareitnews.com/news/darkoverlord-ransomware-accounts-nearly-30-percent-health-data-breaches-july

Office for Civil Rights (OCR). (n.d.). HHS Breach Portal. Retrieved August 8, 2016, from https://ocrportal.hhs.gov/ocr/breach/breach_report.jsf

US Department of Health and Human Services. (2016, Sept. 30). *Enforcement highlights.* Retrieved August 8, 2016, from http://www.hhs.gov/hipaa/for-professionals/compliance-enforcement/data/enforcement-highlights/index.html

US Department of Health and Human Services. (n.d.a). *Addressing gaps in cybersecurity: OCR releases crosswalk between HIPAA Security Rule and NIST cybersecurity framework.* Retrieved August 10, 2016, from http://www.hhs.gov/hipaa/for-professionals/security/nist-security-hipaa-crosswalk/

US Department of Health and Human Services. (n.d.b). *Breach Notification Rule.* Retrieved August 8, 2016, from http://www.hhs.gov/hipaa/for-professionals/breach-notification/index.html

US Department of Health and Human Services. (n.d.c). *Guidance to render unsecured protected health information unusable, unreadable, or indecipherable to unauthorized individuals.* Retrieved August 8, 2016, from http://www.hhs.gov/hipaa/for-professionals/breach-notification/guidance/index.html

What are the penalties for HIPAA violations? (2015, June 14). *HIPAA Journal.* Retrieved from http://www.hipaajournal.com/what-are-the-penalties-for-hipaa-violations-7096/

CHAPTER 10

Performance Standards and Measures

LEARNING OBJECTIVES

- To be able to explain the significant role of health information in national private and public quality improvement initiatives.

- To be able to compare and contrast licensure, certification, and accreditation processes.

- To be able to discuss the role of the Joint Commission and the National Committee for Quality Assurance in ensuring the quality of care in the United States.

- To be able to understand performance measurement development in the United States.

- To be able to identify the roles of specific public and private organizations in the development and endorsement of national performance measures.

- To be able to understand the origins and uses of major health care comparative data sets.

This chapter examines public and private organizations and processes that establish standards for ensuring that **health records** are maintained accurately and completely and that they contain the data and information needed to define and report a wide range of measures to determine the quality and efficiency of health care. These activities are very important and have a significant influence on providers and HIT capabilities, significant enough for us to devote an entire chapter to them.

Health care organizations and health plans use data and information to measure performance against internal and external standards; to compare performance to other like organizations; to demonstrate performance to licensing, certifying, and accrediting bodies; and to demonstrate performance for reimbursement purposes. This chapter begins with an examination of the **licensure, certification,** and **accreditation** of health care facilities and health plans, followed by an overview of key comparative data sets often used by health care organizations in benchmarking performance. The chapter concludes with a description of the national initiatives using **performance measures** to improve the quality and safety of health care, including those affecting provider reimbursement.

In the section titled "Licensure, Certification, and Accreditation," we define these processes, list the accrediting organizations recognized by CMS, and examine the missions and general functions of **the Joint Commission** and the **National Committee for Quality Assurance (NCQA).** These discussions focus on how the licensure, certification, and accreditation processes not only use health information to measure performance but also how they influence the health care information that is collected.

"Measuring the Quality of Care" begins with a historical perspective of major milestones in the national agenda for health care quality improvement, followed by a discussion of the current efforts to improve health care quality and patient safety, focusing on the efforts that involve using health care data and information to measure performance. Quality measures are created and validated by a range of organizations, private and public. However, in the recent years significant progress has been made in aligning these measures across organizations. Another significant movement related to quality measurement in the United States is implementation of value-based reimbursement programs, which are based on established performance criteria. The government plans for significant growth in these programs over the next decade.

LICENSURE, CERTIFICATION, AND ACCREDITATION

Health care organizations, such as hospitals, nursing homes, home health agencies, and the like, must be licensed to operate. If they wish to file

Medicare or Medicaid claims, they must also be certified, and if they wish to demonstrate quality performance, they will undergo an accreditation process. What are these processes, and how are they related? If a health care organization is licensed, certified, and accredited, how will this affect the health care information that it creates, uses, and maintains? In this section we will examine each of these processes, their impact on the health care organizations, and their relationships with one another.

Licensure

Licensure is the process that gives a facility legal approval to operate. As a rule, state governments oversee the licensure of health care facilities, and each state sets its own licensure laws and regulations. All facilities must have a license to operate, and it is generally the state department of health or a similar agency that carries out the licensure function. Licensure regulations tend to emphasize areas such as physical plant standards, fire safety, space allocations, and sanitation. They may also contain minimum standards for equipment and personnel. A few states tie licensure to professional standards and quality of care, but not all. In their licensure regulations, states generally set minimum standards for the content, retention, and authentication of patient medical records. Exhibit 10.1 is an excerpt from the South Carolina licensure regulations for hospitals. This excerpt governs patient medical record content (with the exception of newborn patient records, which are addressed in a separate section of the regulations). Although each state has its own set of medical record content standards, these are fairly typical in scope and content.

An initial license is required before a facility opens its doors, and this license to operate must generally be renewed annually. Some states allow organizations with the Joint Commission or other accreditation to forgo a formal licensure survey conducted by the state; others require the state survey regardless of accreditation status. As we will see in the section on accreditation, the accrediting bodies' standards are more detailed and more stringent than the typical state licensure regulations. Also, most accreditation standards are updated annually; most licensure standards are not.

Certification

Certification gives a health care organization the authority to participate in the federal Medicare and Medicaid programs. Legislation passed in

Exhibit 10.1 Medical Record Content: Excerpt from South Carolina Standards for Licensing Hospitals and Institutional General Infirmaries

601.5 Contents:

A. Adequate and complete medical records shall be written for all patients admitted to the hospital and newborns delivered in the hospital. All notes shall be legibly written or typed and signed. Although use of initials in lieu of licensed nurses' signatures is not encouraged, initials will be accepted provided such initials can be readily identified within the medical record. A minimum medical record shall include the following information:

1. Admission Record: An admission record must be prepared for each patient and must contain the following information, when obtainable: Name; address, including county; occupation; age; date of birth; sex; marital status; religion; county of birth; father's name; mother's maiden name; husband's or wife's name; dates of military service; health insurance number; provisional diagnosis; case number; days of care; social security number; the name of the person providing information; name, address and telephone number of person or persons to be notified in the event of emergency; name and address of referring physician; name, address and telephone number of attending physician; date and hour of admission;

2. History and physical within 48 hours after admission;

3. Provisional or working diagnosis;

4. Pre-operative diagnosis;

1972 mandated that hospitals had to be reviewed and certified to receive reimbursement from Medicare and Medicaid programs (CMS, n.d.a). At that time the Health Care Financing Administration, now the **Centers for Medicare and Medicaid Services (CMS),** developed a set of minimum standards known as the **conditions of participation (CoPs).** CMS contracts with state agencies to inspect facilities to make sure they meet these minimum standards, organized by facility functions and services. See Exhibit 10.2 for the CoP standards section governing medical record content.

5. Medical treatment;

6. Complete surgical record, if any, including technique of operation and findings, statement of tissue and organs removed and post-operative diagnosis;

7. Report of anesthesia;

8. Nurses' notes;

9. Progress notes;

10. Gross pathological findings and microscopic;

11. Temperature chart, including pulse and respiration;

12. Medication Administration Record or similar document for recording of medications, treatments and other pertinent data. Nurses shall sign this record after each medication administered or treatment rendered;

13. Final diagnosis and discharge summary;

14. Date and hour of discharge summary;

15. In case of death, cause and autopsy findings, if autopsy is performed;

16. Special examinations, if any, e.g., consultations, clinical laboratory, x-ray and other examinations.

Source: South Carolina Department of Health and Environmental Control, Standards for Licensing Hospitals and Institutional General Infirmaries, Regulation 61–16 § 601.5 (2010).

Accreditation

Accreditation is an external review process that an organization elects to undergo; it is voluntary and has fees associated with it. The accrediting agency grants recognition to organizations that meet its predetermined performance standards. The review process and standards are devised and regulated by the accrediting agency. By far the best-known health care accrediting agency in the United States is the Joint Commission, but there are others. The National Committee for Quality Assurance (NCQA) is a leading accrediting agency for health plans.

Exhibit 10.2 Medical Record Content: Excerpt from the Conditions of Participation for Hospitals

Sec. 482.24 Condition of participation: Medical record services.

(c)   Standard: Content of record. The medical record must contain information to justify admission and continued hospitalization, support the diagnosis, and describe the patient's progress and response to medications and services.

(1)   All entries must be legible and complete, and must be authenticated and dated promptly by the person (identified by name and discipline) who is responsible for ordering, providing, or evaluating the service furnished.

(i)   The author of each entry must be identified and must authenticate his or her entry.

(ii) Authentication may include signatures, written initials or computer entry.

(2)   All records must document the following, as appropriate:

(i)   Evidence of a physical examination, including a health history, performed no more than 7 days prior to admission or within 48 hours after admission.

(ii) Admitting diagnosis.

(iii) Results of all consultative evaluations of the patient and appropriate findings by clinical and other staff involved in the care of the patient.

(iv) Documentation of complications, hospital acquired infections, and unfavorable reactions to drugs and anesthesia.

(v)   Properly executed informed consent forms for procedures and treatments specified by the medical staff, or by Federal or State law if applicable, to require written patient consent.

(vi) All practitioners' orders, nursing notes, reports of treatment, medication records, radiology, and laboratory reports, and vital signs and other information necessary to monitor the patient's condition.

(vii) Discharge summary with outcome of hospitalization, disposition of case, and provisions for follow-up care.

(viii) Final diagnosis with completion of medical records within 30 days following discharge.

Source: Conditions of Participation: Medical Record Services, 42 C.F.R. §§ 482.24c et seq. (2007).

Although accreditation is voluntary, there are financial and legal incentives for health care organizations to seek accreditation. In order to eliminate duplicative processes, Section 1865 of the Social Security Act "permits providers and suppliers 'accredited' by an approved national **accreditation organization (AO)** to be exempt from routine surveys by State survey agencies to determine compliance with Medicare conditions" (CMS, 2015). This is often referred to as ***deemed status.*** Table 10.1 lists the 2015 approved AOs with corresponding program types and websites.

Table 10.1 2015 approved CMS accrediting organizations

Accrediting Organization	Program Types	Website
Accreditation Association for Ambulatory Health Care (AAAHC)	ASC (ambulatory surgery center)	www.aaahc.org
Accreditation Commission for Health Care, Inc. (ACHC)	HHA (home health agency) Hospice	www.achc.org
American Association for Accreditation of Ambulatory Surgery Facilities (AAAASF)	ASC OPT (outpatient physical therapy) RHC (rural health clinics)	www.aaaasf.org
American Osteopathic Association/Healthcare Facilities Accreditation Program (HFAP)	ASC CAH (critical access hospital) Hospital	www.hfap.org
Center for Improvement in Healthcare Quality (CIHQ)	Hospital	www.cihq.org
Community Health Accreditation Program (CHAP)	HHA Hospice	www.chapinc.org
DNV GL—Healthcare (DNV GL)	CAH Hospital	www.dnvglhealthcare.com
The Compliance Team (TCT)	RHC	www.thecomplianceteam.org
The Joint Commission (TJC)	ASC CAH HHA Hospice Hospital Psychiatric hospital	www.jointcommission.org

Similar to CMS, many states also recognize accreditation in lieu of their own licensure surveys. Other benefits for an organization are that accreditation

- May be required for reimbursement from payers (including CMS)
- Validates the quality of care within the organization
- May favorably influence liability insurance premiums
- May enhance access to managed care contracts
- Gives the organization a competitive edge over nonaccredited organizations

The Joint Commission

The Joint Commission's stated mission is "to continuously improve health care for the public, in collaboration with other stakeholders, by evaluating health care organizations and inspiring them to excel in providing safe and effective care of the highest quality and value" (The Joint Commission, n.d.). The Joint Commission on Accreditation of Hospitals (as the Joint Commission was first called) was formed as an independent, not-for-profit organization in 1951, as a joint effort of the American College of Surgeons, American College of Physicians, American Medical Association, and American Hospital Association. The Joint Commission has grown and evolved to set standards for and accredit nearly twenty-one thousand health care organizations and programs in the United States. In addition to hospitals, the Joint Commission has accreditation programs for health care organizations that offer ambulatory care, behavioral health care, home care, long-term care, and office-based surgery. They also provide an accreditation program for organizations that offer laboratory services (The Joint Commission, 2016, n.d.).

In order to maintain accreditation, a health care organization must undergo an on-site survey by a Joint Commission survey team every three years. Laboratories must be surveyed every two years. This survey is conducted to ensure that the organization continues to meet the established standards. The standards themselves are the result of an ongoing, dynamic process that incorporates the experience and perspectives of health care professionals and others throughout the country. New standards manuals are published annually and health care organizations are responsible for knowing and incorporating any changes as they occur.

Categories of accreditation (The Joint Commission, 2016) that an organization can achieve are the following:

- **Preliminary accreditation:** for organizations that demonstrate compliance with selected standards under the Early Survey Policy, which allows organizations to undergo a survey prior to having the ability to demonstrate full compliance. Organizations that receive preliminary accreditation will be required to undergo a second on-site survey.

- **Accreditation:** for organizations that demonstrate compliance with all standards.

- **Accreditation with follow-up survey:** for organizations that are not in compliance with specific standards and require a follow-up survey within thirty days to six months.

- **Contingent accreditation:** for organizations that fail to address all requirements in an accreditation with follow-up survey decision or for organizations that do not have the proper license or other similar issue at the time of the initial survey. A follow-up survey is generally required within thirty days.

- **Preliminary denial of accreditation:** for organizations for which there is justification for denying accreditation. This decision is subject to appeal.

- **Denial of accreditation:** for organizations that fail to meet standards and that have exhausted all appeals.

The Joint Commission focus on quality of care provided in health care facilities dates back to the early 1900s, when the American College of Surgeons began surveying hospitals and established a hospital standardization program. With the program came the question, how is quality of care measured? One of the early concerns of the standardization program was the lack of documentation in patient records. The early surveyors found that documentation was so poor that they had no way to judge the quality of care provided. The Joint Commission's emphasis on health care information and the documentation of care has continued to the present. Not only do the Joint Commission reporting requirements rely heavily on patient information but also the current survey process uses "tracer methodology," through which the surveyors analyze the organization's systems by tracing the care provided to individual patients. Patient records provide the road maps for the tracer methodology. The absence of quality health records would have a direct impact on the accreditation process. The following sections discuss Joint Commission standards that directly influence the creation, maintenance, and use of health care information. These sections further illustrate how the overall accreditation process relies on the availability of high-quality health care information (The Joint Commission, 2016).

The Joint Commission Record of Care (RC), Treatment, and Services Standards

The **Joint Commission Record of Care (RC), Treatment, and Services standards** provide information about the requirements for the content of a complete health record, regardless of its format. The RC standards for an ambulatory care program dictate that the organization will do the following:

- Maintain complete and accurate clinical record.
- Ensure clinical record entries are authenticated appropriately by authorized persons.
- Ensure documentation in clinical records is timely.
- Audit their clinical records.
- Retain their clinical records according to relevant laws and regulations.
- Ensure clinical records contain specific information that reflects the patient's care, treatment, or services.
- Ensure clinical records accurately reflect operative and high-risk procedures and use of sedation and anesthesia.
- Ensure documentation of proper use of restraints and seclusion.
- Ensure ambulatory care records contain a summary list.
- Ensure qualified staff members receive and record verbal orders. (The Joint Commission, 2014b)

Each RC standard has specific elements that must be addressed. For more information, refer to the most recent edition of the appropriate *Comprehensive Accreditation Manual.* All Joint Commission–accredited organizations have access to the complete manual.

The Joint Commission Information Management Standards

The **Joint Commission Information Management (IM) standards** reflect the Joint Commission's belief that quality information management influences quality care. In the overview of the IM standards, the Joint Commission states, "Every episode of care generates health information *that must be managed systematically*" (emphasis is the authors'). Information is a resource that must be managed similar to any other resource within the organization.

Whether the information management systems employed by the organization are basic or sophisticated, the functions should include features that allow for the following:

- Categorizing, filing, and maintaining all data and information used by the organization
- Accurately capturing health information generated by delivery of care, treatment, and services
- Accessing information by those authorized users who need the information to provide safe, quality care (The Joint Commission, 2014a)

The IM standards apply to noncomputerized systems and systems employing the latest technologies. The first standard within the IM chapter focuses on information planning. The organization's plan for IM should consider the full spectrum of data generated and used by the organization as well as the flow of information within and to and from external organizations. Identifying and understanding the flow of information is critical to meeting the organization's needs for data collection and distribution while maintaining the appropriate level of security (The Joint Commission, 2014a). The remaining IM standards address the requirements for health care organizations:

- Provide continuity of the information management process, including managing system interruptions and maintaining backup systems.
- Ensure the privacy, security, and integrity of health information.
- Manage data collection, including use of standardized data sets and terminology and limiting the use of abbreviations.
- Manage health information retrieval, dissemination, and transmission.
- Provide knowledge-based information resources twenty-four hours a day, seven days a week.
- Ensure the accuracy of the health information. (The Joint Commission, 2011, 2014a)

National Committee for Quality Assurance

The National Committee for Quality Assurance (NCQA) is the leading accrediting body for health plans, including health maintenance organizations (HMOs), Preferred Provider Organizations (PPOs), and Point of Service (POS) plans in the United States. In addition, the NCQA also accredits the following programs:

- Disease management
- Case management
- Wellness and health promotion
- Accountable care organizations
- Wellness and health promotion
- Managed behavioral health care organizations (NCQA, n.d.a)

The full list of NCQA accreditation requirements are published on its website at www.ncqa.org. The 2015 Health Plan Accreditation Program requirements include specific criteria divided into the following sections:

- Quality management and improvement (QI)
- Utilization management (UM)
- Credentialing and recredentialing (CR)
- Members' rights and responsibilities (RR)
- Member connections (MEM)
- Medicaid benefits and services (MED)
- **Health Effectiveness Data and Information Set (HEDIS)** performance measures (see the "Measuring the Quality of Care" section for more information about HEDIS) (NCQA, 2015).

MEASURING THE QUALITY OF CARE

Two landmark Institute of Medicine (IOM) reports, *To Err Is Human: Building a Safer Health System,* published in 2000 (Kohn, Corrigan, & Donaldson), and *Crossing the Quality Chasm: A New Health System for the 21st Century,* published in 2001, are often cited as marking the beginning of the modern era of national health care quality and patient safety initiatives. The two reports led to increased awareness of the severity of patient safety and quality issues and helped frame the national landscape of improvement efforts. *To Err Is Human* estimated that as many as ninety-eight thousand people died in hospitals each year as a result of preventable medical errors. The report found that most errors could be traced to poor processes and systems and recommended development and implementation of improved performance standards, including those associated with licensure, certification, and accreditation. *Crossing the Quality Chasm* specifically outlined six aims for establishing quality health care, stating that health care in the United States should be (CMSS, 2014; Kohn, Corrigan, & Donaldson, 2000; IOM, 2001):

1. Safe
2. Effective
3. Patient-centered
4. Timely
5. Efficient
6. Equitable

One of the challenges to meeting these aims was determining how to measure success in each area. What are the standards and performance measures associated with these important aims?

Types of Measures

Whether at the local organizational level or at a national level, quality improvement requires the identification of standards that define quality care and measurement of performance to determine whether or not the identified standards are met. **Quality measures** are used across the full continuum of care, from individual physicians to health plans. As we will examine in this chapter, there are literally *hundreds of different health care quality measures* in use today. These existing quality measures can generally be categorized into four types: structure, process, outcome, and patient experience. Table 10.2 summarizes the types of measures, descriptions, and examples of each.

Data Sources for Measures

Whether quality measures are applied by an individual physician or by a federal agency, they rely on valid and reliable data. A few of the common sources of health care data used in performance measurement are listed in the following sections.

Administrative Data

Administrative data submitted to private and government payers have the advantage of being easy to obtain. Private and public payers have very large claims databases.

Table 10.2 Major types of quality measures

Type	Description	Example
Structure	Assesses the characteristics of a care setting, including facilities, personnel, and policies related to care delivery	Does an intensive care unit (ICU) have a critical care specialist on staff at all times?
Process	Determines if the services provided to patients are consistent with routine clinical care	Does a doctor ensure that his or her patients receive recommended cancer screenings?
Outcome	Evaluates patient health as a result of the care received	What is the survival rate for patients who experience a heart attack?
Patient Experience	Provides feedback on patients' experiences of care	Do patients report that their provider explains their treatment options in ways that are easy to understand?

Source: Morris (2014).

Disease Registries

Public health agencies, including state and federal agencies collect data on patients with specific conditions. These **disease registries** often go beyond administrative claims data.

Health Records

The EHR is recognized as a rich source of detailed patient information. However, the full potential of the EHR as an easy-to-use source of reliable data has not been reached. More work on standardization and tools for data extraction is needed. Data extraction from paper records is labor intensive and, therefore, expensive to implement. As you have seen in previous chapters, Meaningful Use criteria address the need for EHR data extraction and sharing.

Qualitative Data

Qualitative data from patient surveys or interviews are often used for patient experience measures (Morris, 2014).

Measurement Development

Regardless of the data source, the resulting measures must not only be reliable and valid but also feasible to collect (CMSS, 2015). There are dozens of public and private organizations that develop health care–related performance measures. The following paragraphs identify a few of the key players and their respective role in the development of recognized measures.

The NCQA is responsible for the HEDIS measures, one of the oldest and most widely used sets of health care performance measures in the United States. More than 90 percent of health plans in the United States collect and report HEDIS data. HEDIS data is not only used for accreditation of health plans but also for the basis of health plan comparison and quality improvement.

The Joint Commission also has a long history of developing and using performance measures as a component of accreditation. In 1987, the Joint Commission revamped its accreditation process with the goal of incorporating standardized performance measures. This initiative led to the development of ORYX program. The current ORYX program is closely aligned with CMS quality initiatives, using many of the same measures. Hospitals seeking Joint Commission Accreditation in 2016 were required to report on six of nine sets of chart (paper)-abstracted **clinical quality measures (CQMs)** or six of eight **electronic clinical quality measures (eCQMs)** (The Joint Commission, 2015b).

CQMs are identified and updated by CMS each year. Selected CQMs are used in the **EHR Incentive Programs** for **eligible professionals** and other CMS quality initiatives (discussed following in this chapter). The CMS does not develop all of the CQMs but rather relies on private organizations, such as NCQA, the Joint Commission, the **American Medical Association Physician Consortium for Performance Improvement (AMA-PCPI),** and a host of other health care societies, collaboratives, and alliances, as well as government agencies, such as AHRQ, **Centers for Disease Control and Prevention (CDC),** and **Health Resources and Services Administration (HRSA)** for most of them. Table 10.3 is an excerpt from the CQMs for the 2014 EHR Incentive Programs. Note that each measure is defined by a unique identifier, **National Quality Forum (NQF)** number, a measure description, numerator and denominator statements, measure steward, and **Physicians Quality Reporting System (PQRS) number.** *Note:* The PQRS role in quality improvement and performance measurement is discussed in more detail following in this chapter.

The NQF is a nonprofit, member organization whose mission is "to lead national collaboration to improve health and healthcare quality through measurement" (NQF, n.d.). It was created in 1999 and includes board members from private and public sectors, including providers, purchasers, and representatives from AHRQ, CDC, CMS, and HRSA. The NQF maintains a large, searchable database of performance measures. Measures can be searched on

Table 10.3 Excerpt of CQMs for 2014 EHR Incentive Programs

CMS eMeasure ID	NQF No.	Measure Title and NQS Domain	Measure Description	Numerator Statement	Denominator Statement	Measure Steward	PQRS No.
CMS69v5	0421	Preventive Care and Screening: Body Mass Index (BMI) Screening and Follow-Up Plan; Domain: Population/Public Health	Percentage of patients aged eighteen years and older with a BMI documented during the current encounter or during the previous six months AND with a BMI outside of normal parameters, a follow-up plan is documented during the encounter or during the previous six months of the current encounter. Normal Parameters: Age eighteen years and older BMI = > 18.5 and < 25 kg/m2	Patients with a documented BMI during the encounter or during the previous six months, AND when the BMI is outside of normal parameters, a follow-up plan is documented during the encounter or during the previous six months of the current encounter	All patients eighteen and older on the date of the encounter with at least one eligible encounter during the measurement period	Centers for Medicare & Medicaid Services	128 GPRO PREV-9
CMS132v5	0564	Cataracts: Complications within Thirty Days Following Cataract Surgery Requiring Additional Surgical Procedures	Percentage of patients aged eighteen years and older with a diagnosis of uncomplicated cataract who had cataract surgery and had any of a specified list of surgical procedures in the thirty days following cataract surgery which would indicate the	Patients who had one or more specified operative procedures for any of the following major complications within thirty days following cataract	All patients aged eighteen years and older who had cataract surgery and no significant	PCPI(R) Foundation (PCPI[R])	192

		Domain: Patient Safety	occurrence of any of the following major complications: retained nuclear fragments, endophthalmitis, dislocated or wrong power IOL, retinal detachment, or wound dehiscence	surgery: retained nuclear fragments, endophthalmitis, dislocated or wrong power IOL, retinal detachment, or wound dehiscence	ocular conditions impacting the surgical complication rate		
CMS133v5	0565	Cataracts: 20/40 or Better Visual Acuity within Ninety Days Following Cataract Surgery Domain: Clinical Process/Effectiveness	Percentage of patients aged eighteen years and older with a diagnosis of uncomplicated cataract who had cataract surgery and no significant ocular conditions impacting the visual outcome of surgery and had best-corrected visual acuity of 20/40 or better (distance or near) achieved within 90 days following the cataract surgery	Patients who had best-corrected visual acuity of 20/40 or better (distance or near) achieved within ninety days following cataract surgery	All patients aged eighteen years and older who had cataract surgery	PCPI(R) Foundation (PCPI[R])	191
CMS158v5	N/A	Pregnant Women That Had HBsAg Testing Domain: Clinical Process/Effectiveness	This measure identifies pregnant women who had a HBsAg (hepatitis B) test during their pregnancy	Patients who were tested for hepatitis B surface antigen (HBsAg) during pregnancy within 280 days prior to delivery	All female patients aged twelve and older who had a live birth or delivery during the measurement period	Optum	369

(Continued)

Table 10.3 *(Continued)*

CMS eMeasure ID	NQF No.	Measure Title and NQS Domain	Measure Description	Numerator Statement	Denominator Statement	Measure Steward	PQRS No.
CMS159v5	0710	Depression Remission at Twelve Months Domain: Clinical Process/ Effectiveness	Patients age eighteen and older with major depression or dysthymia and an initial Patient Health Questionnaire (PHQ-9) score greater than nine who demonstrate remission at twelve months (+/- 30 days after an index visit) defined as a PHQ-9 score less than five. This measure applies to both patients with newly diagnoses and existing depression whose current PHQ-9 score indicates a need for treatment.	Patients who achieved remission at twelve months as demonstrated by a twelve month (+/- 30 days grace period) PHQ-9 score of less than five	Patients age eighteen and older with a diagnosis of major depression or dysthymia and an initial PHQ-9 score greater than nine during the index visit	MN Community Measurement	370 GPRO MH-1

Source: CMS (n.d.f).

the NQF website (www.qualityforum.org) by any combination of the following dimensions:

- Endorsement Status (e.g. Endorsed, Not Endorsed)
- Measure Status (Time Limited, Reserved)
- Measure Format (eMeasure, Measure)
- Measure Steward (e.g., NCQA, CMS, The Joint Commission)
- Use in Federal Program (e.g., Meaningful Use, Medicare Shared Savings Program)
- Clinical Condition/Topic Area (e.g., Cancer, Infectious Disease)
- Cross-Cutting Area (e.g., Overuse, Safety, Disparities)
- Care Setting (e.g., Ambulatory Care, Home Health, Hospital)
- National Quality Strategy Priorities (e.g., Affordable Care, Patient Safety)
- Actual/Planned Use (e.g., Public Reporting, Payment Program)
- Data Source (e.g., Administrative Data, Electronic Clinical Data, Healthcare Provider Survey)
- Level of Analysis (e.g., Clinician, Facility, Health Plan)
- Target Population (Children's Health)

Figure 10.1 is a screenshot from the NQF website showing a few of the thousand-plus measures in the database that are classified as Home Health.

Figure 10.1 Screenshot from NQF

	0013	Blood pressure measurement
	0517	CAHPS® Home Health Care Survey (experience with care)
	1632	CARE - Consumer Assessments and Reports of End of Life
	0429	Change in Basic Mobility as Measured by the AM-PAC:
	0430	Change in Daily Activity Function as measured by the AM-PAC:

Source: National Quality Forum (2016). Copyright ©2016 National Quality Forum. Used with permission.

Comparative Health Care Data Sets

Comparative health care data sets and information are often aligned with organizations' quality improvement efforts. An organization might collect data on one or more of the specific performance measures, such as those previously identified, and then use this information to compare its performance to other similar organizations or state average results, for example. The process of comparing one or more performance measures against a standard is called *benchmarking.* Benchmarking may be limited to internally set standards; however, frequently it employs one or more externally generated benchmark or standard.

Providers may select from many publicly and privately available health care data sets for benchmarking purposes. Many of the organizations identified in the previous section not only develop standards but also provide searchable websites that enable consumers and providers to compare results of their measures across multiple organizations. Although each comparative data set is unique, they can be loosely categorized by purpose: patient satisfaction, practice patterns, or clinical data. The following paragraphs identify some of the more well-known and frequently used comparative data sets and list their associated searchable website when applicable.

Patient Satisfaction Data Sets

Patient satisfaction data generally come from survey data. Several private organizations, such as NRC+Picker, Press Ganey, and the health care division of Gallup, provide extensive consulting services to health care organizations across the country. One of these services is to conduct patient satisfaction surveys. Some health care organizations undertake patient satisfaction surveys on their own. The advantage of using a national organization is the comparative database it offers, which organizations can use for benchmarking purposes.

Some of the most widely used groups of patient experience surveys in the public arena were developed under the **Agency for Healthcare Research and Quality (AHRQ) Consumer Assessment of Healthcare Providers and Systems (CAHPS)** program. CAHPS originated in 1995 to assess participants' perspectives on their health plans. Since that time the program has evolved to include the following surveys:

- Health Plan
- Clinician & Group
- Hospital

- Home Health Care
- In-Center Hemodialysis
- Nursing Home
- Surgical Care
- American Indian
- Dental Plan
- Experience of Care and Health Outcomes (for mental health and substance abuse services)

CAHPS surveys are available to any organization. Federal agencies, such as CMS, use the CAHPS survey results, but the results are also used by health systems, physician practices, hospitals, and other health care providers in their quality improvement efforts (AHRQ, 2016). The **Hospital CAHPS (HCAHPS)** results are available to consumers as a part of CMS Hospital Compare (discussed under "Clinical Data Sets") and from the AHRQ website. Information about the CAHPS comparative data and access to the database and chart books is located at http://www.ahrq.gov/cahps/cahps-database/comparative-data/index.html (AHRQ, 2016).

Practice Patterns Data Set

The **Dartmouth Atlas** is a widely used, interactive, online tool that enables health care organizations to compare data across a wide variety of parameters. The project is a privately funded program through the Dartmouth Institute for Health Policy and Clinical Practice, which primarily uses Medicare data to document variations in the use of medical resources across the United States. To access the Dartmouth Atlas, go to http://www.dartmouthatlas.org (The Dartmouth Institute, n.d.).

Clinical Data Sets

The Joint Commission and CMS are committed to the improvement of clinical outcomes, and as a part of that commitment they provide consumers with comparative data that encompasses clinical measures. The Joint Commission's **Quality Check** has evolved since its introduction in 1994 to become a comprehensive guide to health care organizations in the United States. Visitors to www.Qualitycheck.org can search for health care organizations by a variety of parameters, identify accreditation status, and compare hospital performance measures in terms of the Joint Commission's (2015a) National

Patient Safety Goals. The 2016 **National Patient Safety Goals** for Hospitals describes sixteen specific goals, including these:

- Identifying patients correctly
- Improving staff member communication
- Using medicines safely
- Using alarms safely
- Preventing infection
- Identifying patient safety risks
- Preventing mistakes in surgery (The Joint Commission, 2016)

Hospital Compare is the CMS-sponsored interactive, online comparative data set. Located at www.medicare.gov/hospitalcompare, this data set contains information about the quality of care at over four thousand Medicare-certified hospitals. The interactive tool enables consumers to compare clinical and patient satisfaction data. The purpose of the tool is to promote informed decision making by consumers of hospital care and to encourage hospitals to improve the quality of care they provide (CMS, n.d.b). In addition to Hospital Compare, CMS sponsors public reporting of other health care organizations, such as nursing homes, home health agencies, and kidney dialysis facilities (CMS, n.d.d).

Comparative Data for Health Plans

In addition to data sets used by providers, the NCQA website enables consumers to have access to comparative data for health plans through a variety of report cards. The majority of the comparative data is derived from HEDIS and CAHPS. **NCQA health care report cards** are found at http://reportcard.ncqa.org. NCQA also offers a subscription service for a more detailed interactive tool, Quality Compass (NCQA, n.d.b, n.d.c).

FEDERAL QUALITY IMPROVEMENT INITIATIVES

As stated at the beginning of the chapter, the publication of the IOM reports addressing serious quality concerns marked a new era of government initiatives to improve the quality of patient care. Multiple new programs were established and new efforts to link Medicare and Medicaid reimbursement to quality care were undertaken. In this section we will examine the **Patient Safety Act,** the National Quality Strategy, and a selection of related government programs aimed at improving the quality of health care through performance measurement including the related aspects of the Medicare Access & CHIP Reauthorization Act of 2015 (MACRA).

The Patient Safety Act

The IOM *To Err Is Human: Building a Safer Health System* (Kohn, Corrigan, & Donaldson, 2000) outlined serious concerns about and the need to improve the safety and quality of health care in the United States. Despite the ongoing efforts by voluntary accrediting bodies to ensure high-quality care, this report identified a critical need for reporting and analyzing individual facility and aggregate data related to adverse events. To address the need to capture information to improve health care quality and prevent harm to patients, the Patient Safety and Quality Improvement Act of 2005 (Patient Safety Act) was passed by Congress "to promote shared learning to enhance quality and safety nationally." To implement the act, the Department of Health and Human Services issued the Patient Safety Rule (effective January 2009), which authorized the identification of **Patient Safety Organizations (PSOs).** As of August 2016, there were eighty-two PSOs in twenty-eight states. PSOs are responsible for the collection and analysis of health information that is referred to in the Final Rule as patient safety work product (PSWP). The PSWP contains identifiable patient information that is covered by specific privilege and confidentiality protections (AHRQ, n.d.a).

The types of patient safety events that are reported under these protections include the following:

- **Incidents:** patient safety events that reached the patient, whether or not there was harm involved
- **Near misses (or close calls):** patient safety events that did not reach the patient
- **Unsafe conditions:** circumstances that increase the probability of a patient safety event occurring

To facilitate these activities, AHRQ has created **Common Formats,** which are "common definitions and reporting formats to help providers uniformly report patient safety events" (AHRQ, n.d.b).

National Quality Strategy

The requirement for a **National Strategy for Quality Improvement in Health Care (National Quality Strategy)** was established by the Affordable Care Act and subsequently published in 2011. More than three hundred groups and individuals representing all aspects of the health care industry and public provided input. It has subsequently been updated on an annual basis, but the three broad aims and six priorities have remained consistent. The three broad aims used to "guide and assess national efforts to improve health and the quality of health care" (AHRQ, 2011) are as follows:

1. **Better care:** Improve the overall quality by making health care more patient-centered, reliable, accessible, and safe.

2. **Healthy people/healthy communities:** Improve the health of the US population by supporting proven interventions to address behavioral, social, and environmental determinants of health in addition to delivering higher-quality care.

3. **Affordable care:** Reduce the cost of quality health care for individuals, families, employers, and government

To achieve these aims, the National Quality Strategy identifies the following six priorities:

1. Making care safer by reducing harm caused in the delivery of care

2. Ensuring that each person and family are engaged as partners in their care

3. Promoting effective communication and coordination of care

4. Promoting the most effective prevention and treatment practices for the leading causes of mortality, starting with cardiovascular disease

5. Working with communities to promote wide use of best practices to enable healthy living

6. Making quality care more affordable for individuals, families, employers, and governments by developing and spreading new health care delivery models

The strategy goes further by recommending that all sectors of the health care system (individuals, families, payers, providers, employers, and communities) employ one or more of the following "levers" to "align" with the National Quality Strategy (NQS)(AHRQ, 2011):

- **Measurement and feedback:** Provide performance feedback to plans and providers to improve care.

- **Public reporting:** Compare treatment results, costs, and patient experience for consumers.

- **Learning and technical assistance:** Foster learning environments that offer training, resources, tools, and guidance to help organizations achieve quality improvement goals.

- **Certification, accreditation, and regulation:** Adopt or adhere to approaches to meet safety and quality standards.

- **Consumer incentives and benefit designs:** Help consumers adopt healthy behaviors and make informed decisions.

- **Payment:** Reward and incentivize providers to deliver high-quality, patient-centered care.

- **Health information technology:** Improve communication, transparency, and efficiency for better coordinated health and health care.

- **Innovation and diffusion:** Foster innovation in health care quality improvement, and facilitate rapid adoption within and across organizations and communities.

- **Workforce development:** Invest in people to prepare the next generation of health care professionals and support lifelong learning for providers.

CMS Quality Programs

The Centers for Medicare and Medicaid (CMS) released its specific Quality Strategy in 2016, which is based on the NQS. Adhering to the same broad aims in the NQS, CMS developed a strategy to improve health care delivery by the following means:

- Using incentives to improve care
- Tying payment to value through new payment models
- Changing how care is given through
  - Better teamwork
  - Better coordination across health care settings
  - More attention to population health
  - Putting the power of health care information to work (CMS, 2016)

Since 2001, CMS has engaged in a variety of Quality Initiatives, including initiatives that result in public reporting of performance measures as previously discussed. The Physician Quality Reporting System (PQRS) encourages individual "eligible professionals" (EPs) (e.g., physicians) and group practices to assess and report the quality of care provided to their patients. EPs and group practices that do not report on quality measures as outlined for Medicare Part B covered services risk a negative payment adjustment. There are several mechanisms for reporting PQRS data, including EHRs (CMS, n.d.g).

Using PQRS reporting to determine reimbursement for Medicare Part B is one of many mechanisms through which CMS incentivizes improved quality of care. CMS has multiple value-based or pay-for-performance programs aimed at tying reimbursements to demonstration of quality. CMS's original value-based programs were an attempt to link performance on endorsed quality measures to reimbursement. These programs included the following:

- **Hospital Value-Based Purchasing (HVBP)** program rewards acute care hospitals for quality care using incentives.

- **Hospital Readmissions Reduction (HRR)** program rewards acute care hospitals that reduce unnecessary hospital readmissions for certain conditions, such as acute myocardial infarction, health failure, pneumonia, chronic obstructive pulmonary disease, elective hip or knee replacement, and coronary artery bypass surgery.

- **Hospital-Acquired Conditions (HAC)** program determines whether or not an acute care hospital should be paid a reduced amount based on performance across health-acquired infections and unacceptable adverse events.

- **Value Modifier (VM)** program (also known as **Physician Value-Based Modifier** or **PVBM**) rewards physicians (and, beginning in 2018, other primary care professionals, for example, physician assistants and nurse practitioners) for high-quality, lower-cost performance using an adjustment (modifier) for each claim.

Three other value-based programs are applied to end-stage renal disease programs, skilled nursing facilities, and home health programs.

Beyond these traditional value-based programs, CMS encourages innovative, alternative models of care through the CMS Innovation Center. These models are designed to promote lower-cost, higher-quality care. All depend on appropriate reporting of performance measures (CMS, n.d.h).

The Medicare Access and CHIP Reauthorization Act (MACRA)

The Medicare Access and CHIP Reauthorization Act (MACRA) was enacted in 2015. MACRA is one aspect of CMS's push toward improving quality and value. In January 2015, the Department of Health and Human Services announced two goals for value-based payments and **alternative payment models (APMs):**

- **Goal 1:** 30 percent of Medicare payments are tied to quality or value through APMs by the end of 2016; 50 percent by the end of 2018.
- **Goal 2:** 85 percent of Medicare fee-for-service payments are tied to quality or value by the end of 2016; 90 percent by the end of 2018.

They also invited private sector payers to match or exceed these same goals.

MACRA affects physician providers, moving HHS closer to meeting these goals. Key elements to MACRA are the following:

- Changes the way Medicare rewards physicians and practitioners for value over volume
- Streamlines multiple quality programs directed at physicians and practitioners under the new **Merit-based Incentive Payment System (MIPS)**
- Provides bonus payments for physician and practitioners participation in eligible APMs (see Chapter One for examples of APMs)

MIPS will incorporate aspects of three existing quality and value programs: PQRS, Value-based Modifier, and the Medicare EHR Incentive Program. The resulting set of performance measures will be divided into the following categories to calculate a score (between 0 and 100) for eligible professionals. Each category of performance will be weighted as shown in Table 10.4.

Health care providers meeting the established threshold score will receive no adjustment to payment; those scoring below will receive a negative adjustment and those above, a positive adjustment. Exceptional performers may receive bonus payments (CMS, n.d.c, n.d.e).

Table 10.4 MIPS performance categories

Category	Weight (%)
Quality	50
Advancing care information	25
Clinical practice improvement activities	15
Resource use	10

Figure 10.2 Projected timetable for implementation of MACRA

| 2015 and earlier | 2016 | 2017 | 2018 | 2019 | 2020 | 2021 | 2022 | 2023 | 2024 | 2025 | 2026 and later |

MIPS
Quality
Resource Use
Clinical practice Improvement Activities 4% 5% 7%   9%
Meaningful Use of Certified EHR Technology
PQRS, Value Modifier, EHR Incentives

MIPS Payment Adjustment (+/-)

Certain APMs
Qualifying APM Participant
Medicare Payment Threshold
Excluded from MIPS

5% Incentive Payment

Excluded from MIPS

Source: CMS (n.d.e).

The exact implementation dates for MACRA were not set by the publication date for this textbook; however, the projected timetable for implementation of the various aspects of the law is shown in Figure 10.2 (CMS, n.d.c).

SUMMARY

In this chapter we examined how health care organizations and health plans use data and information to demonstrate performance to licensing, certifying, and accrediting bodies; to measure performance against internal and external standards; to compare performance to other similar organizations; and to demonstrate performance for reimbursement purposes. This chapter began with an examination of the licensure, certification, and accreditation of health care facilities and health plans, followed by an overview of key comparative data sets often used by health care organizations in benchmarking performance. The chapter further explored major milestones in the national agenda for health care quality improvement, followed by a discussion of the current efforts to improve health care quality and patient safety, focusing on the efforts that involve using health care data and information to measure performance. The private and public organizations responsible for developing and endorsing national quality measures were introduced, and the progress that has been made in aligning these measures across these organizations was discussed. The chapter concluded with an overview of the significant movement toward value-based reimbursement programs and plans for significant growth in these programs over the next decade.

Clearly, there is a bewildering and complex set of measures with many organizations involved. Consequently, many measures being collected are inconsistent across the organizations requiring them. There are differences of opinion about which measures to be collected and the specific definitions of these measures. Efforts are under way, largely driven by CMS, to align measures to ease the collection burden for health care providers. However, today's reality remains an overwhelmingly complex web of standards and measurement requirements.

EHRs have been cited as the solution for easing the collection burden for health care organizations and providers. However, the most current EHR systems are limited in their ability to collect the required measures. The result is that organizations and providers must resort to manual data collection. In other chapters in this text we have explored reasons for the current limitations of EHRs in this area, including provider resistance because of the time burden. There is a largely unresolved tension in the health care community and HIT industry between the desire to collect accurate and timely measures and the provider resistance to entering the data into the EHR in a standard, retrievable format.

KEY TERMS

Accreditation

Accreditation organization (AO)

Administrative data

Agency for Healthcare Research and
    Quality (AHRQ)

Alternative payment models
    (APMs)

American Medical Association
    Physician Consortium for
    Performance Improvement
    (AMA-PCPI)

Centers for Disease Control and
    Prevention (CDC)

Centers for Medicare and Medicaid
    Services (CMS)

Certification

Clinical quality measures (CQMs)

Common formats

Comparative health care data sets

Conditions of participation (CoPs)

Consumer Assessment of Healthcare
    Providers and Systems (CAHPS)

Dartmouth Atlas

Deemed status

Disease registries

EHR Incentive Programs

Electronic clinical quality measures
    (eCQMs)

Eligible professionals

Health Effectiveness Data and
    Information Set (HEDIS)

Health records

Health Resources and Services
    Administration (HRSA)

Hospital-acquired conditions (HAC)

Hospital CAHPS (HCAHPS)

Hospital Compare

Hospital Readmissions Reduction
    (HRR)

Hospital Value-Based Purchasing
    (HVBP)

The Joint Commission

The Joint Commission Information
    Management (IM) standards

The Joint Commission Record of Care (RC), Treatment, and Services standards

Licensure

The Medicare Access and CHIP Reauthorization Act (MACRA)

Merit-based Incentive Payment System (MIPS)

National Committee for Quality Assurance (NCQA)

National Patient Safety Goals

National Quality Forum (NQF)

National Strategy for Quality Improvement in Health Care (National Quality Strategy)

NCQA health care report cards

Patient Safety Act

Patient Safety Organizations (PSOs)

Performance measures

Physician Value-Based Modifier (PVBM)

Physicians Quality Reporting System (PQRS) number

Qualitative data

Quality Check

Quality measures

Value Modifier (VM)

LEARNING ACTIVITIES

1. Research two local health care organizations—one acute care facility and one other type of organization. Determine each organization's current licensure, accreditation, and certification status. How are these processes related within your state? Do the processes differ between the two types of health care organizations?

2. Visit the Joint Commission website at www.jointcommission.org. What accreditation programs (other than the Hospital Accreditation Program) does the Joint Commission have? List the programs and their respective missions.

3. Visit the NCQA website at www.ncqa.org and look up at least two health plans with which you are familiar. What do the report cards tell you about these plans? Do you find this information useful? Why or why not?

4. Visit the patient safety organization website at www.pso.ahrq.gov. Does your state have a PSO? If not, identify a PSO from a neighboring state. Research the PSO and report on how long it has operated and who its clients are.

5. Use Hospital Compare and the Joint Commission Quality Check to research three hospitals in your region of the country. Write a report outlining your findings. Would any of the information you discovered influence your choice of care for you or your family? Why or why not?

6. Research the current status of the CMS Quality programs discussed in this chapter. Write an update for this section of the chapter.

7. Research the current year's National Quality Strategy. Has it changed since this book was published? List the differences and comment on the changes.

8. Use the NQF website to identify four specific performance measures that are endorsed by NQF for physician practices. Research each measure to identify how each measure is calculated, including the source of the data, the numerator, and the denominator. Do you think these measures are a good reflection of quality practice? Why or why not?

REFERENCES

Agency for Healthcare Research and Quality (AHRQ). (2011). *National quality strategy (NQS).* Retrieved August 31, 2016, from http://www.ahrq.gov/workingforquality/nqs/nqs2011annlrpt.pdf

Agency for Healthcare Research and Quality (AHRQ). (2016, July). *Comparative data.* Retrieved August 31, 2016, from http://www.ahrq.gov/cahps/cahps-database/comparative-data/index.html

Agency for Healthcare Research and Quality (AHRQ). (n.d.a). *About the PSO program.* Retrieved August 31, 2016, from https://pso.ahrq.gov/about

Agency for Healthcare Research and Quality (AHRQ). (n.d.b). *Common formats.* Retrieved August 31, 2016, from https://pso.ahrq.gov/common

Centers for Medicare and Medicaid (CMS). (2015, Sept.). *CMS-approved accrediting organizations contacts for prospective clients.* Retrieved August 30, 2016, from https://www.cms.gov/Medicare/Provider-Enrollment-and-Certification/SurveyCertificationGenInfo/Downloads/Accrediting-Organization-Contacts-for-Prospective-Clients-.pdf

Centers for Medicare and Medicaid (CMS). (2016). *CMS quality strategy 2016.* Retrieved August 31, 2016, from https://www.cms.gov/medicare/quality-initiatives-patient-assessment-instruments/qualityinitiativesgeninfo/downloads/cms-quality-strategy.pdf

Centers for Medicare and Medicaid (CMS). (n.d.a). *Accreditation of Medicare-certified providers & suppliers.* Retrieved August 21, 2016, from https://www.cms.gov/Medicare/Provider-Enrollment-and-Certification/SurveyCertificationGenInfo/Accreditation-of-Medicare-Certified-Providers-and-Suppliers.html

Centers for Medicare and Medicaid (CMS). (n.d.b). *Hospital compare.* Retrieved August 31, 2016, from https://www.medicare.gov/hospitalcompare

Centers for Medicare and Medicaid (CMS). (n.d.c). *MACRA.* Retrieved August 31, 2016, from https://www.cms.gov/Medicare/Quality-Initiatives-Patient-Assessment-Instruments/Value-Based-Programs/MACRA-MIPS-and-APMs/MACRA-MIPS-and-APMs.html

Centers for Medicare and Medicaid (CMS). (n.d.d). *Medicare.* Retrieved August 31, 2016, from https://www.cms.gov/Medicare

Centers for Medicare and Medicaid (CMS). (n.d.e). *The Medicare Access & CHIP Reauthorization Act of 2015: Path to value.* Retrieved August 31, 2016, from https://www.cms.gov/Medicare/Quality-Initiatives-Patient-Assessment-Instruments/Value-Based-Programs/MACRA-MIPS-and-APMs/MACRA-LAN-PPT.pdf

Centers for Medicare & Medicaid Services (n.d.f). *The merit-based incentive payment system: MIPS scoring methodology overview.* Retrieved August 4, 2016, from https://www.cms.gov/Medicare/Quality-Initiatives-Patient-Assessment-Instruments/Value-Based-Programs/MACRA-MIPS-and-APMs/MIPS-Scoring-Methodology-slide-deck.pdf

Centers for Medicare and Medicaid (CMS). (n.d.g). *Physician quality reporting system.* Retrieved August 31, 2016, from https://www.cms.gov/Medicare/Quality-Initiatives-Patient-Assessment-Instruments/PQRS/index.html?redirect=/pqri

Centers for Medicare and Medicaid (CMS). (n.d.h). *Value-based programs.* Retrieved August 31, 2016, from https://www.cms.gov/Medicare/Quality-Initiatives-Patient-Assessment-Instruments/Value-Based-Programs/Value-Based-Programs.html

Council of Medical Specialty Societies (CMSS). (2014, Nov.). *The measurement of health care performance* (3rd ed.). Retrieved August 21, 2016, from http://cmss.org/wp-content/uploads/2015/07/CMSS-Quality-Primer-layout.final.pdf

The Dartmouth Institute (n.d.) *Understanding of the efficiency and effectiveness of the health care system.* Retrieved August 31, 2016, from http://www.dartmouthatlas.org/

Institute of Medicine Committee (IOM) on Quality in America. (2001). *Crossing the quality chasm: A new health system for the 21st century.* Washington, DC: National Academy Press.

The Joint Commission. (2011). *Comprehensive accreditation manual for hospitals.* Oakbrook Terrace, IL: Author.

The Joint Commission. (2014a, Aug.). *Program: Ambulatory. Chapter: information management* (e-dition). Retrieved August 21, 2016, from http://foh.hhs.gov/tjc/im/standards.pdf

The Joint Commission. (2014b, Aug.). *Program: Ambulatory. Chapter: Record of care, treatment and services* (e-dition). Retrieved August 21, 2016, from http://foh.hhs.gov/tjc/roc/standards.pdf

The Joint Commission. (2015a, Nov. 5). *Hospital: 2016 national patient safety goals.* Retrieved August 31, 2016, from https://www.jointcommission.org/hap_2016_npsgs/

The Joint Commission. (2015b, Sept. 2). *Joint Commission measure sets effective January 1, 2016.* Retrieved August 21, 2016, from https://www.jointcommission.org/joint_commission_measure_sets_effective_january_1_2016/

The Joint Commission. (2016, April 27). *Accreditation process overview.* Retrieved August 21, 2016, from https://www.jointcommission.org/accreditation_process_overview/

The Joint Commission. (n.d.). *About the Joint Commission.* Retrieved August 21, 2016, from https://www.jointcommission.org/about_us/about_the_joint_commission_main.aspx

Kohn, L. T., Corrigan, J., & Donaldson, M. S. (2000). *To err is human: Building a safer health system.* Washington, DC: National Academy Press.

Morris, C. (2014, May). *Measuring health care quality: An overview of quality measures* (Issue brief). FamiliesUSA. Retrieved August 21, 2016, from http://familiesusa.org/sites/default/files/product_documents/HIS_Quality Measurement_Brief_final_web.pdf

National Committee for Quality Assurance (NCQA). (2015). *2015 NCQA health plan accreditation standards.* Retrieved August 21, 2016 from http://www.ncqa.org/programs/accreditation/health-plan-hp

National Committee for Quality Assurance (NCQA). (n.d.a). *About NCQA.* Retrieved August 21, 2016, from http://www.ncqa.org/about-ncqa

National Committee for Quality Assurance (NCQA). (n.d.b). *Quality compass.* Retrieved August 21, 2016, from http://www.ncqa.org/tabid/177/Default.aspx

National Committee for Quality Assurance (NCQA). (n.d.c). *Report cards.* Retrieved August 21, 2016, from http://www.ncqa.org/report-cards

National Quality Forum (NQF). (n.d.). *About us.* Retrieved August 31, 2016, from http://www.qualityforum.org/About_NQF/

CHAPTER 11

Health Care Information System Standards

LEARNING OBJECTIVES

- To be able to give examples of the methods by which standards are developed: ad hoc, de facto, government mandate, and consensus.

- To be able to identify and discuss the role of organizations that currently have a significant impact on the adoption of health care information standards in the United States.

- To be able to identify and discuss the role of federal initiatives and legislation that have a significant impact on the adoption of health care information standards in the United States.

- To be able to identify examples within the major types of health care information standards and the organizations that develop or approve them.

- To understand the importance of health care IT standards to the future of the US health care delivery system.

Throughout this text we have examined a variety of different types of **standards** that affect, directly or indirectly, the management of health information systems. In Chapter Ten we examined health care performance standards; Chapter Two looked at data quality standards, Chapter Nine at security standards, and so on. In this chapter we will examine yet another category of standards that affect health care data and information systems: health care information system (HCIS) standards. In all cases the standards examined represent the measuring stick or set of rules against which an entity, such as an organization or system, will compare its structures, processes, or functions to determine compliance. In the case of the HCIS standards discussed in this chapter the aim is to provide a common set of rules by which health care information systems can communicate. Systems that conform to different standards cannot possibly communicate with one another. Portability, **data exchange,** and **interoperability** among different health information systems can be achieved only if they can "communicate." For a simple analogy, think about traveling to a country where you do not speak the language. You would not be able to communicate with that country's citizens without a common language or translator. Think of the common language you adopt as the standard set of rules to which all parties agree to adhere. Once you and others agree on a common language, you and they can communicate. You may still have some problems, but generally these can be overcome.

By nature HCIS standards include technical specifications, which make it less easy for the typical health care administrator to fully understand them. In addition, a complex web of public and private organizations create, manage, and implement HCIS standards, resulting in standards that are not always aligned, making the standards even more difficult to fully grasp. In fact, some may actually compete with one another. In addition to the complex web of standards specifically designed for HCIS, there are many general IT standards that affect health care information systems. Networking standards, such as Ethernet and Wi-Fi, employed by health care organizations are not specific to health care. **Extensible markup language (XML)** is widely accepted as a standard for sharing data using web-based technologies in health care and other industries. There are many other examples that are beyond the scope of this text. Our focus will be on the standards that are specific to HCIS.

With HIPAA came the push for adoption of administrative transaction and data exchange standards. This effort has been largely successful; claims are routinely submitted via standard electronic transaction protocols. However, although real progress has been made in recent years, complete interoperability among health care information systems remains elusive. Chapter Three examined the need for interoperability among health care information systems to promote better health of our citizens; Chapter Two discussed the lack of standardization in EHRs as an issue with using EHR data in research; and Chapter Nine outlined problems associated with misalignment of quality and performance measures, in part because of a lack of interoperability and standardization in EHRs and other health care information systems. Interoperability, as defined by the ONC (2015) in its publication **Connecting Health Care for the Nation: A Shared Nation-wide Interoperability Roadmap,** results from multiple initiatives, including payment, regulatory, and other policy changes to support a collaborative and connected health care system. The best political and social infrastructures, however, will not succeed in achieving interoperability without supportive technologies.

This chapter is divided into three main sections. The first section is an overview of HCIS standards, providing general information about the types of standards and their purposes. The second section examines a few of the major initiatives, public and private, responsible for creating, requiring, or implementing HCIS standards. Finally, the last section of the chapter examines some of the most commonly adopted HCIS standards, including examples of the standards when possible.

HCIS STANDARDS OVERVIEW

Keith Boone, a prolific blogger and writer on all topics related to HIT standards, once wrote, "Standards are like potato chips. You always need more than one to get the job done" (Boone, 2012b). In general, the health care IT community discusses HCIS standards in terms of their specific function, such as privacy and security, EHRs, electronic prescribing (e-prescribing), lab reporting, and so on, but the reality is that achieving one of these or other functions requires multiple standards directed at different levels within the HCIS. For example, there is a need for standards at the level of basic communication across the Internet or other network (Transporting), standards for structuring the content of messages communicated across the network (Data Interchange and Messaging), standards that describe required data elements for a particular function, such as the EHR or clinical summary (Content), and standards for naming or classifying the actual data, such as units of measure, lab tests, diagnoses, and so on (Vocabulary/Terminology). Unfortunately, there is no universal model for categorizing the plethora of HCIS standards. In this chapter we will look at standards described as Data Interchange and Messaging, Content, and Vocabulary/Terminology standards.

Standards, as we have seen, are the sets of rules for what should be included for the needed function and system level. This is only a portion of the challenge in implementing standards. The other challenge is how are the standards used for a particular function or use case? Much of the work today toward achieving interoperability of health care information systems is concerned with the how. Organizations that develop standards may also create specific implementation guides for using the standard in a particular use case. (To further complicate the already complicated standards environment, these implementation guides are sometimes referred to as *standards.*) Other organizations, such as the ONC, develop frameworks for implementing standards, and several government initiatives, such as HIPAA and HITECH, have set requirements for implementing specific standards or sets of standards.

STANDARDS DEVELOPMENT PROCESS

When seeking to understand why so many different IT and health care information standards exist, it is helpful to look first at the **standards development process** that exists in the United States (and internationally). In general the methods used to establish health care IT standards can be divided into four categories (Hammond & Cimino, 2006):

1. **Ad hoc.** A standard is established by the ad hoc method when a group of interested people or organizations agrees on a certain specification without any formal adoption process. The Digital Imaging and Communications in Medicine (DICOM) standard for health care imaging came about in this way.

2. **De facto.** A de facto standard arises when a vendor or other commercial enterprise controls such a large segment of the market that its product becomes the recognized norm. The SQL database language and the Windows operating system are examples of de facto standards. XML is becoming a de facto standard for health care and other types of industry messaging.

3. **Government mandate.** Standards are also established when the government mandates that the health care industry adopt them. Examples are the transaction and code sets mandated by the **Health Insurance Portability and Accountability Act (HIPAA)** regulations.

4. **Consensus.** Consensus-based standards come about when representatives from various interested groups come together to reach a formal agreement on specifications. The process is generally open and involves considerable comment and feedback from the industry. This method is employed by the **standards developing organizations (SDOs)** accredited by the **American National Standards Institute (ANSI)**. Many health care information standards are developed by this method, including Health Level Seven (HL7)

standards and the health-related **Accredited Standards Committee (ASC)** standards.

The relationships among standard-setting organizations can be confusing, to say the least. Not only do many of the acronyms sound similar but also the organizations themselves, as voluntary, member-based organizations, can set their own missions and goals. Therefore, although there is a formally recognized relationship among the **International Organization for Standardization (ISO)**, ANSI, and the SDOs, there is also some overlap in activities. Table 11.1 outlines the relationships among the formal standard-setting organizations and for each one gives a brief overview of important facts and a current website.

Table 11.1 Relationships among standards-setting organizations

Organizations	Facts	Website
International Organization for Standardization (ISO)	• Members are national standards bodies from many different countries around the world. • Oversees the flow of documentation and international approval of standards development under the auspices of the its member bodies	www.iso.org
American National Standards Institute (ANSI)	• US member of ISO • Accredits standards development organizations (SDOs) from a wide range of industries, including health care • Does not develop standards but accredits the organizations that develop standards • Publishes more than ten thousand standards developed by accredited SDOs	www.ansi.org
Standards Developing Organizations (SDOs)	• Must be accredited by ANSI • Develop standards in accordance with ANSI criteria • Can use the label "Approved American National Standard" • Approximately two hundred SDOs are accredited; twenty of these produce 90 percent of the standards.	www.standardsportal .org

Source: ANSI (n.d.a, n.d.b, n.d.c); ISO (n.d.).

All the ANSI-accredited SDOs must adhere to the guidelines established for accreditation; therefore, they have similar standard-setting processes. According to ANSI, this process includes the following:

- Consensus on a proposed standard by a group or "consensus body" that includes representatives from materially affected or interested parties
- Broad-based public review and comment on draft standards
- Consideration of and response to comments submitted by voting members of the relevant consensus body and by public review commenters
- Incorporation of approved changes into a draft standard
- Right to appeal by any participant that believes that due process principles were not sufficiently respected during the standards development in accordance with the ANSI-accredited procedures of the standards developer (ANSI, n.d.c)

The IT industry in general has experienced a movement away from the process of establishing standards via the accredited SDOs. The Internet and World Wide Web standards, for example, were developed by groups with much less formal structures. However, the accredited SDOs continue to have a significant impact on the IT standards for the health care industry.

Boone (2012a) lists the following organizations as major developers of HIT standards in the United States, which includes a mix of accredited SDOs and other developers. Each organization's specific areas for standard development are indicated in parentheses. ANSI-accredited SDOs are indicated with an "*."

- International Standards Organization (ISO) [various]
- **ASTM International (ASTM)** [various]*
- Accredited Standards Committee (ASC) X12 [Insurance Transactions]*
- **Health Level Seven International (HL7)** [various]*
- **Digital Imaging and Communication in Medicine (DICOM)** [Imaging]
- **National Council for Prescription Drug Programs (NCPDP)** [ePrescribing]
- Regienstrief (LOINC) [Laboratory Vocabulary]

- **International Health Terminology SDO (IHTSDO)** [Clinical Terminology]

In addition, Boone (2012a) identifies the following "other" organizations as having a major impact on HIT:

- World Wide Web Consortium (W3C) [XML, HTML]
- Internet Engineering Task Force (IETF) [Internet]
- Organization for the Advancement of Structured Information Standards (OASIS) [Business use of XML]

He further identifies key groups known as "profiling bodies" (Boone, 2012a) that use existing standards to create comprehensive implementation guides. Two examples of profiling bodies are **Integrating the Healthcare Enterprise (IHE)** and the ONC, which focus on guidance for implementing clinical interoperability standards.

PERSPECTIVE
European Committee for Standardization (CEN)

Although the focus of this chapter is standards developed within the United States, it is important to recognize there are other standards organizations worldwide. For example, the **European Committee for Standardization (CEN)** was created in Brussels in 1975. In 2010 CEN partnered with another European standards developing organization, the European Committee for Electrotechnical Standardization (CENELEC), to form the **CEN-CENELEC Management Centre (CCMC)** in Brussels, Belgium. The CCMC current membership includes national standards bodies from thirty-three European countries (CEN-CENELEC, n.d.).

The Technical Committee within CEN that oversees health care informatics standards is CEN TC 251, which consists of two working groups:

- WG1: Enterprise and Information
- WG2: Technology and Applications

Source: CEN (n.d.).

FEDERAL INITIATIVES AFFECTING HEALTH CARE IT STANDARDS

There are many federal initiatives that affect health care IT standards. In this section we look at federal initiatives for health care IT standards as a part of HIPAA, **CMS e-prescribing**, CMS EHR Incentive Program, and the **Office of the National Coordinator for Health Information Technology (ONC)**, including the Interoperability Roadmap.

HIPAA

In August 2000, the US Department of Health and Human Services published the final rule outlining the standards to be adopted by health care organizations for electronic transactions and announced the **designated standard maintenance organizations (DSMOs)**. In publishing this rule, which has been modified as needed, the federal government mandated that health care organizations adopt certain standards for electronic transactions and standard code sets for these transactions and identified the standards organizations that would oversee the adoption of standards for HIPAA compliance. The DSMOs have the responsibility for the development, maintenance, and modification of relevant electronic data interchange standards. HIPAA transaction standards apply to all covered entities' **electronic data interchange (EDI)** related to claims and encounter information, payment and remittance advice, claims status, eligibility, enrollment and disenrollment, referrals and authorizations, coordination of benefits, and premiums payment. The current HIPAA transaction standards are ASC X12N version 5010 (which accommodates ICD-10) along with NCPDP D.0 for pharmacy transactions (CMS, 2016b). In addition to these transaction standards, several standard code sets were established for use in electronic transactions, including ICD-10-CM, ICD-10-PCS, HCPCS, CPT, and **Code on Dental Procedures and Nomenclature (CDT)** (CMS, 2016a).

Centers for Medicare and Medicaid E-prescribing

The Medicare Prescription Drug, Improvement, and Modernization Act of 2003 (MMA) established a Voluntary Prescription Drug Benefit program. There is no requirement in this act that providers write prescriptions electronically, but those who choose to do so must comply with specific e-prescribing standards. The current published CMS e-prescribing standards consist of three sets of existing health care IT standards as "foundation" standards, which include NCPDP's **SCRIPT Standard for e-Prescribing,** ASC X12N standard for

Health Care Eligibility Benefit and Response, and NCPDP's telecommunications standard. In addition, the final rule identifies three additional electronic tools to be used in implementing e-prescribing:

- NCPDP Formulary and Benefit Standard Implementation Guide, which provides information about drugs covered under the beneficiary's benefit plan
- NCPDP SCRIPT Medication History Transactions, which provides information about medications a beneficiary has been taking
- Fill Status Notification (RxFill), which allows prescribers to receive an electronic notice from the pharmacy regarding the beneficiary's prescription status (CMS, 2013)

Centers for Medicare and Medicaid EHR Incentive Programs

As discussed previously, the Medicare and Medicaid EHR Incentive Programs were established as a part of the HITECH Act to encourage eligible providers (EPs) and eligible hospitals (EHs) to demonstrate Meaningful Use of certified EHR technology. EHR certification for Stage 1 and Stage 2 Meaningful Use requires EPs and EHs to meet specific criteria. Certification requirements are organized according to objectives, measures, specific criteria, and standards. Not all criteria include specific standards, but many do. Examples of standards required by 2014 certification rules include using the HL7 Implementation Guide for CDA in meeting the criteria for providing patients the ability to view online, download, and transmit information about a hospital. Other standards include SNOMED CT, which is required for coding a patient's smoking status, **RxNorm,** which is required for medications, and LOINC, which is required for laboratory tests, among others (HealthIT.gov, 2014).

Office of the National Coordinator for Health Information Technology

As discussed in previous chapters the Office of the National Coordinator for Health Information Technology (ONC) was established in 2004 and charged with providing "leadership for the development and nationwide implementation of an interoperable health information technology infrastructure to improve the quality and efficiency of health care" (HHS, 2008). In 2009, the role of the ONC was strengthened when the HITECH Act legislatively mandated ONC to provide this leadership and oversight (HHS, 2012). Today, the ONC is "the principal federal entity charged with coordination of nationwide

Exhibit 11.1 Excerpt from ONC 2016 Interoperability Standards Advisory

Section I: Best Available Vocabulary/Code Set/Terminology Standards and Implementation Specifications

I-A: Allergies

Interoperability Need: Representing patient allergic reactions

Type	Standard/ Implementation Specification	Standards Process Maturity	Implementation Maturity	Adoption Level	Federally Required	Cost	Test Tool Availability
Standard	SNOMED CT	Final	Production		No	Free	N/A

Limitations, Dependencies, and Preconditions for Consideration:

- SNOMED CT may not be sufficient to differentiate between an allergy or adverse reaction, or the level of severity

Applicable Value Set(s):

Value Set Problem urn:oid:2.16.840.1.113883.3.88.12.3221.7.4

Interoperability Need: Representing patient allergens: medications

Type	Standard/ Implementation Specification	Standards Process Maturity	Implementation Maturity	Adoption Level	Federally Required	Cost	Test Tool Availability
Standard	RxNorm	Final	Production		Yes	Free	N/A
Standard	NDF-RT	Final	Production	Unknown	No	Free	N/A

Source: ONC (2016).

efforts to implement and use the most advanced health information technology and the electronic exchange of health information" (HealthIT.gov, n.d.).

Current ONC initiatives, in addition to implementing HITECH, include implementation of health care IT standards for interoperability. In Chapter Three, the ONC Interoperability Roadmap was introduced and key milestones related to payment reform and outcomes were outlined. The Roadmap also outlines key milestones for the development and implementation of technologies to support interoperability (ONC, 2015). Beginning in 2015, the ONC published its first **Interoperability Standards Advisory,** which has been subsequently updated annually. This Advisory document outlines the ONC-identified "best available" standards and implementation specifications for clinical IT interoperability. The identified standards and specifications in the 2016 Advisory are grouped into three sections:

- Best Available Vocabulary/Code Set/Terminology Standards and Implementation Specifications, which address the "semantics," or standard meanings of codes and terms needed for interoperability

- Best Available Content/Structure Standards and Implementation Specifications, which address the "syntax," or rules by which the common data elements can be shared to achieve interoperability

- Best Available Standards and Implementation Specification for Services, which address infrastructure components needed to achieve interoperability (ONC, 2016)

Each specific standard is identified and defined by six characteristics: process maturity, implementation maturity, adoption level, federal requirement status, cost, and whether a testing tool is available. The Advisory also includes hyperlinks to the standards and implementation guides cited. Exhibit 11.1 is an excerpt from the 2016 Advisory.

OTHER ORGANIZATIONS INFLUENCING HEALTH CARE IT STANDARDS

The following organizations certainly do not represent the full list of bodies that are involved with health care IT standards development and implementation. However, they do represent a few of the most significant nongovernment contributors. ASTM International and HL7 International are accredited SDOs with standards specifically addressing health care information. IHE is a recognized profiling body influencing the implementation of interoperability standards.

ASTM International

ASTM International was formerly known as the American Society for Testing and Materials. ASTM International has more than thirty thousand members from across the globe, and they are responsible for publishing more than twelve thousand standards. ASTM standards range from those that dictate traffic paint to cell phone casings (ASTM, n.d.a, n.d.b). The ASTM Standards for Healthcare Services, Products and Technology include medical device standards and health information standards. The health information standards are managed by the ASTM Committee E31, which focuses on "the development of standards that help doctors and health care practitioners preserve and transfer patient information using EHR technologies" (ASTM, 2014). Of particular note, the E31 standards include the continuity of care record (CCR) discussed further on in this chapter.

HL7 International

HL7 International was founded in 1987. It is an ANSI-accredited SDO "dedicated to providing a comprehensive framework and related standards for the exchange, integration, sharing, and retrieval of electronic health information that supports clinical practice and the management, delivery and evaluation of health services" (HL7, n.d.). The HL7 standards related to interoperability and listed on its website as "Primary Standards," or most used, include the following:

- **Version 2 and 3 HL7 messaging standards,** interoperability specifications for health and medical transactions; these are the standards commonly referred to as HL7
- **Clinical Document Architecture (CDA),** a document markup standard for clinical information exchange among providers based on version 3 of HL7
- **Continuity of Care Document (CCD),** a joint effort with ASTM providing complete guidance for implementation of CDA in the United States
- **Clinical Context Object Workgroup (CCOW),** interoperability standards for visually integrating applications "at the point of use"

These primary standards are not the only ones developed by HL7 International. The organization also publishes Functional EHR and PHR specifications; Arden Syntax, a markup language for sharing medical information; and

GELLO, a query language for medical records. One of most promising of the HL7 International standards is **Fast Healthcare Interoperability Resources (FHIR).** FHIR is built on HL7 but is considered easier to implement because it uses web-based technologies (Ahier, 2015). Several of the HL7 standards, including FHIR, will be explained in greater detail further on in this chapter.

IHE

Integrating the Healthcare Enterprise (IHE) has developed a series of profiles to guide health care documentation sharing. These profiles are not standards but rather include very specific guidance for how existing standards can be implemented to meet clinical needs (IHE, n.d.b). The current IHE profiles are organized as follows:

- Anatomic Pathology
- Cardiology
- Eye Care
- IT Infrastructure
- Laboratory
- Pathology and Laboratory Medicine
- Patient Care Coordination
- Patient Care Device
- Pharmacy
- Quality, Research, and Public Health
- Radiation Oncology
- Radiology

As an example, the IHE Patient Care Coordination Profile group includes twenty individual profiles, and each profile is further identified by its current implementation stage (IHE, n.d.a).

HEALTH IT STANDARDS

The development and implementation of health care IT standards is complex and constantly evolving. The preceding sections of this chapter are intended to provide some insight into the processes of the organizations involved in standards development. The following sections examine examples of the actual standards. This is by no means an exhaustive list of health care IT standards but rather samplings of a few that are commonly used or significant in other ways.

VOCABULARY AND TERMINOLOGY STANDARDS

One of the most difficult problems in exchanging health care information and creating interoperable EHRs is coordinating the vast amount of health information that is generated in diverse locations for patients and populations. The **vocabulary and terminology standards** discussed in this section serve similar purposes—to create a common language that enables different information systems or vendor products to communicate unambiguously with one another. In a very simplified example, a standard vocabulary would ensure that the medical term *myocardial infarction*, for example, is mapped to the term *heart attack* and that both terms share exactly the same attributes. An effective standard vocabulary must also standardize the very complex hierarchy and syntax of the language used in the health industry. This is a complicated and detailed endeavor to say the least. So it is not surprising that, to date, no single vocabulary has emerged to meet all the information exchange needs of the health care sector.

The most widely recognized coding and classification systems—ICD, Current Procedural Terminology (CPT), and diagnosis related groups (DRGs)— were discussed in Chapter Two. Although these systems and the other coding systems discussed in this section do not meet the criteria for full clinical vocabularies, they are used to code diagnoses and procedures and are the basis for information retrieval in health care information systems. Most were originally developed to facilitate disease and procedure information retrieval, but they have been adopted to code for billing services as well. Several of the most commonly used classification systems are actually incorporated across more robust standard vocabularies such as SNOMED CT and UMLS.

The code sets required by HIPAA include the following:

- HCPCS (ancillary services or procedures) (see Chapter Two)
- CPT-4 (physicians procedures) (see Chapter Two)
- CDT (dental terminology)
- ICD-10 (see Chapter Two)
- NDC (national drug codes)

The HITECH Meaningful Use final rule also includes ICD-10 as its classification standard.

The National Committee on Vital and Health Statistics (NCVHS) has the responsibility, under a HIPAA mandate, to recommend uniform data standards for patient medical record information (PMRI). Although no single vocabulary has been recognized by NCVHS as the standard, they have recommended the following as a core set of PMRI terminology standards:

- **Systematized Nomenclature of Medicine—Clinical Terms (SNOMED CT)**
- **Logical Observation Identifiers Names and Codes (LOINC)** laboratory subset
- Several federal drug terminologies, including RxNorm (NCVHS, 2003)

The HITECH Meaningful Use final rule and the ONC Advisory include these standards and the standard for **clinical vaccines administered (CVX).**

In this section we will describe SNOMED CT, LOINC, CVX, and RxNorm, along with the National Library of Medicine's Unified Medical Language (UMLS) (of which RxNorm is one component), which has become the standard for bibliographical searches in health care and has the potential for other uses as well.

Code on Dental Procedures and Nomenclature

The American Dental Association (ADA) publishes the CDT, *Code on Dental Procedures and Nomenclature.* This set of codes is designed to support accurate recording and reporting of dental treatments. The ADA strives to maintain an up-to-date set of codes that reflect actual practice (ADA, n.d.). The code set is divided into twelve sections, as follows (Washington Dental Service, 2012):

I. Diagnostic (D0000–D0999)

II. Preventative (D1000–D1999)

III. Restorative (D2000–D2999)

IV. Endodontics (D3000–D3999)

V. Periodontics (D4000–D4999)

VI. Prosthodontics (D5000–D5899)

VII. Maxillofacial prosthetics (D5900–D5999)

VIII. Implant services (D6000–D6199)

IX. Prosthodontics (D6200–D6999)

X. Oral and maxillofacial surgery (D7000–7999)

XI.   Orthodontics (D8000–8999)

XII.   General Services (D9000–D9999)

National Drug Codes

The **National Drug Code (NDC)** is the universal product identifier for all human drugs. The Drug Listing Act of 1972 requires registered drug companies to provide the Food and Drug Administration (FDA) a current listing of all drugs "manufactured, prepared, propagated, compounded, or processed by it for commercial distribution" (FDA, 2016). The FDA, in turn, assigns the unique, three-segment NDC (listed as package code in the following example) and maintains the information in the National Drug Code Directory. The NDC Directory is updated twice each month. Data maintained for each drug include up to sixteen fields. The information for the common over-the-counter drug Tylenol PM (Extra Strength), for example, is as follows:

Product NDC: 50580–176

Product Type Name: Human OTC Drug Proprietary Name: Tylenol PM (Extra Strength)

Non-proprietary Name: Acetaminophen and Diphenhydramine Hydrochloride

Dosage Formulation: Tablet, Coated Route Name: Oral

Start Marketing Date: 12–01–1991 End Marketing Date: <blank field>

Marketing Category Name: OTC Monograph Final Application Number: part338

Labeler Name: McNeil Consumer Healthcare Div. McNeil-PPC, Inc Substance Name: Acetaminophen; Diphenhydramine Hydrochloride Strength Number/Unit: 500 mg/1, 25 mg/1

Pharm Class: Histamine H1 Receptor Antagonists [MoA], Histamine-1 Receptor Antagonist [EPC]

Package Code: 50580–176–10

Package Description: 1 Bottle, Plastic in 1 Carton (50580–176–10) > 100 tablet, coated in 1 Bottle, Plastic

DEA classification: <blank> (US FDA, 2016)

Systematized Nomenclature of Medicine—Clinical Terms

Systematized Nomenclature of Medicine—Clinical Terms (SNOMED CT) is a comprehensive clinical terminology developed specifically to facilitate the electronic storage and retrieval of detailed clinical information. It is the result of collaboration between the College of American Pathologists (CAP) and the United Kingdom's National Health Service (NHS). SNOMED CT merges CAP's SNOMED Reference Terminology, an older classification system used to group diseases, and the NHS's Clinical Terms Version 3 (also known as Read Codes), an established clinical terminology used in Great Britain and elsewhere. As a result, SNOMED CT is based on decades of research. As of April 2007 SNOMED is owned, maintained, and distributed by the International Health Terminology Standards Development Organization (IHTSDO), a nonprofit association based in Denmark. The National Library of Medicine is the US member of the IHTSDO and distributes SNOMED CT at no cost within the United States (IHTSDO, n.d.; NLM, 2016b).

Logical Observation Identifiers Names and Codes

The Logical Observation Identifiers Names and Codes (LOINC) system was developed to facilitate the electronic transmission of laboratory results to hospitals, physicians, third-party payers, and other users of laboratory data. Initiated in 1994 by the Regenstrief Institute at Indiana University, LOINC provides a standard set of universal names and codes for identifying individual laboratory and clinical results. These standard codes enable users to merge clinical results from disparate sources (Regenstrief Institute, n.d.).

LOINC codes have a fixed length field of seven characters. Current codes range from three to seven characters long. There are six parts in the LOINC name structure: component/analyte, property, time aspect, system, scale type, and method. The syntax for a name follows this pattern (Case, 2011):

LOINC Code: Component: Property Measured: Timing: System: Scale: Method

Example

5193–8:Hepatitis B virus surface Ab: ACnc:Pt:Ser:Qn:EIA

Clinical Vaccines Administered

The Centers for Disease Control and Prevention (CDC) National Center of Immunization and Respiratory Diseases (NCIRD) developed the Clinical Vaccines Administered (CVX) as standard codes and terminology for use with HL7 messaging standards. Table 11.2 is an excerpt from the full CVX table.

Table 11.2. Excerpt from CVX (clinical vaccines administered)

Short Description	Full Vaccine Name	CVX Code	Status	Last Date Updated	Notes
adenovirus types 4 and 7	adenovirus, type 4 and type 7, live, oral	143	Active	3/20/2011	This vaccine is administered as two tablets.
anthrax	anthrax vaccine	24	Active	5/28/2010	
BCG	Bacillus Calmette-Guerin vaccine	19	Active	5/28/2010	
DTaP, IPV, Hib, HepB	Diphtheria and Tetanus Toxoids and Acellular Pertussis Absorbed, Inactivated Poliovirus, Haemophilus b Conjugate (Meningococcal Outer Membrane Protein Complex), and Hepatitis B (Recombinant) Vaccine	146	Pending	9/21/2015	Note that this vaccine is different from CVX 132.
influenza, seasonal, injectable	influenza, seasonal, injectable	141	Active	7/17/2013	This is one of two codes replacing CVX 15, which is being retired.
influenza, live, intranasal	influenza virus vaccine, live, attenuated, for intranasal use	111	Inactive	5/28/2010	

Source: CDC (2016).

RxNorm

The National Library of Medicine (NLM) produces RxNorm, which serves two purposes: as "a normalized naming system for generic and brand name drugs and as a tool for supporting semantic interoperation between drug terminologies and pharmacy knowledge–based systems" (NLM, 2016a). The goal of RxNorm is to enable disparate health information systems to communicate with one another in an unambiguous manner.

There are twelve separate RxNorm data files that are released on a monthly basis. The files show this information:

- Drug names and unique identifiers
- Relationships
- Attributes
- Semantic types
- Data history (three files)
- Obsolete data (three files)
- Metadata (two files)

The following example from the first RxNorm data file represents the "concept," Azithromycin 250 MG Oral Capsule, with the unique identifier 141962 (NLM, 2016a):

```
141962|ENG||||||944489|944489|141962||RXNORM|SCD|141962|
    Azithromycin 250 MG Oral Capsule||N||
```

Unified Medical Language System

The NLM began the **Unified Medical Language System (UMLS)** project in 1986, and it is ongoing today. The purpose of the UMLS project is "to facilitate the development of computer systems that behave as if they 'understand' the meaning of the language of biomedicine and health. The UMLS provides data for system developers as well as search and report functions for less technical users" (NLM, 2016b).

The UMLS has three basic components, called *knowledge sources:*

- **UMLS Metathesaurus**, which contains concepts from more than one hundred source vocabularies. All the common health information vocabularies, including SNOMED CT, ICD, and CPT, along with approximately one hundred other vocabularies, including RxNorm, are incorporated into the metathesaurus. The metathesaurus project's goal is to incorporate and map existing vocabularies into a single system.
- **UMLS Semantic Network**, which defines 133 broad categories and dozens of relationships between categories for labeling the biomedical domain. The semantic network contains information about the categories (such as "Disease or Syndrome" and "Virus") to which

metathesaurus concepts are assigned. The semantic network also outlines the relationships among the categories (for example, "Virus" causes "Disease or Syndrome").

- **SPECIALIST Lexicon and Lexical Tools.** The **SPECIALIST lexicon** is a dictionary of English words, common and biomedical, which exist to support natural language processing.

The UMLS products are widely used in NLM's own applications, such as PubMed, and they are available to other organizations free of charge, provided the users submit a license agreement (NLM, 2016b). Currently, components of UMLS are incorporated into other standards and profiles for health care IT interoperability.

DATA EXCHANGE AND MESSAGING STANDARDS

The ability to exchange and integrate data among health care applications is critical to the success of any overall health care information system, whether an organizational, regional, or national level of integration is desired. Although there is some overlap, these standards differ from the vocabulary standards because their major purpose is to standardize the actual "messaging" between health care information systems. Messaging standards are key to interoperability. In this section we will look at a few of the standards that have been developed for this purpose. There are others, and new needs are continually being identified. However, the following groups of standards are recognized as important to the health care sector, and together they provide examples of broad standards addressing all types of applications and specific standards addressing one type of application:

- Health Level Seven Messaging standards (HL7)
- Digital Imaging and Communications in Medicine (DICOM)
- National Council for Prescription Drug Programs (NCPDP)
- ANSI **ASC X12N standards**

Two other groups of standards discussed in this section actually combine some features of messaging standards and content standards:

- Continuity of Care Document (CCD)
- Fast Health Interoperability Resources (FHIR)

HIPAA specifically requires covered entities to comply with specific ANSI X12N and NCPCP. HITECH and the ONC Advisory also cite specific messaging standards and the CCD. FHIR is currently under development by HL7 International and is being cited by health care IT professionals as a major advancement toward true interoperability.

Health Level Seven Standards

Two versions of HL7 messaging standards, Version 2 and Version 3, are listed by HL7 International as "primary," or commonly used. HL7 v2 remains popular in spite of the development of HL7 v3. HL7 v2 was first introduced in 1987 and has become the "workhorse of electronic data exchange" (HL7, n.d.). HL7 v3 incorporates the root elements of XML and, as such, is a significant change from early versions. See the HL7 Perspective for an example of HL7 v3.

Digital Imaging and Communications in Medicine Standards

The growth of digital diagnostic imaging (such as CT scans and MRIs) gave rise to the need for a standard for the electronic transfer of these images between devices manufactured by different vendors. The American College of Radiology (ACR) and the National Electrical Manufacturers Association (NEMA) published the first standard, a precursor to the current Digital Imaging and Communications in Medicine (DICOM) standard, in 1985. The goals of DICOM are to "achieve compatibility and to improve workflow efficiency between imaging systems and other information systems in healthcare environments worldwide." It is used by all of the major diagnostic medical imaging vendors, which translates to its use in nearly every medical profession that uses images (DICOM, 2016).

National Council for Prescription Drug Program Standards

The National Council for Prescription Drug Programs (NCPDP), an ANSI-accredited SDO with more than 1,600 members representing the pharmacy services industry, has developed a set of standards for the electronic submission of third-party drug claims (NCPDP, 2012). These standards not only include the telecommunication standards and batch standards required by HIPAA but also the SCRIPT standard required for e-prescribing, among others. Of note, the SCRIPT standard currently incorporates the RxNorm as its standardized medication nomenclature. The NCPDP Provider Identification

The following object identifiers (OIDs) are used within the Good Health Hospital (GHH):

- GHH Placer Order IDs: 2.16.840.1.113883.19.1122.14
- GHH Lab Filler Order IDs: 2.16.840.1.113883.19.1122.4
- The code system for the observation within the GHH is LOINC: 2.16.840.1.113883.6.1
- The HL7 Confidentiality Code system: 2.16.840.1.113883.5.25

The HL7 v3 Message: Domain Content Excerpt

The "Domain Content" starts with its own root element: observationEvent. The elements within specify the type of observation, the ID, the time of the observation, statusCode, and the results. The value for the actual result is shown in the value element. The interpretationCode element shows that the value has been interpreted as high (H), while referenceRange provides the normal values for this particular observation.

```
<observationEvent>
<id root="2.16.840.1.113883.19.1122.4" extension="1045813"
assigningAuthorityName="GHH LAB Filler Orders"/>
<code code="1554-5" codeSystemName="LN"
codeSystem="2.16.840.1.113883.6.1"
```

Number is a unique identifier of more than seventy-five thousand pharmacies. Table 11.3 presents excerpts from the NCPDP Data Dictionary, which outlines a few of the Transmission Header Segment requirements. The entire data dictionary table is more than seventy pages long (CMS, 2002).

ANSI ASC X12N Standards

The ANSI Accredited Standards Committee (ASC) X12 develops standards in X12 and XML formats for the electronic exchange of business information. One ASC X12 subcommittee, X12N, has been specifically designated to deal

```
displayName="GLUCOSE∧POST 12H CFST:MCNC:PT:SER/PLAS:QN"/>
<statusCode code="completed"/>
<effectiveTime value="200202150730"/>
<priorityCode code="R"/>
<confidentialityCode code="N" codeSystem="2.16.840.1.113883.5.25"/>
<value xsi:type="PQ" value="182" unit="mg/dL"/>
<interpretationCode code="H"/>
<referenceRange>
<interpretationRange>
<value xsi:type="IVL_PQ">
<low value="70" unit="mg/dL"/>
<high value="105" unit="mg/dL"/>
</value>
<interpretationCode code="N"/>
</interpretationRange>
</referenceRange>
</assignedEntity>
</author>
```

Source: Spronk (2007). http://www.ringholm.de/docs/04300_en.htm. Used under CC BY-SA 3.0, https://creativecommons.org/licenses/by-sa/3.0/. Used with permission.

with electronic data interchange (EDI) standards in the insurance industry, and this subcommittee has a special health care task group, known as TG2. According to the X12 TG2 website, "the purpose of the Health Care Task group shall be the development and maintenance of data standards (both national and international) which shall support the exchange of business information for health care administration. Health care data includes, but is not limited to, such business functions as eligibility, referrals and authorizations, claims, claim status, payment and remittance advice, and provider directories" (ASC X12, n.d.). To this end ASC X12N has developed a set of standards that are monitored and updated through ASC X12N work groups.

Table 11.3 Excerpt from NCPDP data dictionary

NCPDP Data Dictionary Name	Field Number	NCPDP Definition of Field	Version D.0 Format	Valid Values per the Standard
Service Provider ID Qualifier	202-B2	Code qualifying the Service Provider ID	X(02)	Blank=Not Specified 01=National Provider Identifier (NPI) 02=Blue Cross 03=Blue Shield 04=Medicare 05=Medicaid 06=UPIN 07=NCPDP Provider ID 08=State License 09=Champus 10=Health Industry Number (HIN) 11=Federal Tax ID 12=Drug Enforcement Administration (DEA) 13=State Issued 14=Plan Specific 15=HCID (HC IDea) 99=Other
Service Provider ID	201-B1	ID assigned to pharmacy or provider	X(15)	N/A
Date of Service	401-D1	Identifies the date the prescription was filled or professional service rendered or subsequent payer began coverage following Part A expiration in a long-term care setting only	9(08)	Format=CCYYMMDD

Source: CMS (2002).

Table 11.4. X12 TG2 work groups

Work Group Number	Work Group Name
WG1	Health Care Eligibility
WG2	Health Care Claims
WG3	Claim Payments
WG4	Enrollments
WG5	Claims Status
WG9	Patient Information
WG10	Health Care Services Review
WG15	Provider Information
WG20	Insurance—824 Implementation Guide
WG21	Health Care Regulation Advisory/Collaboration

Source: ASC X12 (n.d.).

Table 11.4 lists the current X12 work group areas. A portion of the X12 5010 Professional Claim standard is shown in Exhibit 11.2. The standard for Professional Claim alone is more than ninety pages in length.

Continuity of Care Document (CCD)

The Continuity of Care Document (CCD) is a standard for the electronic exchange of patient summary information, so-called transportable patient care information. The current CCD standard is actually a merger of two other standards: the HL7 Clinical Document Architecture (CDA) standard and the ASTM Continuity of Care Record (CCR). There has been some discussion among experts about the CCR and CCD being competing standards, but HL7 has taken the position that CCD is an implementation of CCR and simply an evolution of the CCR (Rouse, 2010). Although discussed in this section, the CCD standard is not solely a content standard; it includes elements of a data exchange standard. It has an XML-based specification for exchanging patient summary data, but it also includes a standard outline of the summary content. The content sections of the CCD include the following:

- Payers
- Advance Directives
- Support

Exhibit 11.2 X12 5010 professional claim standard

Element Identifier	Description	ID	Min. Max.	Usage Reg.	Loop	Loop Repeat	Values
						5010	
				837-P 5010			
ISA	**INTERCHANGE CONTROL HEADER**		1	**R**	—	1	
ISA01	Authorization Information Qualifier	ID	2-2	R			00, 03
ISA02	Authorization Information	AN	10-10	R			
ISA03	Security Information Qualifier	ID	2-2	R			00, 01
ISA04	Security Information	AN	10-10	R			
ISA05	Interchange ID Qualifier	ID	2-2	R			01, 14, 20, 27, 28, 29, 30, 33, ZZ
ISA06	Interchange Sender ID	AN	15-15	R			
ISA07	Interchange ID Qualifier	ID	2-2	R			01, 14, 20, 27, 28, 29, 30, 33, ZZ
ISA08	Interchange Receiver ID	AN	15-15	R			
ISA09	Interchange Date	DT	6-6	R			YYMMDD
ISA10	Interchange Time	TM	4-4	R			HHMM

Segment	Description	Type	Min-Max	Req		Value
ISA11	Interchange Control Standards ID		1-1	R		
ISA12	Interchange Control Version Number	ID	5-5	R		00501
ISA13	Interchange Control Number	N0	9-9	R		
ISA14	Acknowledgement Requested	ID	1-1	R		0, 1
ISA15	Usage Indicator	ID	1-1	R		P, T
ISA16	Component Element Separator	AN	1-1	R		
GS	**FUNCTIONAL GROUP HEADER**		**1**	**R**	——	**1**
GS01	Functional Identifier Code	ID	2-2	R		
GS02	Application Sender Code	AN	2-15	R		
GS03	Application Receiver Code	AN	2-15	R		
GS04	Date	DT	8-8	R		CCYYMMDD
GS05	Time	TM	4-8	R		HHMM
GS06	Group Control Number	N0	1-9	R		
GS07	Responsible Agency Code	ID	1-2	R		X
GS08	Version Identifier Code	AN	1-12	R		005010X222

Source: ASC X12 (n.d.).

- Functional Status
- Problems
- Family History
- Social History
- Allergies
- Medications
- Medical Equipment
- Immunizations
- Vital Signs
- Results
- Procedures
- Encounters
- Plan of Care (Dolin, 2011)

Fast Health Interoperability Resources (FHIR)

Fast Health Interoperability Resources (FHIR) is currently being tested (as of this text's publication date) by a range of health care IT professionals. So far, the testing has led to predominantly positive results, with many citing FHIR as having the potential to truly accelerate health care IT interoperability. The difference between FHIR and other standards is that it goes beyond the function of a traditional messaging system and includes modern web services to exchange clinical information. FHIR builds on the HL7 Clinical Document Architecture (CDA) and HL7 messaging, However, unlike CDA, FHIR enables granular pieces of information rather than an entire summary document to be shared (Ahier, 2015). According to Ahier (2015), FHIR offers easy-to-use tools not only to build faster and more efficient data exchange mechanisms but also to use personal health care information to create "innovative new apps" with the potential to create a "plug and play platform . . . similar to the Apple app store."

HEALTH RECORD CONTENT AND FUNCTIONAL STANDARDS

Health record content and functional standards are not the same as messaging or data exchange standards. These standards outline what should be included in an EHR or other clinical record. They do not include technical specifications but rather the EHR content requirements. As mentioned previously, the CCD and FHIR have content standards within them, along with messaging standards. HL7 EHR-S (Electronic Health Record-System) Functional Model is an example of a comprehensive **EHR content and functional standard** that does not include technical specifications.

HL7 EHR-S Functional Model

The **HL7 Health Record-System (EHR-S) Functional Model,** Release 2 was published by Health Level Seven International in 2014. The purpose of this functional model is to outline important features and functions that should be contained in an EHR. Targeted users of the functional model include vendors and care providers, and it has been recognized by the ISO as an international standard (ISO 10781). The stated benefits of the functional model are as follows:

- Provide an international standard for global use.
- Enable a consistent framework for the development of profiles that are conformant to the base model.
- Support the goal of interoperability.
- Provide a standard that is easily readable and understandable to an "everyday person," which enables a user to articulate his or her business requirements (HL7, 2014).

The EHR-S Functional Model is divided into seven sections:

1. Overarching (OV)
2. Care Provision (CP)
3. Care Provision Support (CPS)
4. Population Health Support (POP)
5. Administrative Support (AS)
6. Record Infrastructure (RI)
7. Trust Infrastructure (TI)

Each function within the model is identified by section and described by specific elements. Table 11.5 is an example of the function list for managing a problem list. *Note:* The list type indicates Header (H), Function (F), or Conformance Criteria (C).

Table 11.5. Excerpt from the HL7 EHR-S Functional Model

ID	Type	Name	Statement	Description	Conformance Criteria
CP.1	H	Manage Clinical History	Manage the patient's clinical history lists used to present summary or detailed information on patient health history.	Patient Clinical History lists are used to present succinct snapshots of critical health information including patient history, allergy intolerance and adverse reactions, medications, problems, strengths, immunizations, medical equipment/devices, and patient and family preferences.	
CP.1.4	F	Manage Problem List	Create and maintain patient-specific problem lists.	A problem list may include but is not limited to chronic conditions, diagnoses, or symptoms, injury/poisoning (both intentional and unintentional), adverse effects of medical care (e.g., drugs, surgical), functional limitations, visit or stay-specific conditions, diagnoses, or symptoms	
CP.1.4	C				1. The system SHALL provide the ability to manage, as discrete data, all active problems associated with a patient.
CP.1.4	C				2. The system SHALL capture and render a history of all problems associated with a patient.
CP.1.4	C				3. The system SHALL provide the ability to manage relevant dates including the onset date and resolution date of problem.

Source: HL7 EHR-System Functional Model, Release 2. (2014). Retrieved September 6, 2016, from http://www.hl7.org/implement/standards/product_brief.cfm?product_id=269. Used with permission.

SUMMARY

Multiple standard-setting organizations have roles in standards development, leading to a somewhat confusing array of current health care IT standards that address code sets, vocabularies and terminology, data exchange and messaging, and content and function. The standards developing organizations and standards discussed in this chapter, along with other general IT standards, enable health care information systems to be interoperable, portable, and to exchange data. The future of our health care system relies on having interoperable EHRs and other health care information systems. Clearly, this will not be realized without standards. The government, as well as the private sector, is actively engaged in promoting the development of best practices for implementing health care IT standards. HIPAA and CMS, for example, have had a significant impact on the adoption of specific health care information standards that focus on code set, terminology, and transactions. The ONC is charged with coordinating the national efforts for achieving interoperability among health care information systems, which has led to their publication of the Interoperability Roadmap and annual Interoperability Standards Advisories. Both of these tools will likely have a significant impact on the direction of national standards development and cooperation among the many standards developing organizations.

KEY TERMS

Accredited Standards Committee (ASC)

Ad hoc standards development process

American National Standards Institute (ANSI)

ASC X12N standards

ASTM International (ASTM)

CEN-CENELEC Management Centre (CCMC)

Clinical Context Object Workgroup (CCOW)

Clinical Document Architecture (CDA)

Clinical vaccines administered (CVX)

CMS e-prescribing

Code on Dental Procedures and Nomenclature (CDT)

Connecting Health Care for the Nation: A Shared Nationwide Interoperability Roadmap

Consensus standards development process

Continuity of Care Document (CCD)

Data exchange

De facto standards development process

Designated standard maintenance organizations (DSMOs)

Digital Imaging and Communication in Medicine (DICOM)

EHR content and functional standard

Electronic data interchange (EDI)

European Committee for
    Standardization (CEN)
Extensible markup language (XML)
Fast Healthcare Interoperability
    Resources (FHIR)
Government mandate standards
    development process
Health Level Seven International (HL7)
Health Insurance Portability and
    Accountability Act (HIPAA)
HL7 Health Record-System (EHR-S)
    Functional Model
HL7 messaging standards
Integrating the Healthcare Enterprise
    (IHE)
International Health Terminology
    SDO (IHTSDO)
International Organization for
    Standardization (ISO)
Interoperability
Interoperability Standards Advisory
Logical Observation Identifiers Names
    and Codes (LOINC)

National Council for Prescription
    Drug Programs (NCPDP)
National Drug Code (NDC)
Office of the National Coordinator
    for Health Information Technology
    (ONC)
RxNorm
SCRIPT Standard for e-Prescribing
SPECIALIST lexicon
Standards
Standards developing organizations
    (SDOs)
Standards Development Process
Systematized Nomenclature of
    Medicine—Clinical Terms
    (SNOMED CT)
UMLS Metathesaurus
UMLS Semantic Network
Unified Medical Language System
    (UMLS)
Vocabulary and terminology
    standards

LEARNING ACTIVITIES

1. Standards development is a dynamic process. Select one or more of the standards listed in this chapter and conduct an Internet search for information on that standard. Has the standard changed? What are the current issues concerning the standard?

2. Visit a hospital IT department and speak with a clinical analyst or other person who works with clinical applications. Investigate the standards that the hospital's applications use. Discuss any issues concerning use of these standards.

3. Visit the ONC website at HealthIT.gov. Identify the current efforts of the ONC to promote adoption of health care IT standards for interoperability. What impact do you believe these initiatives will have? Why?

4. As you reflect on the information from in this chapter and your own research, compare and contrast the intent of code set, vocabulary and

terminology, data exchange, messaging, and content and functional health care IT standards. How are these types of standards different? How are they related? Are all needed for complete interoperability? Why or why not?

5. Some health care IT professionals believe that the technology currently exists for achieving interoperability among health care information systems, particularly EHRs. They contend that the remaining barriers are nontechnical. Do you agree with this sentiment? Why or why not? Support your answer.

REFERENCES

Accredited Standards Committee X12 (ASC X12). (n.d.). *X12N/TG2: Health care purpose and scope.* Retrieved September 6, 2016, from http://www.wpc-edi.com/onlyconnect/TG2.htm

Ahier, B. (2015, Jan. 6). *FHIR and the future of interoperability.* Retrieved November 10, 2016, from http://www.healthcareitnews.com/news/fhir-and-future-interoperability

American Dental Association (ADA). (n.d.). *Code on dental procedures and nomenclature (CDT code).* Retrieved September 7, 2016, from http://www.ada.org/en/publications/cdt/

American National Standards Institute (ANSI). (n.d.a). *About ANSI.* Retrieved September 7, 2016, from https://www.ansi.org/about_ansi/overview/overview.aspx?menuid=1

American National Standards Institute (ANSI). (n.d.b). *Resources: Standards developing organizations (SDOs).* Retrieved September 7, 2016, from https://www.standardsportal.org/usa_en/resources/sdo.aspx

American National Standards Institute (ANSI). (n.d.c). *Standards activities overview.* Retrieved September 7, 2016, from https://www.ansi.org/standards_activities/overview/overview.aspx?menuid=3

ASTM International. (2014, Nov.). *ASTM standards for healthcare services, products and technology.* Retrieved September 5, 2016, from http://www.astm.org/ABOUT/images/Medical_sector.pdf

ASTM International. (n.d.a). *ASTM video.* Retrieved September 5, 2016, from https://www.astm.org/about-astm-corporate.html

ASTM International. (n.d.b). *Standards & publications.* Retrieved September 6, 2016, from https://www.astm.org/Standard/standards-and-publications.html

Boone, K. W. (2012a, April 9). *Health IT standards 101.* Retrieved September 7, 2016, from http://www.healthcareitnews.com/blog/health-it-standards-101

Boone, K. W. (2012b, March 26). *An informatics model for HealthIT standards* [Web log post]. Retrieved September 22, 2016, from http://motorcycleguy.blogspot .com/2012/03/informatics-model-for-healthit.html

Case, J. (2011). *Using RELMA or . . . In search of the missing LOINC* [PowerPoint]. Retrieved March 2012 from http://loinc.org/slideshows/lab-loinc-tutorial

CEN CENELEC. (n.d.). *About us.* Retrieved September 7, 2016, from http://www .cencenelec.eu/aboutus/Pages/default.aspx

Centers for Disease Control and Prevention (CDC). (2016, June 21). IIS: HL7 standard code set CVX—Vaccines administered. *Vaccines and Immunizations.* Retrieved September 6, 2016, from http://www2a.cdc.gov/vaccines/iis/ iisstandards/vaccines.asp?rpt=cvx

Centers for Medicare and Medicaid (CMS). (2002). NCPDP flat file format. *NCPDP reference manual.* Retrieved September 6, 2016, from http://www.cms.gov/ Medicare/Billing/ElectronicBillingEDITrans/downloads/NCPDPflatfile.pdf

Centers for Medicare and Medicaid (CMS). (2013, April 2). *Adopted standard and transactions, adopted part D: E-prescribing standards.* Retrieved September 5, 2016, from https://www.cms.gov/Medicare/E-Health/Eprescribing/Adopted-Standard-and-Transactions.html

Centers for Medicare and Medicaid (CMS). (2016a, June 23). *Adopted standards and operating rules.* Retrieved September 5, 2016, from https://www.cms.gov/ Regulations-and-Guidance/Administrative-Simplification/HIPAA-ACA/ AdoptedStandardsandOperatingRules.html

Centers for Medicare and Medicaid (CMS). (2016b, June 21). *Standards-setting and related organizations.* Retrieved September 5, 2016, from https://www.cms.gov/ Regulations-and-Guidance/Administrative-Simplification/HIPAA-ACA/ StandardsSettingandRelatedOrganizations.html

Department of Health and Human Services (HHS). (2008). *The ONC-coordinated federal health information technology strategic plan: 2008–2012.* Retrieved August 2008 from http://www.hhs.gov/healthit/resources/ HITStrategicPlanSummary.pdf

Department of Health and Human Services (HHS). (2012). *About ONC.* The Office of the National Coordinator for Health Information Technology. Retrieved March 2012 from http://healthit.hhs.gov/portal/server.pt/community/healthit_ hhs_gov_onc/1200

DICOM. (2016). *Strategic document.* DICOM: Digital Imaging and Communications in Medicine. Retrieved September 6, 2016, from http://dicom.nema.org/dicom/ geninfo/Strategy.pdf

Dolin, B. (2011). *CDA and CCD for patient summaries.* Retrieved November 10, 2016, from https://www.hl7.org/documentcenter/public_temp_143D9F91-1C23-BA17-0C15A882DDE6815D/calendarofevents/himss/2012/ CDA%20and%20CCD%20for%20Patient%20Summaries.pdf

European Committee for Standardization (CEN). (n.d.). *CEN/TC 251: Health informatics.* Retrieved September 7, 2016, from https://standards.cen.eu/dyn/www/f?p=204:29:0::::FSP_ORG_ID,FSP_LANG_ID:6232,25&cs=1FFF281A84075B985DD039F95A2CAB820#1

Food and Drug Administration (FDA). (2016, April 22). *National drug code directory.* Retrieved September 7, 2016, from http://www.fda.gov/Drugs/InformationOnDrugs/ucm142438.htm

Hammond, W., & Cimino, J. (2006). Standards in biomedical informatics. In E. Shortliff & J. Cimino (Eds.), *Biomedical informatics* (pp. 265–311). New York, NY: Springer-Verlag.

HealthIT.gov (2014). *Meaningful use table series.* Retrieved September 22, 2016, from https://www.healthit.gov/sites/default/files/meaningfulusetablesseries1_110112.pdf

HealthIT.gov. (n.d.). *About ONC.* Retrieved September 5, 2016, from https://www.healthit.gov/newsroom/about-onc

Health Level Seven International (HL7). (2014). *HL7 EHR-System Functional Model, release 2.* Retrieved September 6, 2016, from http://www.hl7.org/implement/standards/product_brief.cfm?product_id=269

Health Level Seven International (HL7). (n.d.). *HL7 version 2 product suite.* Retrieved September 6, 2016, from http://www.hl7.org/implement/standards/product_brief.cfm?product_id=185

Integrating the Healthcare Enterprise (IHE). (n.d.a.). *IHE patient care coordination profiles.* Retrieved November 10, 2016, from http://wiki.ihe.net/index.php/Profiles#IHE_Patient_Care_Coordination_Profiles

Integrating the Healthcare Enterprise (IHE). (n.d.b.). *Profiles.* Retrieved November 10, 2016, from https://www.ihe.net/Profiles/

International Health Terminology Standards Development Organization (IHTSDO). (n.d.). *History of SNOMED CT.* Retrieved September 7, 2016, from http://www.ihtsdo.org/snomed-ct/what-is-snomed-ct/history-of-snomed-ct

International Organization for Standardization (ISO). (n.d.). *About ISO.* Retrieved September 7, 2016, from http://www.iso.org/iso/home/about.htm

National Committee on Vital and Health Statistics (NCVHS). (2003, Nov. 5). *Letter to the secretary: Recommendations for PMRI terminology standards.* Retrieved March 2012 from http://www.ncvhs.hhs.gov/031105lt3.pdf

National Council for Prescription Drug Programs (NCPDP). (2012). *About.* Retrieved March 2012 from http://www.ncpdp.org/about.aspx

National Library of Medicine (NLM). (2016a, Jan. 4). *RxNorm overview.* Unified Medical Language System (UMLS). Retrieved September 6, 2016, from https://www.nlm.nih.gov/research/umls/rxnorm/overview.html

National Library of Medicine (NLM). (2016b, July 13). *SNOMED CT.* Retrieved September 7, 2016, from https://www.nlm.nih.gov/healthit/snomedct/

Office of the National Coordinator for Health Information Technology (ONC). (2015). *Connecting health and care for the nation: A shared nationwide interoperability roadmap.* Retrieved August 3, 2016, from https://www.healthit.gov/sites/default/files/nationwide-interoperability-roadmap-draft-version-1.0.pdf

Office of the National Coordinator for Health Information Technology (ONC). (2016). *2016 interoperability standards advisory: Best available standards and implementation specifications.* Retrieved September 5, 2016, from https://www.healthit.gov/sites/default/files/2016-interoperability-standards-advisory-final-508.pdf

Regenstrief Institute, Inc. (n.d.). *About LOINC.* Retrieved September 7, 2016, from https://loinc.org/background

Rouse, M. (2010, May). *Continuity of care document.* SearchHealthIT. Retrieved March 2012 from http://searchhealthit.techtarget.com/definition/Continuity-of-Care-Document-CCD

Spronk, R. (2007). *HL7 message examples: Version 2 and version 3.* Retrieved from http://www.ringholm.de/docs/04300_en.htm

United States Food & Drug Administration (US FDA). (2016). *National drug code directory.* Retrieved November 10, 2016, from http://www.fda.gov/Drugs/InformationOnDrugs/ucm142438.htm

Washington Dental Service. (2012). *CDT procedure code information.* Retrieved March 2012 from http://wwwldeltadentalwa.com/Dentist/Public/ResourceCenter/CDT%20Procedure%20Codes.aspx

Senior-Level Management Issues Related to Health Care Information Systems Management

CHAPTER 12

IT Alignment and Strategic Planning

LEARNING OBJECTIVES

- To be able to understand the importance of an IT strategic plan.
- To review the components of the IT strategic plan.
- To be able to understand the processes for developing an IT strategy.
- To be able to discuss the challenges of developing an IT strategy.
- To describe the Gartner Hype Cycle recognizing the wide range of emerging technologies at various stages of maturity.

Information technology (IT) investments serve to advance organizational performance. These investments should enable the organization to reduce costs, improve service, enhance the quality of care, and, in general, achieve its strategic objectives. The goal of **IT alignment** and strategic planning is to ensure a strong and clear relationship between IT investment decisions and the health care organization's overall strategies, goals, and objectives. For example, an organization's decision to invest in a new claims adjudication system should be the clear result of a goal of improving the effectiveness of its claims processing process. An organization's decision to implement a care coordination application should be a consequence of its population health management strategy.

Developing a sound alignment can be very important for one simple reason—if you define the IT agenda incorrectly or even partially correctly, you run the risk that significant organizational resources will be misdirected; the resources will not be put to furthering strategically important areas. This risk has nothing to do with how well you execute the IT direction you choose. Being on time, on budget, and on specification is of little value to the organization if it is doing the wrong thing!

IT PLANNING OBJECTIVES

The IT strategic planning process has several objectives:

- To ensure that information technology plans and activities align with the plans and activities of the organization; in other words, the IT needs of each aspect of organizational strategy are clear, and the portfolio of IT plans and activities can be mapped to organizational strategies and operational needs

- To ensure that the alignment is comprehensive; in other words, each aspect of strategy has been addressed from an IT perspective that recognizes not all aspects of strategy have an IT component, and not all components will be funded

- To identify non-IT organizational initiatives needed to ensure maximum leverage of the IT initiative (for example, process reengineering)

- To ensure that the organization has not missed a strategic IT opportunity, such as those that might result from new technologies

- To develop a tactical plan that details approved project descriptions, timetables, budgets, staffing plans, and plan risk factors

- To create a communication tool that can inform the organization of the IT initiatives that will and will not be undertaken

- To establish a political process that helps ensure the plan results have sufficient organizational support

At the end of the alignment and strategic-planning process, an organization should have an outline that at a high level resembles Table 12.1. With this outline, leadership can see the IT investments needed to advance each of the organization's strategies. For example, the goal of improving the quality of patient care may lead the organization to invest in databases to measure and report quality, predictive algorithms to identify patients at risk of readmission, and the EHR.

In many ways the content of Table 12.1 is deceiving. It presents a tidy, orderly linkage between the IT agenda and the strategies of the organization. One might assume this linkage is established through a linear, rational, and straightforward series of steps. But the process of arriving at a series of connections similar to those in Table 12.1 is complex, iterative, and at times driven by politics and instincts.

Table 12.1 IT initiatives linked to organizational goals

Goal	IT Initiatives
Research and education	Research patient data registry
	Genetics and genomics platform
	Grants management
Patient care: quality improvement	Quality measurement databases
	Order entry
	Electronic health record
Patient care: sharing data across the system	Enterprise master person index
	Clinical data repository
	Common infrastructure
Patient care: non-acute services	Nursing documentation
	Transition of care
Financial stability	Revenue system enhancements
	Payroll-personnel system
	Cost accounting

The development of well-aligned IT strategies has been notoriously difficult for many years, and there appears to be no reason such an alignment will become significantly easier over time.

OVERVIEW OF STRATEGY

Strategy is the determination of the basic long-term goals and objectives of an organization, the adoption of the course of action, and the allocation of resources necessary to carry out those actions (Chandler, 1962). Strategy seeks to answer questions such as, where does this organization need to go, and how will it get there? Where should the organization focus its management attention and expenditures?

The development of an organization's strategy has two major components: formulation and implementation (Henderson & Venkatraman, 1993).

Formulation

Formulation involves making decisions about the mission and goals of the organization and the activities and initiatives it will undertake to achieve them. Formulation could involve determining the following:

- Our mission is to provide high-quality medical care.
- We have a goal of reducing the cost of care while at least preserving the quality of that care.
- One of our greatest leverage points lies in reducing inappropriate and unnecessary care.
- To achieve this goal, we will emphasize reducing the number of inappropriate radiology procedures.
- We will carry out initiatives that enable us to intervene at the time of procedure ordering if we need to suggest a more cost-effective modality.

We can imagine other goals directed toward achieving this mission. For each goal, we can envision multiple leverage points, and for each leverage point, we may see multiple initiatives. The result is an inverted tree that cascades from our mission to a series of initiatives.

Formulation involves understanding competing ideas and choosing between them. In our example, we could have arrived at a different set of goals and initiatives.

We could have decided to improve quality with less emphasis on care costs. We could have decided to focus on reducing the cost per procedure. We could have decided to produce retrospective reports of radiology use by provider and used this feedback to lead to ordering behavior change rather than intervening at the time of ordering.

In IT, we also have a need for formulation. In keeping with an IT mission to use the technology to support improvement of the quality of care, we may have a goal to integrate our clinical application systems. To achieve this goal, we may decide to follow any of the following initiatives:

- Provide a common way to access all systems (single sign-on).
- Interface existing heterogeneous systems.
- Require that all applications use a common database.
- Implement a common suite of clinical applications from one vendor.

Implementation

Implementation involves making decisions about how we structure ourselves, acquire skills, establish organizational capabilities, and alter organizational processes to achieve the goals and carry out the activities we have defined during formulation of our strategy. For example, if we have decided to reduce care costs by reducing inappropriate procedure use, we may need to implement one or more of the following:

- An organizational unit of providers with health services research training to analyze care practices and identify deficiencies
- A steering committee of clinical leadership to guide these efforts and provide political support
- A provider order entry system to provide real-time feedback on order appropriateness
- Data warehouse technologies to support analyses of utilization

Using our clinical applications integration example, we may come to one of the following determinations:

- We need to acquire interface engine technology, adopt HL7 standards, and form an information systems department that manages the technology and interfaces applications.
- We need to engage external consulting assistance for the selection of a clinical application suite and hire a group to implement the suite.

The implementation component of strategy development is not the development of project plans and budgets. Rather, it is the identification of the capabilities, capacities, and competencies the organization will need if it is to carry out the results of the formulation component of strategy.

Vectors for Arriving at IT Strategy

The IT strategy is developed using some combination of four **IT strategy vectors:**

- Organizational strategies
- Continuous improvement of core processes and information management
- Examination of the role of new information technologies
- Assessment of strategic trajectories

By a vector we mean the choice of perspectives and approaches through which an organization determines its IT investment decisions. For example, the first vector (derived from organization strategies) involves answering a question such as, "Given our strategy of improving patient safety, what IT applications will we need?" However, the third vector (determined by examining the role of new information technologies) involves answering a question such as, "There is a great deal of discussion about cloud-based applications. Does this approach to delivering applications provide us with ways to be more effective at addressing some of our organization challenges?" Figure 12.1 illustrates the convergence of these four vectors into a series of iterative leadership discussions and debates. These debates lead to an IT agenda.

Figure 12.1 Overview of IT strategy development

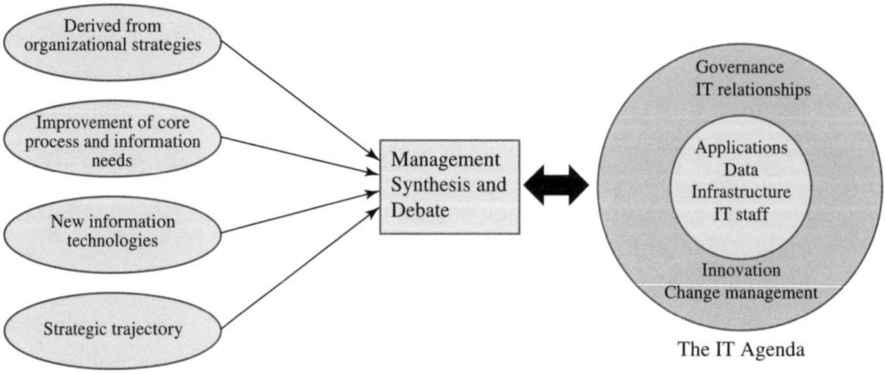

IT Strategies Derived from Organizational Strategies

The first vector involves deriving the IT agenda directly from the organization's goals and plans. For example, an organization may decide it intends to become the low-cost provider of care. It may decide to achieve this goal through implementation of disease management programs, the reengineering of inpatient care, and the reduction of unit costs for certain tests and procedures it believes are inordinately expensive.

The IT strategy development then centers on answering questions such as, "How do we apply IT to support disease management?" The answers might involve web-based publication of disease management protocols for use by providers, business intelligence technology to assess the conformance of care practice to the protocols, provider documentation systems based on disease guidelines, and CPOE systems that employ the disease guidelines to influence ordering decisions. An organization may choose all or some of these responses and develop various sequences of implementation. Nonetheless, it has developed an answer to the question of how to apply IT in support of disease management.

Most of the time the linkage between organizational strategy and IT strategy involves developing the IT ramifications of organizational initiatives, such as adding or changing services and products, growing market share, improving service, streamlining processes, or reducing costs. At times, however, an organization may decide it needs to change or add to its core characteristics or culture. The organization may decide it needs its staff members to be more care-quality or service-delivery or bottom-line oriented. It may decide it needs to decentralize or recentralize decision making. It may decide to improve its ability to manage knowledge, or it may not. These characteristics (and there are many others) can point to initiatives for IT.

In cases in which characteristics are to be changed, IT strategies must be developed to answer questions such as, "What is our basic IT approach to supporting a decentralized decision-making structure?" The organization might answer this question by permitting decentralized choices of applications as long as those applications meet certain standards. (For example, they may run on a common infrastructure or support common data standards.) It might answer the question of how IT supports an emphasis on knowledge management by developing an intranet service that provides access to preferred treatment guidelines.

IT Strategies to Continuously Improve Core Processes and Information Management

All organizations have a small number of core processes and information management tasks that are essential for the effective and efficient functioning of the organization. For a hospital these processes might include ensuring patient access to care, ordering tests and procedures, and managing the revenue cycle. For a restaurant these processes might include menu design, food preparation, and dining room service. For a health plan, information management needs might point to a requirement to understand the costs of care or the degree to which care practices vary by physician.

Using the vector of continuous improvement of core processes and information management to determine IT strategies involves defining the organization's core processes and information management needs. The organization measures the performance of core processes and uses the resulting data to develop plans to improve its performance. The organization defines core information needs, identifies the gap between the current status and its needs, and develops plans to close those gaps. These plans will often point to an IT agenda. This vector may be a result of a strategy discussion, although this is not always the case. An organization may make ongoing efforts to improve processes regardless of the specifics of its strategic plan. For example, every year it may establish initiatives designed to reduce costs or improve services. The organization has decided that, regardless of a specific strategy, it will not thrive if core processes and information management are something other than excellent.

Table 12.2 illustrates a process orientation. It provides an organization with data on the magnitude of some problems that plague the delivery

Table 12.2 Summary of the scope of outpatient care problems

For every:	There appear to be:
1,000 patients coming in for outpatient care	14 patients with life-threatening or serious ADEs
1,000 outpatients who are taking a prescription drug	90 patients who seek medical attention because of drug complications
1,000 prescriptions written	40 prescriptions with medical errors
1,000 women with a marginally abnormal mammogram	360 who will not receive appropriate follow-up care
1,000 referrals	250 referring physicians who have not received follow-up information four weeks later
1,000 patients who qualified for secondary prevention of high cholesterol	380 will not have an LDL-C on record within three years

of outpatient care. These problems afflict the processes of referral, results management, and test ordering. The organization may decide to make IT investments in an effort to reduce or eliminate these problems. For example, strengthening the decision support for e-prescribing could reduce the prevalence of adverse drug events (ADEs). Abnormal test results could be highlighted in the EHR to help ensure patient follow-up.

When this vector is used, the IT agenda is driven at least in part by a relentless year-in, year-out focus on improving core processes and information management needs.

IT Strategies That Rely on New IT Capabilities

The third vector involves considering how new IT capabilities may enable a new IT agenda or significantly alter the current agenda. For example, telemedicine capabilities may enable the organization to consider a strategy of extending the reach of its specialists across its catchment area to improve its population health efforts. Data-mining algorithm advances might enable an organization to assess different treatment approaches to determine which approaches lead to the best outcomes.

In this vector, the organization examines new applications and new base technologies and tries to answer the question, "Does this application or technology enable us to advance our strategies or improve our core processes in new ways?" For example, advances in sensors and mobile applications might lead the organization to think of new approaches to providing feedback to the chronically ill patient. Holding new technologies up to the spotlight of organizational interest can lead to decisions to invest in a new technology.

An extreme form of this mechanism occurs when a new technology or application suggests that fundamental strategies (or even the organization's existence) may be called into question or may need to undergo significant transformation. In general these strategies lead to a decision to adopt a new business model. A business model is the combination of an organization's decisions about what it will do, how it will do it, and why "the what and how" are of such value that customers will pay them.

For example, Uber's business model is that it will get you from point A to point B (the what) but it will do so in a way that involves "renting" capacity from drivers already on the road and making the process of ordering a ride and paying for a ride very easy (the how). The what for Uber is no different than that for a traditional taxi company but the how is very different. Uber's superior business model was made possible by new information technologies—the web, mobile devices, and advanced analytics.

PERSPECTIVE
Internet of Things

The Internet of Things is a class of information technology that has several components; things (people, buildings, equipment, etc.); sensors attached to the things (sensors that measure heat, acidity, movement, etc.); processors that read and interpret sensor data; and a network (the Internet usually) that connects sensors and processors to cloud-based (usually) analytics.

There are several potential uses of the Internet of Things in health care:

- Monitor equipment utilization and performance; for example, is a part in the MRI about to fail?
- Supply management; for example, where is a supply in its transit to the hospital?
- Monitoring of environmental data; for example, what is the humidity outside?
- Monitoring the physiological status of a patient; for example, is the patient's blood sugar level too low?
- Process orchestration; for example, is the orderly who needs to take the patient to radiology on her way?

In an IT strategy discussion, these questions could be raised:

- What is the Internet of Things?
- What are the possible uses and are those uses mature?
- Does the Internet of Things help us advance strategies or suggest new strategies?
- If so, what do we do?

IT Strategies Based on Assessment of Strategic Trajectories

Organization and IT strategies invariably have a fixed time horizon and fixed scope. These strategies might cover a period of time two to three years into the future. They outline a bounded set of initiatives to be undertaken in that time period. Assessment of strategic trajectories asks the questions, What do we think we will be doing after that time horizon and scope? Do we think we will be doing very different kinds of things, or will we be carrying out initiatives similar to the ones we are pursuing now?

For example, we might be planning to implement a broad portfolio of health care information technology. The organization believes that through medical advances and preventive care the number of patients older than one hundred will increase dramatically. The strategic trajectory discussion asks, "Does this increase in longevity have significant implications for the types of health care that we deliver and hence on the types of information technology that we implement?"

Or we might be in the process of using IT to support joint clinical programs with other hospitals in the area. These efforts would be greatly helped by the availability of broad interoperability. However, such pervasive interoperability has proved elusive and may be elusive for a decade. How would pervasive interoperability affect our IT strategy?

The strategic trajectory discussion can be highly speculative. It might be so forward looking and speculative that the organization decides not to act today on its discussion. Yet it can also point to initiatives to be undertaken within the next year to better understand this possible future and to prepare the organization's information systems for it. For example, if we believe our information systems will eventually need to store large amounts of genetic information, it would be worth understanding whether the new population health systems we will be selecting soon will be capable of storing and analyzing these data.

THE IT ASSEST

The discussion of vectors and alignment up to this point has focused generally on the development of an application agenda as the outcome. In other words, the completion of the IT strategy discussion is an inventory of systems, such as the EHR system, customer relationship management system, and an enterprise data warehouse, that are needed to further overall organizational strategies. However, the application inventory is a component of the larger idea of the IT asset. These areas are discussed in the following sections.

The **IT asset** is composed of those IT resources that the organization has or can obtain and that are applied to further the goals, plans, and initiatives of the organization. The IT strategy discussion identifies specific changes or enhancements to the composition of the asset—for example, the implementation of a new application—and general properties of the asset that must exist—for example, high reliability of the infrastructure. The IT asset has four components: applications, infrastructure, data, and IT staff members.

Applications

Applications are the systems that users interact with: for example, scheduling, billing, and EHR systems. In addition to developing an inventory of applications, the organization may need to develop strategies regarding properties of the overall portfolio of applications.

For example, if the organization is an integrated delivery system, decisions will need to be made about the degree to which applications should be the same across the organization. E-mail systems ought to be the same, but is there a strategic reason to have the same pharmacy system across all hospitals? Should an organization buy or build its applications? Building applications is risky and often requires skills that most health care organizations do not possess. However, internally developed applications can be less expensive and can be tailored to an organization's needs.

Strategic thinking may center on the form and rigor of the justification process for new applications. Formal return on investment analyses may be emphasized so that all application decisions will emphasize cost reduction or revenue gain. Or the organization may decide to have a decision process that takes a more holistic approach to acquisition decisions, so that factors such as improving quality of care must also be considered.

In general, strategy discussions surrounding the application asset as a whole focus on, in addition to the application inventory, a few key areas:

- **Sourcing.** What are the sources for our applications? And what criteria determine the source to be used for an application? Should we get all applications from the same vendor or will we use a small number of approved vendors?

- **Application uniformity.** For large organizations with many subsidiaries or locations, to what degree should our applications be the same at all locations? If some have to be the same but some can be different, how do we decide where we allow autonomy? This discussion often involves a trade-off between local autonomy and the central desire for efficiency and consistency.

- **Application acquisition.** What processes and steps should we use when we acquire applications? Should we subject all acquisitions to rigorous analyses? Should we use a request for proposal for all application acquisitions? This discussion is generally an assessment of the extent to which the IT acquisition process should follow the degree of rigor applied to non-IT acquisitions (of diagnostic equipment, for example).

Infrastructure

Infrastructure needs may arise from the strategic-planning process. An organization desiring to extend its IT systems to community physicians will need to ensure that it can deliver low-cost and secure network connections. Organizations placing significant emphasis on clinical information systems must ensure very high reliability of their infrastructure; computerized provider order entry systems cannot go down.

In addition to initiatives designed to add specific components to the infrastructure—for example, new software to monitor network utilization—architecture strategies will focus on the addition or enhancement of broad infrastructure capabilities and characteristics.

Capabilities are defined by completing this sentence: "We want our applications to be able to . . ." Organizations might complete that sentence with phrases such as "be accessed from home," "have logic that guides clinical decision making," or "share a pool of consistently defined data."

Characteristics refer to broad properties of the infrastructure, such as reliability, security, agility, supportability, integratability, and potency. An organization may be heading into the implementation of mission-critical systems and hence must ensure very high degrees of reliability in its applications and infrastructure. The organization may be concerned about the threats posed by ransomware and denial of service attacks and decide to strengthen the security of its infrastructure. The asset plans in these cases involve discussions and analyses that are intended to answer the question, What steps do we need to take to significantly improve the reliability of our systems or improve security?

Data

Data and information were discussed in Chapter Two. Strategies concerning data may center on the degree of data standardization across the organization, accountability for data quality and stewardship, data sources, and determination of database management and analyses technologies.

Data strategy conversations may originate with questions such as, We need to better understand the costs of our care. How do we improve the linkage between our clinical data and our financial data? Or, we have to develop a much quicker response to outbreaks of epidemics. How do we link into the city's emergency rooms and quickly get data on chief complaints?

In general, strategies surrounding data focus on acquiring new types of data, defining the meaning of data, determining the organizational function responsible for maintaining that meaning, integrating existing sets of data, and obtaining technologies used to manage, analyze, and report data.

IT Staff Members

IT staff members are the analysts, programmers, and computer operators who, day in and day out, manage and advance information systems in an organization. IT staff members were discussed in Chapter Eight. IT strategy discussions may highlight the need to add IT staff members with specific skills, such as mobile application developers and population health implementation staff members. Organizations may decide that they need to explore outsourcing the IT function in an effort to improve IT performance or obtain difficult-to-find skills. The service orientation of the IT group may need to be improved.

In general, the IT staff member strategies focus on the acquisition of new skills, the organization of the IT staff, the sourcing of the IT staff, and the characteristics of the IT department—is it, for example, innovative, service oriented, and efficient?

A NORMATIVE APPROACH TO DEVELOPING ALIGNMENT AND IT STRATEGY

You may now be asking yourself, how do I bring all of this together? In other words, is there a suggested approach an organization can take to develop its IT strategy that takes into account these various vectors? And by the way, what does an IT strategic plan look like?

Across health care organizations the approaches taken to developing, documenting, and managing an IT strategy are quite varied. Some organizations have well-developed, formal approaches that rely on the deliberations of multiple committees and leadership retreats. Other organizations have remarkably informal processes. A small number of medical staff members and administrative leaders meet in informal conversations to define the organization's IT strategy. In some cases the strategy is developed during a specific time in the year, often preceding development of the annual budget. In other organizations, IT strategic planning goes on all the time and permeates a wide range of formal and informal discussions.

There is no single right way to develop an IT strategy and to ensure alignment. However, the process of developing IT strategy should be similar in approach and nature to the process used for overall strategic planning. If the organization's core approach to strategy development is informal, its approach to IT strategy development should also be informal.

Recognizing this variability, a normative approach to the development of IT strategy can be described.

Strategy Discussion Linkage

Organizational strategy is generally discussed in senior leadership meetings. These meetings may focus specifically on strategy, or strategy may be a regular agenda item. These meetings may be supplemented with retreats centered on strategy development and with task forces and committees that are asked to develop recommendations for specific aspects of the strategy. (For example, a committee of clinical leadership members might be asked to develop recommendations for improving patient safety.) These discussions will examine the organization's external environment—such as changes in reimbursement and competitive position—and internal environment—such as operational efficiency, financial health, and clinical strengths. This examination invariably results in the identification of gaps between the organization's desired position and role and its current status. This examination usually includes a review of the status and capabilities of the organization's IT capabilities and application portfolio.

Regardless of their form, the organization's CIO should be present at such meetings or kept informed of the discussion and its conclusions. If task forces and committees supplement strategy development, an IT manager should be asked to be a member. The CIO (or the IT member of a task force) should be expected to develop an assessment of the IT ramifications of strategic options and to identify areas where IT can enable new approaches to carrying out the strategy.

The CIO will not be the only member of the leadership team who will perform this role. Chief financial officers (CFOs), for example, will frequently identify the IT ramifications of plans to improve the revenue cycle. However, the CIO should be held accountable for ensuring the linkage does occur.

As strategy discussions proceed, the CIO must be able to summarize and critique the IT agenda that should be put in place to carry out the various aspects of the strategy. Exhibit 12.1 displays an IT agenda that might emerge. Exhibit 12.2 displays a health plan IT agenda that could result from a strategy designed to improve patient access to health information and self-service administrative tasks for a health plan.

Exhibit 12.1 IT initiatives necessary to support a strategic goal for a provider

Article I. Strategic Goal

Improve service to outpatients

Article II. Problem

- Patients have to call many locations to schedule a series of appointments and services.
- The quality of the response at these locations is highly variable.
- Locations inconsistently capture necessary registration and insurance information.
- Some locations are over capacity, whereas others are underutilized.

Article III. IT Solution

- Common scheduling system for all locations
- A call center for "one-stop" access to all outpatient services
- Development of master schedules for common service groups such as preoperative testing
- Integration of scheduling system with electronic data interchange connection to payers for eligibility determination, referral authorization, and copay information
- Patient support material, such as maps and instructions, to be mailed to patients

IT Liaisons

All major departments and functions (for example, finance, nursing, and medical staff administration) should have a senior IT staff person who serves as the function's point of contact. Because these functions examine ways to address their needs (for example, lower their costs and improve their services), the IT staff person can work with them to identify IT activities necessary to carry out their endeavors. This identification often emerges with recommendations to implement new applications that advance the performance of a function, such as a medication administration record application to improve the nursing workflow. Exhibit 12.3 provides an example of output from a nursing leadership discussion on improving patient safety through the use of a nursing documentation system.

Exhibit 12.2 IT initiatives necessary to support a strategic goal for a health plan

Article IV. Strategic Goal

- Improve service to subscribers
- Reduce costs

Article V. Problem

- Subscribers have difficulty finding high-quality health information.
- The costs of performing routine administrative transactions such as change of address and responding to benefits questions is increasing.
- Subscriber perceptions of the quality of service in performing these transactions is low.

Article VI. IT Solution

- A plan portal that provides:
  - o Health content from high-quality sources
  - o Access to chronic disease services and discussion groups
  - o Subscriber ability to use self-service to perform routine administrative transactions
  - o Subscriber access to benefit information
  - o Functions that enable subscribers to ask questions
  - o Plan ratings of provider quality
- A plan-sponsored provider portal that enables:
  - o Subscribers to conduct routine transactions with their provider, such as requesting an appointment or renewing a prescription
  - o Electronic visits for certain conditions such as back pain
  - o Subscribers to ask care questions of their provider

New Technology Review

The CIO should be asked to discuss, as part of the strategy discussion or in a periodic presentation in senior leadership forums, new technologies and their possible contributions to the goals and plans of the organization. These presentations may lead to suggestions that the organization form a task force

Exhibit 12.3 System support of nursing documentation

Section 6.1. Problem Statement

- Both the admitting physician(s) and nurse document medication history in their admission note.
- Points of failure have been noted:
  - o Incompleteness due to time or recall constraints, lack of knowledge, or lack of clear documentation requirements
  - o Incorrectness due to errors in memory, transcription between documents, and illegibility
  - o Multiple inconsistent records due to failure to resolve conflicting accounts by different caregivers
- Most of the clinical information required to support appropriate clinician decision making is obtained during the history-taking process.

Section 6.2. Technology Interventions and Goals

- A core set of clinical data should be made available to the clinician at the point of decision making:
  - o Demographics
  - o Principle diagnoses and other medical conditions
  - o Drug allergies
  - o Current and previous relevant medications
  - o Laboratory and radiology reports
- Required information should be gathered only once:
  - o Multidisciplinary system of structured, templated documentation
  - o Clinical decision support rules, associated to specific disciplines, should guide gathering
  - o Workflow should support the mobile care giver with integrated wireless access to clinical information
- Needed applications could be implemented in phases:
  - o Nursing admission assessment
  - o Multidisciplinary admission assessment
  - o Planning and progress
  - o Nursing discharge plan
  - o Multidisciplinary discharge plan

Table 12.3 Assessment of telehealth strategic opportunities

Type of Telehealth	Potential Strategic Value	Level of Support of Organization's Strategy
Semi-urgent care	Enables patients to reach a clinician at any time to get advice on addressing low acuity health issues, for example, a modest fever of a child	Moderate
Remote patient monitoring	Supports efforts to manage patient's with a chronic disease	High
Fitness monitoring	Provides information on a patient's exercise program	Low
Visit substitution	Supports conducting visits, for example, surgery follow-up through video rather than requiring a face-to-face visit	High
Clinician consultation	Enables clinicians to seek a consult from a remote specialist	High
Critical care	Provides ability to perform remote stroke assessments and ICU monitoring	Moderate

to closely examine a new technology. For example, a multidisciplinary task force could be formed to examine the ability of telehealth to support the organization's strategies. Table 12.3 provides an overview of different types of telehealth and an overall assessment of strategic importance.

Synthesis of Discussions

The CIO should be asked to synthesize or summarize the conclusions of these discussions. This synthesis will invariably be needed during development of the annual budget. And the synthesis will be a necessary component of the documentation and presentation of the organization's strategic plan. Table 12.4 presents an example of such a synthesis.

The organization should expect the process of synthesis will require debate and discussion; for example, trade-offs will need to be reviewed, priorities set, and the organization's willingness to implement embryonic technologies determined. This synthesis and prioritization process can occur during the course of leadership meetings, through the work of a committee charged to develop an initial set of recommendations, and during discussions internal to the IT management team.

Table 12.4 Summary of IT strategic planning

Strategic Challenge	IT Agenda
Capacity and growth management	Emergency department tracking Inpatient electronic bed board Ambulatory clinic patient tracking
Quality and safety	Inpatient order entry Anticoagulation therapy unit Online discharge summaries Medication administration record
Performance improvement	Registration system overhaul Anatomic pathology Pharmacy Order communication Transfusion and donor services
Budget management and external reviews	Disaster recovery Joint Commission preparation Privacy policy review

An example of an approach to prioritizing recommendations is to give each member of the committee $100 to be distributed across the recommendations. The amount a member gives to each recommendation reflects his or her sense of its importance. For example, a member could give one recommendation $90 and another $10 or give five recommendations $20 each. In the former case, the committee member believes that only two recommendations are important and that the first recommendation is nine times more important than the second. In the latter case, the member believes that five recommendations are of equal importance. The distributed dollars are summed across the members, with a ranking of recommendations emerging.

The leadership should not feel compelled to accept the ranking as a definitive output. Rather, the process of scoring will reveal that members of the leadership team will rate recommendations differently. For example, some members will rate a project as having a high contribution to patient quality and others will view that contribution as low. The discussion that investigates these discrepancies can help the team understand the recommendation more fully and lead to a consensus that strengthens political support for the recommendation. Moreover, if the leadership team decides to approve a recommendation with a low score, it should ask itself why it views the recommendation as more important than the score would suggest.

For an example of the scoring of proposed IT initiatives, see Figure 12.2. It lists categories of organizational goals (for example, enhance patient care), along with goals within the categories. The leadership of the organization, through a series of meetings and presentations, has scored the contribution of the IT initiative to the strategic goals of the organization. The contribution to each goal may be critical (must do), high, moderate, or none. These scores are based on data but nonetheless are fundamentally judgment calls. The scoring and prioritization will result in a set of initiatives deemed to be the most important. The IT staff members will then construct preliminary budgets, staff needs, and timelines for these projects.

Figure 12.3 provides an overview of the timeline for these initiatives and the cost of each. Management will discuss various timeline scenarios, consider project interdependence, and ensure that the IT department and the

Figure 12.2 IT initiative priorities

	Enhances Patient Care	Strengthens Community Outreach	Strengthens Physician Integration	Strengthens Employee Support	Enhances Operational Efficiency	Minimizes Investment Level	Invests in Current Scalable Technology	Supports Growth with Strong ROI	Addresses Significant System Deficiency	Addresses Compliance Issues (MUST DO)	Mandatory Technology Building Block	Overall Priority
	Service		People		Financial		Growth		Quality and Safety		Infra-structure	Overall Priority
Clinical Applications												
1. Physician Order Entry	×		×		×				×	×		Start Now
2. Patient Care Documentation	×				×				×	×		Plan It
3. Clinical Data Repository			×		×			×	×			Start Now
4. Computerized Medical Record			×		×							Delay It
5. PACS (Phase I)	×				×				×			Start Now
6. Expand Physician Practice Mgmt			×		×	×		×				Plan It
7. Departmental Systems												Ongoing
Data Integration												
8. Integration Engine							×		×		×	Plan It
Administrative and Financial Systems												
9. General Financial					×		×					Plan It
10. Materials Management				×	×		×					Plan It
11. Scheduling Application		×		×	×				×			Plan It
12. Decision Support System					×	×			×			Start Now
Emerging Technologies												
13. Wireless LAN and WAN			×		×		×	×				Plan It
14. Voice Recognition			×		×		×					Start Now
Infrastructure												
15. Server Consolidations or Upgrades											×	Plan It
16. Network Upgrades											×	Ongoing
17. Security: SSO, HIPAA, Policies					×				×	×	×	Plan It
Governance												
18. Project and Change Mgmt Office			×	×	×						×	Start Now
19. US Governance (Steering, Bus, Liaisons, SLAs)				×	×	×						Ongoing

Key: Moderate | High | Must Do

Figure 12.3 IT plan timetable and budget

Hospital IT Migration Path	Priority	Funded	FY2015 Capital (in $1000) Actual	FY2016 Capital Expense (in $1000) Low	High	FY2017 Capital Expense (in $1000) Low	High	FY2018 Capital Expense (in $1000) Low	High	Annual Recurring Operate	Timeline / FTE Staffing (FY15 Q4; FY2016 Q1–Q4; FY2017 Q1–Q4; FY2018 Q1–Q4)
Clinical Applications											
1. Physician Order Entry	Start Now	Funded	$ 200		$ 1,800					$ 270	1 4 4 4
2. Patient Care Documentation	Plan It			$ 333	$ 467	$ 167	$ 233			$ 70	1 3 3
3. Clinical Data Repository	Start Now				$ 25					$ 4	0.5 1 1 1 1
4. Computerized Medical Record	Delay It					$ 50	$ 125	$ 150	$ 375		
5. PACS (Phase I)	Start Now			$ 500	$ 500					$ 75	0.5 1
6. Expand of Physician Practice Mgmt	Plan It					$ 50	$ 150				1 1 1 1
7. Departmental Systems	Ongoing			$ 167	$ 333	$ 167	$ 333	$ 167	$ 333	$ 50	1 1 1 1 1 1 1 1 1 1 1 1
Data Integration											
8. Integration Engine	Plan It			$ 100	$ 200						1 1
Administrative and Financial Systems											
9. General Financials	Plan It					$ 300	$ 500				1 2 2
10. Materials Management	Plan It					$ 200	$ 333	$ 100	$ 167		1 2 2
11. Scheduling Application	Plan It					$ 75	$ 150	$ 225	$ 450		1 2 2 2
12. Decision Support System	Start Now	$ 100		$ 50						8	
Emerging Technologies											
13. Wireless LAN & WAN	Plan It					$ 167	$ 667	$ 83	$ 333	$ 75	0.5 0.5 0.5
14. Voice Recognition	Start Now	Pending		$ 100	$ 300					$ 45	0.5 0.5 0.5 0.5
Infrastructure											
15. Server Consolidations / Upgrades	Plan It			$ 250	$ 500					$ 75	0.5 0.5 0.8
16. Network Upgrades	Ongoing	Funded	$ 100	$ 33	$ 133	$ 33	$ 133	$ 33	$ 133	$ 20	1 1 1 1 1 1 1 1 1 1 1 1
17. Security - SSO, HIPAA, Policies	Plan It			$ 33	$ 67	$ 17	$ 33			$ 10	1 0.5 0.5
Governance											
18. Project / Change Mgmt Office	Start Now	Funded		$ 10	$ 20					$ 3	1 1 1 1
19. US Governance (Steering, Bus. Liasons, SLA's)	Ongoing	N/A		N/A	N/A	N/A	N/A	N/A	N/A	N/A	1 3 3 3 3 3 3 3 3 3 3 3

Note: Annual recurring is the ongoing operating cost of the system

On the right of the figure, the approximate project timeline can be seen. The numbers below the timeline (0.5 and 1) indicate the number of IT staff members needed to implement the project.

organization are not overwhelmed by too many initiatives to complete all at once. The organization will use the budget estimates to determine how much IT it can afford. Often there is not enough money to pay for all the desired IT initiatives, and some initiatives with high and moderate scores will be deferred or eliminated as projects. The final plan, including timelines and budgets, will become the basis for assessing progress throughout the year.

Overall, a core role of the organization's CIO is to work with the rest of the leadership team to develop the process that leads to alignment and strategic linkage.

Once all is said and done, the alignment process should produce these results:

- An inventory of the IT initiatives that will be undertaken (These initiatives may include new applications and projects designed to improve the IT asset.)
- A diagram or chart that illustrates the linkage between the initiatives and the organization's strategy and goals
- An overview of the timeline and the major interdependencies between initiatives
- A high-level analysis of the budget needed to carry out these initiatives
- An assessment of any material risks to carrying out the IT agenda and a review of the strategies needed to reduce those risks

It is important to recognize the amount and level of discussion, compromise, and negotiation that go into the strategic alignment process. Producing these results without going through the preceding thoughtful process will be of little real benefit.

IT STRATEGY AND ALIGNMENT CHALLENGES

Creating IT strategy and alignment is a complicated and critical organizational process. The following sections present a series of observations about that process.

Planning Methodologies

Formal processes and methodologies that help organizations develop IT plans, whether based on derived linkage or the examination of more fundamental characteristics of organizations, can be very helpful. If well executed, they can do all of the following:

- Lead to the identification of a portfolio of IT applications and initiatives that are well linked to the organization's strategy.
- Identify alternatives and approaches that might not have been understood without the process.
- Contribute to a more thorough analysis of the major aspects of the plan.
- Enhance and ensure necessary leadership participation and support.
- Help the organization be more decisive.

- Ensure the allocation of resources among competing alternatives is rational and politically defensible.
- Enhance communication of the developed plan.

In addition to formal IT strategic planning methodologies, organizations will often use strategy frameworks that help them frame issues and opportunities. For example, Porter's Competitive Forces Model (Porter, 1980) identifies strategic options such as competing on cost, differentiating based on quality, and attempting to raise barriers to the entry of other competitors. By using this model, the organization will make choices about its overall competitive position.

Models such as these help the leadership engage in a broader and more conceptual approach to strategy development.

Persistence of the Alignment Problem

Despite the apparent simplicity of the normative process we have described and the many examinations of the topic by academics and consultants, achieving IT alignment has been a top concern of senior organizational leadership for several decades. For example, a survey of CIOs from across multiple industries found improving IT alignment with business objectives to be the number one IT top management priority in 2007 (Alter, 2007). A survey of CIOs in 2015 (Information Management, 2016) found alignment to be, once again, the top concern. There are several reasons for the persistent difficulty of achieving alignment (Bensaou & Earl, 1998):

- Business strategies are often not clear or are volatile.
- IT opportunities are poorly understood and new technologies emerge constantly.
- The organization is unable to resolve the different priorities of different parts of the organization.

Weill and Broadbent (1998) note that effective IT alignment requires organizational leadership to clearly understand and strategically and tactically integrate (1) the organization's strategic context (its strategies and market position), (2) the organization's environment, (3) the IT strategy, and (4) the IT portfolio (for example, the current applications, technologies, and staff skills). Understanding and integrating these four continuously evolving and complex areas is exceptionally difficult.

At least two more reasons can be added to this listing of factors that make alignment difficult. First, the organization may find it has not achieved the gains apparently achieved by others it has heard or read about, nor have the vendors' promises of the technologies materialized. Second, the value of IT, particularly infrastructure, is often difficult to quantify, and the value proposition is fuzzy and uncertain; for example, what is the value of improved security of applications?

In both these cases the organization is unsure whether the IT investment will lead to the desired strategic gain or value. This is not strictly an alignment problem. However, alignment does assume the organization believes it has a reasonable ability to achieve desired IT gains.

The Limitations of Alignment

Although alignment is important, it will not guarantee effective application of IT. Planning methodologies and effective use of vectors cannot, by themselves, overcome weaknesses in other factors that can significantly diminish the likelihood that IT investments will lead to improved organization performance. These weaknesses include poor relationships between IT staff members and the rest of the organization, incompetent leadership, weak financial conditions, and ill-conceived IT governance mechanisms. IT strategy also cannot overcome unclear overall strategies and cannot necessarily compensate for material competitive weaknesses.

If one has mediocre painting skills, a class on painting technique will make one a better painter but will not turn one into Picasso. Similarly, superb alignment techniques will not turn an organization limited in its ability to implement IT effectively into one brilliant at IT use. Perhaps this reason, more than any other, is why the alignment issue persists as a top-ranked IT issue. Organizations are searching for IT excellence in the wrong place; it cannot be delivered purely by alignment prowess.

Alignment at Maturity

Organizations that have a history of IT excellence appear to evolve to a state in which their alignment process has become deeply intertwined with the normal management strategy and operations discussions. A study by Earl (1993) of organizations in the United Kingdom with a history of IT excellence found that their IT planning processes had several characteristics.

IT Planning Was Not a Separate Process

IT planning and the strategic discussion of IT occurred as an integral part of the organization's strategic planning processes and management discussions.

In these organizations, management did not think of separating out an IT discussion during the course of strategy development any more than it would run separate finance or human resource planning processes. IT planning was an unseverable, intertwined component of the usual management conversation. This would suggest not having a separate IT steering committee.

IT Planning Had Neither a Beginning nor an End

In many organizations, IT planning processes start in a particular month every year and are completed within a more or less set period. In the studied organizations, the IT planning and strategy conversation went on all the time. This does not mean that an organization doesn't have to have a temporally demarked, annual budget process. Rather, it means that IT planning is a continuous process that reflects the continuous change in the environment.

IT Planning Involved Shared Decision Making and Shared Learning

IT leadership informed organizational leadership of the potential contribution of new technologies and the constraints of current technologies. Organizational leadership ensured that IT leadership understood the business plans, strategies, and their constraints. The IT budget and annual tactical plan resulted from shared analyses of IT opportunities and a set of IT priorities.

The IT Plan Emphasized Themes

A provider organization may have themes of improving care quality, reducing costs, and improving patient service. During the course of any given year, IT will have initiatives that are intended to advance the organization along these themes. The mixture of initiatives will change from year to year, but the themes endure for many years. Because themes endure year after year, organizations develop competence in these themes. They become, for example, progressively better at managing costs and improving patient service. This growing prowess extends into IT. Organizations become more skilled at understanding which IT opportunities hold the most promise and at managing implementation of these applications. And the IT staff members become more skilled at knowing how to apply IT to support such themes as improving care quality and at helping leadership assess the value of new technologies and applications.

IT Strategy Is Not Always Necessary

There are many times in IT activities when the goal, or the core approach to achieving the goal, is not particularly strategic, and **strategy formulation** and **strategy implementation** are not needed. Replacing an inpatient pharmacy system, enhancing help desk support, and upgrading the network, although requiring well-executed projects, do not always require leadership to engage in conversations about organizational goals or to take a strategic look at organizational capabilities and skills.

There are many times when it is unlikely that the way an organization achieves a goal will create a distinct competitive advantage. For example, an organization may decide it needs to provide personal health records to patients, but it does not expect that that application, or its implementation, will be so superior to a competitor's personal health record that an advantage accrues to the organization.

Much of what IT does is not strategic, nor does it require strategic thinking. Many IT projects do not require thoughtful discussions of fundamental approaches to achieving organizational goals or significant changes in the IT asset.

The Challenge of Emerging Technology

The information technology industry in general and the health information technology industry in particular are ever-changing and evolving. New technologies are being introduced every day. How does a health care executive know when to support the adoption of the "latest and greatest" technologies? When does the organization acknowledge its current technologies are out-of-date and need upgrading? How much of the current literature about new technologies is "hype"? Which new technologies are likely to survive to become industry standards?

In this textbook we cover specific methods for selecting health care information systems to meet the health care organizations' operational needs. The questions posed here are more general in nature and relate to the technologies on which these systems are built. Take, for example, the use of smartphones and tablets by health care providers.

Individuals adopted those technologies for personal use with significant spillover into the work environment. Now hospitals and other health care organizations are purchasing these devices as a part of their overall information system infrastructure and are facing the challenges associated with incorporating these devices into their overall systems. At what point should the health care executives have known that these technologies were here to stay and were something to be managed? Do the early adopters of the technologies have an advantage or a disadvantage in the market?

There are no easy answers to these questions, but Gartner, Inc., has developed a useful framework for health care executives to think about when considering adopting new technologies. The hype cycle presents a view of how a technology will evolve over time. The stated purpose is to "provide a sound source of insight to manage its deployment within the context of . . . specific business goals." The hype cycle (Figure 12.4) supports organizations in their decisions to adopt the technology early or wait for further maturation. There are five key phases to the cycle:

1. **Technology trigger.** A potential technology breakthrough kicks things off. Early proof-of-concept stories and media interest trigger significant publicity. Often no usable products exist and commercial viability is unproven.

2. **Peak of inflated expectations.** Early publicity by proponents of the technology reaches a crescendo; often with little practical experience using the technology. Some companies take action; many do not.

3. **Trough of disillusionment.** Interest wanes as experiments and implementations fail to deliver on the hype of the peak. The technology is often immature and users of the technology are

Figure 12.4 Hype cycle for emerging technologies, 2014

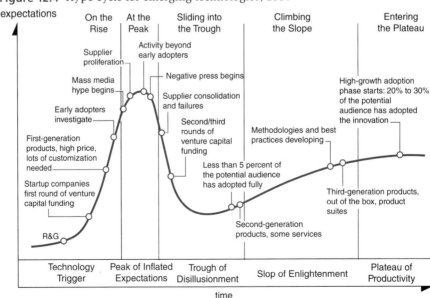

Source: Gartner (2014). Used with permission.

just beginning to learn how to apply the technology to further organizational goals. Producers of the technology shake out or fail. Investments continue only if the surviving vendors improve their products to the satisfaction of early adopters.

4. **Slope of enlightenment.** More instances of how the technology can benefit the enterprise start to crystallize and become more widely understood. Second- and third-generation mature products appear from technology providers. More enterprises fund pilots; conservative companies remain cautious. The real value of the technology begins to emerge.

5. **Plateau of productivity.** Mainstream adoption starts to take off. Criteria for assessing vendor and product viability are more clearly defined. The technology's broad market applicability and relevance are clearly paying off.

In the strategic discussion of new technologies it is prudent to identify where the technology sits on the hype cycle. It may be premature to invest at scale in technologies that are the peak of inflated expectations. The organization may be well served to let the market evolve and the products mature before it initiates significant investment.

However, the organization may decide that the technology, although immature and cloaked in a fog of hype, has significant potential and that there is merit to conducting pilots so that the organization begins to understand the potential of the technology and develop prowess in its use. For example, the Internet of Things mentioned previously is solidly at the peak of inflated expectations. However, the organization's strategy may identify this class of technologies as a potentially very important contributor to its goal of monitoring the health of people with a chronic disease. Hence the organization will pilot the technology to better understand the impact of the technology in improving disease management.

SUMMARY

The development of IT alignment and strategic linkage is a complex undertaking. Four vectors, each complex, must converge. The difficulty of this undertaking is manifest in the frequent citing of IT alignment in surveys of major organizational issues and problems. There are no simple answers to this problem. At the end of the day, good alignment requires talented leaders (including the CIO) who have effective debates and discussions regarding strategies and who have very good instincts and understandings about the organization's strategy and the potential contribution of IT.

On the Rise

- FHIR
- Blue Button+
- Real-time health care system
- Voice user interface

At the Peak

- Natural-language processing (clinical enterprise)
- E-prescribing of controlled substances
- Logical data warehouse
- C-CDA
- Clinical communications and collaboration
- Consent management
- Enterprise file synchronization and sharing
- Enterprise fraud and misuse management
- Secure text messaging
- Health care master data management
- IT GRCM

Sliding into the Trough

- Continua
- Business continuity management planning
- Unified communications
- Semantic interoperability/healthcare
- Legacy decommissioning

It appears that organizations that are mature in their IT use have evolved these IT alignment processes to the point at which they are no longer distinguishable as separate processes. This observation should not be construed as advice to cease using planning approaches or disband effective IT steering committees. Such an evolution, to the degree that it is normative, may occur naturally, just as kids will eventually grow up (at least most of them will).

- End-user experience monitoring
- ICD-10 (US)
- Direct messaging
- HIE
- GS1 Healthcare (GDSN)
- HL7 Infobutton

Climbing the Slope

- Desktop virtualization
- Patient self-service kiosks
- Positive patient identification
- Vendor-neutral archive
- Enterprise mobility services
- Information life cycle management
- IHE XDS.b
- Location- and condition-sensing technologies
- User administration/provisioning
- Enterprise content management
- Patient portals

Entering the Plateau

- Strong authentication for enterprise access
- Medical device connectivity

Source: Gartner (2015). Used with permission.

KEY TERMS

IT alignment	*Strategy formulation*
IT asset	*Strategy implementation*
IT strategy vectors	

LEARNING ACTIVITIES

1. Describe how a population health system can advance the strategies of a health care provider organization.

2. Describe how a customer relationship management system can advance the strategies of a payer organization.

3. Pick an example of a new technology, such as the Internet of Things. Discuss how this technology might leverage the strategy of a provider or a payer organization.

4. If a health care organization has a strategy of lowering its costs of care, what types of IT applications might it consider? If the organization has a strategy of improving the quality of its care, what types of IT applications might it consider? Compare the two lists of applications.

REFERENCES

Alter, A. (2007, Dec.). Top trends for 2008. *CIO Insight, 88,* 37–40.

Bensaou, M., & Earl, M. (1998). The right mind-set for managing information technology. *Harvard Business Review, 76*(5), 119–128.

Chandler, A. (1962). *Strategy and structure. Cambridge, MA: MIT Press.*

Earl, M. (1993). Experiences in strategic information systems planning. *MIS Quarterly, 17*(1), 1–24.

Gartner. (2014, Aug.). *Hype cycle for emerging technologies, 2014. Retrieved May 2016 from* http://www.gartner.com/newsroom/id/2819918

Gartner. (2015, July). *Hype cycle for healthcare provider technologies and standards, 2015. Retrieved May 2016 from* https://www.gartner.com/doc/3086917/hype-cycle-healthcare-provider-technologies

Henderson, J., & Venkatraman, N. (1993). Strategic alignment: Leveraging information technology for transforming organizations. *IBM Systems Journal, 32*(1), 4–16.

Information Management. (2016). *Top 10 CIO concerns.* Retrieved April 2016 from http://www.information-management.com/gallery/data-in-2016-top-10-cio-concerns-10027647-1.html

Porter, M. (1980). *Competitive strategy. New York, NY: Free Press.*

Weill, P., & Broadbent, M. (1998). *Leveraging the new infrastructure.* Boston, MA: Harvard Business School Press.

CHAPTER 13

IT Governance and Management

LEARNING OBJECTIVES

- To be able to understand the scope and importance of IT governance.
- To review the IT roles and responsibilities of users, the IT department, and senior management.
- To be able to discuss the components of an IT budget and the processes for developing the budget.
- To review the factors that enable sustained excellence in the application of IT.
- To understand how IT can contribute to an organization's IT competitiveness.

In this chapter we discuss an eclectic but important set of information technology (IT) management processes, structures, and issues. Developing, managing, and evolving IT management mechanisms is often a central topic for organizational leadership. In this chapter we will cover the following areas:

- **IT governance.** IT governance is composed of the processes, reporting relationships, roles, and committees that an organization develops to make decisions about IT resources and activities and to manage the execution of those decisions. These decisions involve issues such as setting priorities, determining budgets, defining project management approaches, and addressing IT problems.

- **IT budget.** Developing the IT budget is a complex exercise. Organizations always have more IT proposals than can be funded. Some proposals are strategically important and others involve routine maintenance of existing infrastructure, making proposal comparison difficult. Although complex and difficult, the effective development of the IT budget is a critical management responsibility.

- **Management role in major IT initiatives.** Senior management has an extremely important role in ensuring that major IT initiatives succeed and result in desired organizational performance gains. In other chapters of this book, management process for system selection, implementation, and value realization were discussed. In this section we discuss risk factors facing major initiatives and steps management can take to mitigate those risks.

- **IT effectiveness.** Over the years several organizations have demonstrated exceptional effectiveness in applying IT: American Express, Bank of America, Uber, Amazon, Schwab, and American Airlines. This chapter discusses what the management of these organizations did that led to such effectiveness. It also examines the attributes of IT-savvy senior leadership.

- **IT to improve an organization's competitive position.** IT is often used as a means to improve an organization's ability to compete. In this section we will discuss lessons learned from other industries from their efforts to use IT as a competitive asset.

IT GOVERNANCE

IT governance refers to the principles, processes, and organizational structures that govern the IT resources (Drazen & Straisor, 1995). When solid governance exists, the organization is able to give a coherent answer to the following questions:

- Which committees and processes are used to define the IT strategy?
- Who sets priorities for IT, and how are those priorities set?
- Who is responsible for implementing information system plans, and what principles will guide the implementation process?
- How are IT responsibilities distributed between IT and the rest of the organization and between centralized and decentralized (local) IT groups in an integrated delivery system?
- How are IT budgets developed?

At its core, governance involves the following functions:

- Determining the distribution of the responsibility for making decisions, the scope of the decisions that can be made by different organizational functions, and the processes to be used for making decisions
- Defining the roles that various organizational members and committees fulfill for IT—for example, which committee should monitor progress in an EHR implementation and what is the role of a department head during the implementation of a new system for his or her department?
- Developing IT-centric organizational processes for making decisions in key areas such as these:
  - o IT strategy development
  - o IT prioritization and budgeting
  - o IT project management
  - o IT architecture and infrastructure management
- Defining policies and procedures that govern the use of IT—for example, if a user wants to buy a new network for use in his or her department, what policies and procedures govern that decision?

Developing and maintaining an effective and efficient IT governance structure is a complex exercise. Moreover, governance is never static. Continuous refinements may be needed as the organization discovers imperfections in roles, responsibilities, and processes.

PERSPECTIVE
The Foundation of IT Governance

Peter Weill and Jeanne Ross have identified five major areas that form the foundation of IT governance. The organization's governance mechanisms need to create structures and processes for these areas.

- **IT principles:** high-level statements about how IT is used in the business
- **IT architecture:** an integrated set of technical choices to guide the organization in satisfying business needs. The architecture is a set of policies, procedures, and rules for the use of IT and for evolving IT in a direction that improves IT support for the organization.
- **IT infrastructure strategies:** strategies for the existing technical infrastructure (and IT support staff) that ensure the delivery of reliable secure and efficient services
- **Business application needs:** processes for identifying the needed applications
- **IT investment and prioritization:** mechanism for making decisions about project approvals and budgets

Source: Weill and Ross (2004, p. 27).

Governance Characteristics

Well-developed governance mechanisms have several characteristics.

- **They are perceived as objective and fair.** No organizational decision-making mechanisms are free from politics, and some decisions will be made as part of side deals. It is exceptionally rare for all managers of an organization to agree with any particular decision. Nonetheless, organizational participants should generally view governance as fair, objective, well-reasoned, and having integrity. The ability of governance to govern is highly dependent on the willingness of organizational participants to be governed.
- **They are efficient and timely.** Governance mechanisms should arrive at decisions quickly, and governance processes should be efficient, removing as much bureaucracy as possible.

- **They make authority clear.** Committees and individuals who have decision authority should have a clear understanding of the scope of their authority. Individuals who have IT roles should understand those roles. The organization's management must have a consistent understanding of its approach to IT governance. There always will be occasions when decision rights are murky, roles are confusing, or processes are unnecessarily complex, but these occasions should be few.

- **They can change as the organization,** its environment, and its understanding of technology changes. For example, efforts to implement regional interoperability between EHRs will require new governance mechanisms that bring representatives from the partnering organizations together to deal with inter-organizational IT issues such as the allowable uses of shared data.

Governance mechanisms evolve as IT technology and the organization's use of that technology evolve.

IT, User, and Senior Management Responsibilities

Effective application of IT involves the thoughtful distribution of **IT responsibilities** among the IT department, users of applications and IT services, and senior management. In general, these responsibilities address decision-making rights and roles. Although different organizations will arrive at different distributions of these responsibilities, and an organization's distribution may change over time, there is a fairly normative distribution (Applegate, Austin, & McFarlan, 2007).

IT Department Responsibilities

The IT department should be responsible for the following:

- Developing and managing the long-term architectural plan and ensuring that IT projects conform to that plan.
- Developing a process to establish, maintain, and evolve IT standards in several areas:
  - o Telecommunications protocols and platforms
  - o Client devices, such as workstations and mobile devices, and client software configurations

- o Server technologies, middleware, and database management systems
- o Programming languages
- o IT documentation procedures, formats, and revision policies
- o Data definitions (this responsibility is generally shared with the organization function, such as finance and health information management, that manages the integrity and meaning of the data)
- o IT disaster and recovery plans
- o IT security policies and incident response procedures

- Developing procedures that enable the assessment of sourcing options for new initiatives, such as building versus buying new applications or leveraging existing vendor partner offerings versus utilizing a new vendor when making an application purchase
- Maintaining an inventory of installed and planned systems and services and developing plans for the maintenance of systems or the planned obsolescence of applications and platforms
- Managing the professional growth and development of the IT staff [members]
- Establishing communication mechanisms that help the organization understand the IT agenda, challenges, and services and new opportunities to apply IT
- Maintaining effective relationships with preferred IT suppliers of products and services (Applegate, Austin, & McFarlan, 2007, p. 429)[1]

The scope and depth of these responsibilities may vary. Some of the responsibilities of the IT group may be delegated to others. For example, some non-IT departments may be permitted to have their own IT staff members and manage their own systems. This should be done only with the approval of senior management. And the IT department should be asked to provide oversight of the departmental IT group to ensure that professional standards are maintained and that no activities that comprise the organization's systems are undertaken. For example, the IT department can ensure that virus control procedures and software are effectively applied.

In general, the IT department is responsible for making sure that individual and organizational information systems are reliable, secure, efficient, current, and supportable. IT is also usually responsible for managing the relationship with suppliers of IT products and services and ensuring that the processes that lead to new IT purchases are rigorous.

User Responsibilities

IT users (primarily middle managers and supervisors) have several IT-related **user responsibilities:**

- Understanding the scope and quality of IT activities that are supporting their area or function

- Ensuring that the goals of IT initiatives reflect an accurate assessment of the function's needs and challenges and that the estimates of the function's resources (personnel time, funds, and management attention) needed by IT initiatives—to support the implementation of a new system, for example—are realistic

- Developing and reviewing specifications for IT projects and ensuring that ongoing feedback is provided to the IT organization on implementation issues, application enhancements, and IT support, ensuring, for example, that the new application has the functionality needed by the user department

- Ensuring that the applications used by a department are functioning properly, such as by periodically testing the accuracy of system-generated reports and checking that passwords are deleted when staff [members] leave the organization

- Participating in developing and maintaining the IT agenda and priorities (Applegate, Austin, & McFarlan, 2007, p. 431)[2]

These responsibilities constitute a minimal set. In Chapters Six and Seven, we discussed an additional, and more significant, set of responsibilities during the selection and implementation of new applications.

Senior Management Responsibilities

The primary IT **senior management responsibilities** are as follows:

- Ensuring that the organization has a comprehensive, thoughtful, and flexible IT strategy

- Ensuring an appropriate balance between the perspectives and agendas of the IT organization and the users—for example, the IT organization may want a new application that has the most advanced technology, [and] the user department wants the application that has been used in the industry for a long time

- Establishing standard processes for budgeting, acquiring, implementing, and supporting IT applications and infrastructure
- Ensuring that IT purchases and supplier relationships conform to organizational policies and practices—for example, contracts with IT vendors need to use standard organizational contract language
- Developing, modifying, and enforcing the responsibilities and roles of the IT organization and users
- Ensuring that the IT applications and activities conform to all relevant regulations and required management controls and risk mitigation processes and procedures
- Encouraging the thoughtful review of new IT opportunities and appropriate IT experimentation (Applegate, Austin, & McFarlan, 2007, p. 432)[3]

Although organizations will vary in the ways they distribute decision-making responsibility and roles and the ways in which they implement them, problems may arise when the distribution between groups is markedly skewed (Applegate, Austin, & McFarlan, 2007).

Too much user responsibility can lead to a series of uncoordinated and undermanaged user investments in information technology. This can result in these problems:

- An inability to achieve integration between highly heterogeneous systems
- Insufficient attention to infrastructure, resulting in application instability
- High IT costs because of insufficient economies of scale, significant levels of redundant activity, and the cost of supporting a high number of heterogeneous systems
- A lack of, or uneven, rigor applied to the assessment of the value of IT initiatives—for example, insufficient homework may be done and an application selected that has serious functional limitations

Too much IT responsibility can lead to these problems:

- Too much emphasis on technology, to the detriment of the fit of an application with the user function's need: for example, when a promising application does not completely satisfy the IT department's technical standards, IT will not allow its acquisition

PERSPECTIVE
Principles for IT Investments and Management

Charlie Feld and Donna Stoddard have identified three principles for effective IT investments and management. They note that the responsibility for developing and implementing these principles lies with the organization's senior leadership.

1. **A long-term IT renewal plan linked to corporate strategy.** Organizations need IT plans that are focused on achieving the organization's overall strategy and goals. The organization must develop this IT renewal plan and remain focused, often over the course of many years, on its execution.

2. **A simplified, unifying corporate technology platform.** This IT platform must be well architected and be defined and developed from the perspective of the overall organization rather than the accumulation of the perspectives of multiple departments and functions.

3. **A highly functional, performance-oriented IT organization.** The IT organization must be skilled, experienced, organized, goal-directed, responsive, and continuously work on establishing great working relationships with the rest of the organization.

Source: Feld and Stoddard (2004, p. 73).

- A failure to achieve the value of an application because of user resistance to a solution imposed by IT: "We in the IT department have decided that we know what you need. We don't trust your ability to make an intelligent decision."
- Too much rigor applied to IT investment decisions; excessive bureaucracy can stifle innovation
- A very high proportion of the IT budget devoted to infrastructure to the detriment of application initiatives as the IT department seeks to achieve ever greater (though perhaps not necessary) levels of reliability, security, and agility
- Reduction in business innovation when IT is unwilling to experiment with new technologies that might have stability and supportability problems

Either extreme can clearly create problems. And no compromise position will make the IT department and the IT users happy with all facets of the outcome. An outcome of "the best answer we can develop but not an answer that satisfies all" is an inevitable result of the leadership discussion of responsibility and role distribution.

Specific Governance Structures

In any organization there may be a plethora of committees and a series of complex reporting relationships and accountabilities, all of which need to operate with a fair degree of harmony in order for governance to be effective. Among them should be five core structures for governing IT:

- A board committee responsible for IT
- A senior leadership forum that guides the development of the IT agenda, finalizes the IT budget, develops major IT-centric policies, and addresses any significant IT issue that cannot be resolved elsewhere
- Initiative- and project-specific committees and roles (this was discussed in the chapters on implementation and value)
- IT liaison relationships
- A chief information officer (CIO) and other IT staff members (described in Chapter Eight)

The Board

The health care organization's board holds the fundamental accountability for the performance of the organization, including the IT function. The board must decide how it will carry out its responsibility with respect to IT.

At a minimum this responsibility involves receiving a periodic update (perhaps annually) at a board meeting from the CIO about the status of the IT agenda and the issues confronting the effective use of IT. In addition, financial information system controls and IT risk mitigation are often identified and discussed by the board's audit committee, and the IT budget is discussed by the finance committee.

Some organizations create an IT committee on the board. Realizing that the usual board agenda might not always allow sufficient time for discussion of important IT issues and that not all board members have deep experience in IT, the board can appoint a committee of board members who are seasoned IT professionals (IT academics, CIOs of regional organizations, and leaders in the IT industry). The committee, chaired by a trustee, need not be composed entirely of board members. IT professionals who are not on the board may serve as members, too. This committee informs the board of its assessments of a wide range of IT challenges and initiatives and makes recommendations about these issues.

The charter for such a committee might charge the committee to do the following:

- Review and critique IT application, technical, and organizational strategies.
- Review and critique overall IT tactical plans and budgets.
- Discuss and provide advice on major IT issues and challenges.
- Explore opportunities to leverage vendor partnerships.

Senior Leadership Organizational Forum

Most health care organizations have a committee called something similar to the executive committee. Composed of the senior leadership of the organization, this committee is the forum in which strategy discussions occur and major decisions regarding operations, budgets, and initiatives are made. It is highly desirable to have the CIO be a member of this committee.

Major IT decisions should be made at the meetings of this committee. These decisions will cover a gamut of topics, such as approving the outcome of a major system selection process, defining changes in direction that may be needed during the course of significant implementations, setting IT budget targets, and ratifying the IT component of the strategic-planning efforts.

This role does not preclude the executive committee from assigning IT-related tasks or discussions to other committees. For example, a medical staff leadership committee may be asked to develop policies regarding physician documentation of the problem list. A committee of department heads may be asked to select a new application to support registration and scheduling. A committee of human resource staff members may be charged with developing policies regarding organizational staff member use of social media sites.

The executive committee, major departments and functions, and several high-level committees will regularly be confronted with IT topics and issues that do not arise from the organization's IT plan and agenda. For example, a board member may ask if the organization should outsource its IT function. Several influential physicians may suggest that the organization assess a new information technology that seems to be getting a lot of hype. The CEO may ask how the organization should (or whether it should) respond to an external event: for example, a new Institute of Medicine report. The organization may need to address new regulations: for example, rules being issued by CMS.

Some organizations create an **IT steering committee** and charge this committee with addressing all IT issues and decisions. The use of such committees is uneven in health care organizations. Approximately half have such a committee.

IT Liaison Relationships

All major functions and departments of the organization—for example, finance, human resources, member services, medical staff affairs, and nursing—should have an IT liaison. The IT liaison is responsible for the following:

- Developing effective working relationships with the leadership of each major function
- Ensuring that the IT issues and needs of these functions are understood and communicated to the IT department and the executive committee
- Working with function leadership to ensure appropriate IT representation on function task forces and committees that are addressing initiatives that will require IT support
- Ensuring that the organization's IT strategy, plans and policies, and procedures are discussed with function leadership

The IT liaison role is an invaluable one. It ensures that the IT department and the IT strategy receive needed feedback and that function leaders understand the directions and challenges of the IT agenda. It also promotes an effective collaboration between IT and the other functions and departments.

Variations

The specific governance structures just described are typical in medium-sized and large provider or payer organizations. In other types of health care settings, these structures will be different.

A medium-sized physician group might not have a separate board. The physicians and the practice manager might make up the board and the senior leadership forum. The group might not need a CIO. Instead the practice administrator might manage contracts and relationships with companies that

PERSPECTIVE
Improving Coordination and Working Relationships

Carol Brown and Vallabh Sambamurthy have identified five mechanisms used by IT groups to improve their coordination and working relationships with the rest of the organization.

1. **Integrators** are individuals who are responsible for linking a particular organization department or function with the IT department. An integrator might be a CIO who is a participant in senior management forums. An integrator might also be an IT person who is responsible for working with the finance department on IT initiatives that are centered on that function; such a person might have a title such as manager, financial information systems.

2. **Groups** are committees and task forces that regularly bring IT staff [members] and organization staff [members] together to work collectively on IT issues. These groups could include, for example, the information systems steering committee or a standing joint meeting between IT and nursing to address current IT issues and review the status of ongoing IT initiatives.

3. **Processes** are organizational approaches to management activity such as developing the IT budget, selecting new applications, and implementing new systems. These processes invariably involve both IT and non-IT staff [members].

4. **Informal relationship building** includes a series of activities such as one-on-one meetings, IT staff presentations at department head meetings, and co-location of IT staff [members] and user staff [members].

5. **Human resource practices** include training IT staff [members] on team building, offering user feedback to IT staff [members] during their reviews, and having IT staff [members] spend time in a user area observing work.

Source: Brown and Sambamurthy (1999, p. 68).

provide practice management systems and support workstations and printers. The practice administrator also might perform all user liaison functions.

A division within a state department of public health would not have a board, but it should have a forum where division leadership can discuss IT issues. IT decisions might be made there or at meetings of the leadership of the overall department. Similarly, the CIO for the department might not have organized IT in a way that results in a division CIO. And the staff members of the department CIO might provide user liaison functions for the division.

Despite these variations, effective management of IT still requires

- A senior management forum where major IT decisions are made
- A person responsible for day-to-day management of the IT function and for ensuring that an IT strategy exists
- Mechanisms for ensuring that IT relationships have been established with major organizational functions

In addition, although the structures will vary, the guidance for the respective roles of the IT group, users, and management remains the same. The desirable attributes of the person responsible for IT are unchanged. And the properties of good governance do not change.

IT BUDGET

Developing budgets is one of the most critical management undertakings; it is the process that makes strategy real because it involves the commitment of resources. The budget process forces management to make choices between initiatives and investments and requires analysis of the scope and impact of any initiative—for example, it forces answers to questions such as, do we really believe that this initiative enables us to reduce supply costs by 3 percent?

Developing the **IT budget** is challenging for several reasons:

- The IT projects proposed at any one time are eclectic. In addition to the IT initiatives proposed as a result of the alignment and strategic planning process, other initiatives may be put forward by clinical or administrative departments that desire to improve some aspect of their performance. Also on the table may be IT projects designed to improve infrastructure—for example, a proposal to upgrade servers. These initiatives will all be different in character and in the return they offer, making them difficult to compare.
- Dozens, if not hundreds, of IT proposals may be made, making it challenging to fully understand all the requests.
- The aggregate request for capital and operating budgets can be too expensive. It is not unusual for requests to total three to four times

more money than the organization can afford. Even if it wanted to fund all of the requests, the organization doesn't have enough money to do so.

And yet the budget process requires that the organization grapple with these complexities and arrive at a budget answer.

Basic Budget Categories

To facilitate the development of the IT budget, the organization should develop some basic categories that organize the budget discussion.

Capital and Operating

The first category distinguishes between capital and operating budgets. Financial management courses are the best place to learn about these two categories. In brief, however, capital budgets are the funds associated with purchasing and deploying an asset. Common capital items in IT budgets are hardware and applications. Operating budgets are the funds associated with using and maintaining the asset. Common operating items in IT budgets are hardware maintenance contracts and the salaries of IT analysts. In an analogous fashion, the purchase of a car is a capital expense. Gasoline and tune-ups are operating expenses. Both capital and operating budgets are prepared for IT initiatives.

Support, Ongoing, and New IT

Support refers to those IT costs (staff members, hardware, and software licenses) necessary to support and maintain the applications and infra- structure that are in place now. Software maintenance contracts ensure that applications receive appropriate upgrades and bug fixes. Staff members are needed to run the computer room and perform minor enhancements. Disk drives may need to be replaced. Failure to fund support activities can make it much more difficult to ensure the reliability of systems or to evolve appli- cations to accommodate ongoing needs—for example, adding a new test to the dictionary for a laboratory system or introducing a new plan type into the patient accounting system.

Ongoing projects are those application implementations begun in a prior year and still under way. The implementation of a patient accounting system or a care coordination application can take several years. Hence a capital and operating budget is needed for several years to continue the implementation.

New projects are just that—there is a proposal for a new application or infrastructure application. The IT strategy may call for new systems to support nursing. Concerns over network security may lead to requests for new software to deter the efforts of hackers.

Improve Current Operations or Strategic Plan

Proposals may be directed to improving current operations, perhaps by responding to new regulations or streamlining the workflow in a department. Proposals may also be explicitly linked to an aspect of the health care organization's strategic plan—they might call for applications to support a strategic emphasis on disease management, for example.

Budget Targets

During the budget process, organizations define targets for the budget overall and for its components. For example, the organization might state that it would like to keep the overall growth in its operating budget to 2 percent but is willing to allow 5 percent growth in the IT operating budget. The organization might also direct that within that overall 5 percent growth, the budget for support should not grow by more than 3 percent, but the budget for new projects and ongoing projects combined can grow by 11 percent. Table 13.1 illustrates the application of overall and selective operating budget targets.

Similarly, targets can be set for the capital budget. For example, perhaps it will be decided that the capital budget for support should remain flat but that given the decision to invest in an EHR system, the overall capital budget will increase to accommodate the capital required by the EHR investment.

IT Budget Development

In addition to formulating the categories just described, organizational leadership will need to develop the process through which the IT budget is discussed, prioritized, and approved. In other words, it must answer the

Table 13.1 Target increases in an IT operating budget

	Support Operations	Strategic Initiatives	Overall Target
Ongoing and new	9%	15%	11%
Support	3%	3%	3%
OVERALL TARGET	4%	7%	5%

governance question, what processes will we use to decide which projects will be approved subject to our targets? An example of a budget process is outlined in this section and illustrated in Figure 13.1.

This process example has five components.

First, the IT department submits an operating budget to support the applications and infrastructure that will be in place as of the beginning of the fiscal year (the support budget). This budget might be targeted to a 3 percent increase over the support budget for the prior fiscal year. The 3 percent increase reflects inflation, salary increases, a recognition that new systems were implemented during the fiscal year and will require support, and an acknowledgment that infrastructure (workstations, remote locations, and storage) consumption will increase. A figure for capital to support applications and infrastructure is also submitted, and it might be targeted to be the same as that budgeted in the prior fiscal year. If the support operating and capital budgets achieve their targets, there is minimal management discussion of those budgets.

Second, IT leadership reviews the strategic IT initiatives (new and ongoing) with the senior leadership of the organization. This review may occur in a forum such as the executive committee. This committee, mindful of its targets, determines which strategic initiatives will be funded. If the budget being sought to support strategic IT initiatives is large or a major increase over the previous year, there may be discussions about the budget with the board.

Third, the organization must decide which new and ongoing initiatives that improve current operations—for example, a new clinical laboratory or contract management system—will be funded. These discussions must occur in the forum where the overall operations budget is discussed, generally organizational meetings that routinely discuss operations and that include among

Figure 13.1 IT budget decision-making process

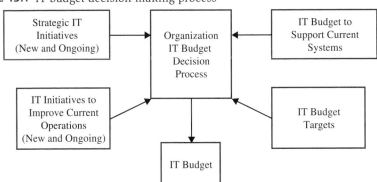

their members the managers of major departments and functions. Budget requests for new IT applications are reviewed in the same conversation that discusses budget requests for new clinical services or improvement of the organization's physical plant.

Fourth, the IT strategy budget discussion and the IT operations budget discussion follow a set of ground rules:

- The IT budget is discussed in the same conversations that discuss non-IT budget requests. This will result in trade-offs between IT expenditures and other expenditures. This integration forces the organization to examine where it believes its monies are best spent, asking, for example, Should we invest in this IT proposal or should we invest in hiring staff members to expand a clinical service? Following this process also means that IT requests and other budget requests are treated no differently.

- The level of analytical rigor required of the IT projects is the same as that required of any other requested budget item.

- When appropriate, a sponsor—for example, a clinical vice president or a CFO—defends the IT requests that support his or her department in front of his or her colleagues. The IT staff members or CIO should be asked to defend infrastructure investments—for example, major changes to the network—but should not be asked to defend applications.

The ground rule that sponsors should present their own IT requests deserves a bit more discussion, because the issue of who defends the request has several important ramifications, particularly for initiatives designed to improve current operations. Having this ground rule has the following results:

- **It forces assessment of trade-offs between IT and non-IT investments.** The sponsor will determine whether to present the IT proposal or some other, perhaps non-IT, proposal. Sponsors are choosing which investments are the most important to them.

- **It forces accountability for investment results.** The sponsor and his or her colleagues know that if the IT proposal is approved, there will be less money available for other initiatives. The defender also knows that the value being promised must be delivered or his or her credibility in next year's budget discussion will be diminished.

- **It improves management comfort when dealing with IT proposals.** Managers can be more comfortable with the IT proposal if one of their operations colleagues is defending it. The defender also learns how to be comfortable when presenting IT proposals.

- **It gets IT out of the role of defending other people's operation improvement initiatives.** However, the IT function must still support the budget requests of others by providing data on the costs and capabilities of the proposed applications and the time frames and resources required to implement them. If the IT function believes that the proposed initiative lacks merit or is too risky, IT staff members need to ensure that this opinion is heard during the budget approval process.

In the fifth and final step of the process, the operations and strategic budget recommendations are reviewed and discussed at an executive committee meeting. The executive committee can accept the recommendations, request further refinement (perhaps cuts) of the budget, or determine that a discussion of the budget is required at an upcoming board meeting.

MANAGEMENT ROLE IN MAJOR IT INITIATIVES

The failure rate of IT initiatives is surprisingly high. Project failure occurs when a project is significantly over budget, takes much longer than the estimated timeline, or has to be terminated because so many problems have occurred that proceeding is no longer judged to be viable. Cook (2007) finds that 35 percent of IT projects were successful, whereas 19 percent failed. The remaining 46 percent delivered a useful product but suffered from budget overruns, prolonged timetables, and application feature shortfalls.

Cash, McFarlan, and McKenney (1992) note that two major categories of risk confront significant IT investments: strategy failures and implementation failures. The project failure rates suggest that management should be more worried about IT implementation than IT strategy. IT strategy is sexier and more visionary than implementation. However, a very large number of strategies and visions go nowhere or are diminished because the organization is unable to implement them.

It is rare that leaders plan to fail. And yet they often do things or don't do things that increase the likelihood that a major initiative will fail. At times they don't appreciate the myriad ways that projects can go south and hence they fail to take steps to mitigate those risk factors. In the sections that follow we discuss factors that imperil implementations, factors that can be managed.

Lack of Clarity of Purpose

Any project or initiative is destined for trouble if its objectives and purpose are unclear. Sometimes the purpose of a project is only partially clear. For example, an organization may have decided that it should implement an EHR in an effort to "improve the quality and efficiency of care." However, it is not really clear to the leadership and staff members how the EHR will be used to improve care. Will problems associated with finding a patient's record be solved? Will the record be used to gather data about care quality? Will the record be used to support outpatient medication ordering and reduce medication error rates?

All these questions can be answered yes, but if the organization never gets beyond the slogan of "improve the quality and efficiency of care," the scope of the project will be murky. The definition of care improvement is left up to the project participant to interpret. And the scope and timetable of the project cannot possibly be precise because project objectives are too fuzzy.

Lack of Belief in the Project

At times the objectives are very clear, but the members of the organization are not convinced that the project is worth doing at all. Because the project will change the work life of many members and require that they participate in design and implementation, they need to be sufficiently convinced that the project will improve their lives or is necessary if the organization is to thrive. They will legitimately ask, what's in it for me? Unconvinced of the need for the project, they will resist it. A resistant organization will likely doom any project. Projects that are viewed as illegitimate by a large portion of the people in an organization rarely succeed.

Insufficient Leadership Support

The organization's leaders may be committed to the undertaking yet not demonstrate that commitment. For example, leaders may not devote sufficient time to the project or may decide to send subordinates to meetings. This broadcasts a signal to the organization that the leaders have other, "more important" things to do. Tough project decisions may get made in a way that shows the leaders are not as serious as their rhetoric, because when push came to shove, they caved in.

Members of the leadership team may have voted yes to proceed with a project, but their votes may not have included their reservations about the utility of the project or the way it was put together. Once problems are encountered in the project (and all projects encounter problems), this qualified leadership support evaporates, and the silent reservations become public statements such as, "I knew that this would never work."

Organizational Inertia

Even when the organization is willing to engage in a project, inertia can hinder it. People are busy. They are stressed. They have jobs to do. Some of the changes are threatening. Staff members may believe these changes leave them less skilled or with reduced power. Or they may not have a good understanding of their work life after the change, and they may imagine that an uncertain outcome cannot be a good outcome.

Projects add work on top of the workload of often already overburdened people. Projects add stress for often already stressed people. As a result, despite the valiant efforts of leadership and the expenditure of significant resources, a project may slowly grind to a halt because too many members find ways to avoid or not deal with the efforts and changes the initiative requires. Bringing significant change to a large portion of the organization is very hard because, if nothing else, there is so much inertia to overcome.

Organizational Baggage

Organizations have baggage. Baggage comes in many forms. Some organizations have no history of competence in making significant organizational change. They have never learned how to mobilize the organization's members. They do not know how to handle conflict. They are unsure how to assemble and leverage multidisciplinary teams. They have never mastered staying the course over years during the execution of complex agendas. These organizations are "incompetent," and this incompetence extends well beyond IT, although it clearly includes IT initiatives.

An organization may have tried initiatives "like this" before and failed. The proponents of the initiative may have failed at other initiatives. Organizations have very long memories, and their members may be thinking something like, "The same clowns who brought us that last fiasco are back with an even 'better' idea." The odor from prior failures significantly taints the credibility of newly proposed initiatives and helps to ensure that organizational acceptance will be weak.

Lack of an Appropriate Reward System

Aspects of organizational policies, incentives, and practices can hinder a project. The organization's incentive system may not be structured to reward multidisciplinary behavior—for example, physicians may be rewarded for research prowess or clinical excellence but not for sitting on committees to design new clinical processes. An integrated delivery system may have encouraged its member hospitals to be self-sufficient. As a result, management practices that involve working across hospitals never matured, and the organization does not know how (even if it is willing) to work across hospitals.

Lack of Candor

Organizations can create environments that do not encourage healthy debate. Such environments can result when leadership is intolerant of being challenged or has an inflated sense of its worth and does not believe that it needs team effort to get things done. The lack of a climate that encourages conflict and can manage conflict means that initiative problems will not get resolved. Moreover, organizational members, not having had their voices heard, will tolerate the initiative only out of the hope that they will outlast the initiative and the leadership.

Sometimes the project team is uncomfortable delivering bad news. Project teams will screw up and make mistakes. Sometimes they really screw up and make really big mistakes. Because they may be embarrassed or worried that they will be admonished, they hide the mistakes from the leadership and attempt to fix the problems without "anyone having to know." This attempt to hide bad news is a recipe for disaster. It is unrealistic to expect problems to go unnoticed; invariably the leadership team finds out about the problem and its trust in the project team erodes. At times leadership has to look in the mirror to see if its own intolerance for bad news in effect created the problem.

Project Complexity

Project complexity is determined by many factors:

- The number of people whose work will be changed by the project and the depth of those changes
- The number of organizational processes that will be changed and the depth of those changes
- The number of processes linking the organization and other organizations that will be changed and the depth of those changes
- The interval over which all this change will occur: for example, will it occur quickly or gradually?

If the change is significant in scale, scope, and depth, then it becomes very difficult (often impossible) for the people managing the project to truly understand what the project needs to do. The design will be imperfect. The process changes will not integrate well. And many curves will be thrown in the project's way as the implementation unfolds and people realize their mistakes and understand what they failed to understand initially.

Sometimes complex projects disappear in an organizational mushroom cloud. The complexity overwhelms the organization and causes the project to crash suddenly. More common is "death by ants"—no single bite (or project problem) will kill the project, but a thousand will. The organization is overwhelmed by the thousand small problems and inefficiencies and terminates the undertaking.

Managers should remember that complexity is relative. Organizations generally have developed a competency to manage projects up to a certain level and type of complexity. Projects that require competency beyond that level are inherently risky. A project that is risky for one organization may not be risky for another. For example, an organization that typically manages projects that cost $2 million, take ten person-years of effort, and affect three hundred people will struggle with a project that costs $20 million and takes one hundred person-years of effort (Cash, McFarlan, & McKenney, 1992).

Failure to Respect Uncertainty

Significant organizational change brings a great deal of uncertainty with it. The leadership may be correct in its understanding of where the organization needs to go and the scope of the changes needed. However, it is highly unlikely that anyone really understands the full impact of the change and how new processes, tasks, and roles will really work. At best, leadership has a good approximation of the new organization. The belief that a particular outcome is certain can be a problem in itself.

Agility and the ability to detect when a change is not working and to alter its direction are very important. Detection requires that the organization listens to the feedback of those who are waist-deep in the change and is able to discern the difference between the organizational noise that comes with any change and the organizational noise that reflects real problems. Altering direction requires that the leadership not cling to ideas that cannot work and also be willing to admit to the organization that it was wrong about some aspects of the change.

Initiative Undernourishment

There may be a temptation, particularly as the leadership tries to accomplish as much as it can with a constrained budget, to tell a project team,

"I know you asked for ten people, but we're going to push you to do it with five." The leadership may believe that such bravado will make the team work extra hard and, through heroic efforts, complete the project in a grand fashion.

However, bravado may turn out to be bellicose stupidity. This approach may doom a project, despite the valiant efforts of the team to do the impossible. Another form of undernourishment involves placing staff members other than the best people on the initiative. If the initiative is very important, then it merits using the best people possible and freeing up their time so they can focus on the initiative. An organization's best staff members are always in demand, and there can be a temptation to say that it would be too difficult to pull them away from other pressing issues.

They are needed elsewhere and this decision is difficult. However, if the initiative is critical to the organization, then those other demands are less important and can be given to someone else. Critical organizational initiatives should not be staffed with the junior varsity.

Failure to Anticipate Short-Term Disruptions

Any major change will lead to short-term problems and disruptions in operations. Even though current processes can be made better, they are working and staff members know how to make them work. When processes are changed, there is a shakeout period as staff members adjust and learn how to make the new processes work well. At times, adjusting to the new application system is the core of the disruption. A shakeout can go on for months and degrade organizational performance. Service will deteriorate. Days in accounts receivable will climb. Balls will be dropped in many areas. The organization can misinterpret these problems as a sign that the initiative is failing.

Listening closely to the issues and suggestions of the front line is essential during this time. These staff members need to know that their problems are being heard and that their ideas for fixing these problems are being acted on. People often know exactly what needs to be done to remove system disruptions. Listening to and acting on their advice also improves their buy-in to the change.

Although working hard to minimize the duration and depth of disruption, the organization also needs to be tolerant during this period and to appreciate the low-grade form of hell that staff members are enduring. It is critical that this period be kept as short and as pain free as possible. If the disruption lasts too long, staff members may conclude that the change is not working and abandon their support.

Lack of Technology Stability and Maturity

Information technology may be obviously immature. New technologies are being introduced all the time, and it takes time for them to work through their kinks and achieve an acceptable level of stability, supportability, and maturity. Some forms of social networking are current examples of information technologies that are in their youth.

Organizations can become involved in projects that require immature technology to play a critical role. This clearly elevates the risk of the project. The technology will suffer from performance problems, and the organization's IT staff members and the technology supplier may have a limited ability to identify and resolve technology problems. Organizational members, tired of the instability, become tired of the project and it fails.

In general, it is not common, nor should it often be necessary, for a project to hinge on the adequate performance of new technology. A thoughtful assessment that a new technology has potentially extraordinary promise and that the organization can achieve differential value by being an early adopter should precede any such decision. Even in these cases, pilot projects that provide experience with the new technology while limiting the scope of its implementation (which minimizes potential damage) are highly recommended.

Projects can also get into trouble when the amount of technology change is extensive. For example, the organization may be attempting to implement, over a short period of time, applications from several different vendors that involve different operating systems, network requirements, security models, and database management systems. This broad scope can overwhelm the IT department's ability to respond to technology misbehavior.

How to Avoid These Mistakes

Major IT projects fail in many ways. However, a large number of these failures can be mitigated by management attention to risk factors. Few management teams and senior leaders start IT projects hoping that failure is the outcome. Summarizing our discussion in this section produces a set of recommendations that can help organizations reduce the risk of IT initiative failure:

- Ensure that the objectives of the IT initiative are clear.
- Communicate the objectives and the initiative, and test the degree to which organizational members have bought into them.
- Publicly demonstrate conviction by "being there" and showing resolve during tough decisions.

- Respect organizational inertia, and keep hammering away at it.
- Distance the project from any organizational baggage, perhaps through a thoughtful choice of project sponsors and managers.
- Change the reward system if necessary to create incentives for participants to work toward project success.
- Accept and welcome the debate that surrounds projects, invite bad news, and do not hang those who make mistakes.
- Address complexity by breaking the project into manageable pieces, and test for evidence that the project might be at risk from trying to do too much all at once.
- Realize that there is much you do not know about how to change the organization or the form of new processes; be prepared to change direction and listen and respond to those who are on the front line.
- Supply resources for the project appropriately, and assign the project to your best team.
- Try to limit the duration and depth of the short-term operational disruption, but accept that it will occur.
- Ensure and communicate regular, visible progress.
- Be wary of new technology and projects that involve a broad scope of information technology change.

These steps, along with solid project management, can dramatically reduce the risk that an IT project will fail. However, these steps are not foolproof. Major IT projects, particularly those accompanied by major organizational change, will always have a nontrivial level of risk.

There will also be times when a review of the failure factors indicates that a project is too risky. The organization may not be ready; there may be too much baggage, too much inertia to overcome; the best team may not be available; the organization may not be good at handling conflict; or the project may require too much new information technology. Projects with considerable risk should not be undertaken until progress has been made in addressing the failure factors. Management of IT project risk is a critical contributor to IT success.

IT EFFECTIVENESS

Several studies have examined organizations that have been particularly effective in the use of IT (McAfee & Brynjolfsson, 2008; McKenney, Copeland, & Mason, 1995; Ross, Beath, & Goodhue, 1996; Sambamurthy & Zmud, 1996;

Weill & Broadbent, 1998). Determining effectiveness is difficult, and these studies have defined organizations that show **effectiveness in IT** in a variety of ways. Among them are organizations that have developed information systems that defined an industry (as Amazon has altered the retail industry, for example), organizations that have a reputation for being effective over decades (such as Bank of America), and organizations that have demonstrated exceptional IT innovation (Amazon.com for example).

The studies have attempted to identify those organizational factors or attributes that have led to or created the environment in which effectiveness has occurred. In other words, the studies have sought to answer the question, what are the organizational attributes that result in some organizations developing truly remarkable IT prowess?

If an organization understands these attributes and desires to be very effective in its use of IT, then it is in a position to develop strategies and approaches to create or modify its own attributes. For example, one attribute is having strong working relationships between the IT function and the rest of the organization. If an organization finds that its own relationships are weak or dysfunctional, strategies and plans can be created to improve them.

The studies suggest that organizations that aspire to high levels of effectiveness and innovation in their application of IT must take steps to ensure that the core capacity of the organization to achieve such effectiveness is developed. It is a critical IT responsibility of organizational leadership to continuously (year in and year out) identify and accomplish the steps needed to improve overall effectiveness in IT. The development of this capacity is a challenge different from the challenge of identifying specific opportunities to use IT in the course of improving operations or enhancing management decision making. For an analogy, consider running. A runner's training, injury management, and diet are designed to ensure the core capacity to run a marathon. This capacity development is different from developing an approach to running a specific marathon, which must consider the nature of the course, the competing runners, and the weather.

Although having somewhat different conclusions (resulting in part from somewhat different study questions), the studies have much in common regarding capacity development.

Individuals and Leadership Matter

It is critical that the organization possess talented, skilled, and experienced individuals. These individuals will occupy a variety of roles: CEO, CIO, IT staff members, and user middle managers. These individuals must be strong contributors.

Although such an observation may seem trite, too often organizations, dazzled by the technology or the glorified experiences of others, embark on technology crusades and substantive investments that they have insufficient talent or leadership to effect well. The studies found that leadership is essential. Leaders must understand the vision, communicate the vision, be able to recruit and motivate a team, and have the staying power to see large IT implementations through several years of work with disappointments, setbacks, and political problems along the way.

Relationships Are Critical

Not only must the individual players be strong but also the team must be strong. There are critical senior executive, IT executive, and project team roles that must be filled by highly competent individuals, and great chemistry must exist between the individuals in these distinct roles. Substitutions among team members, even when involving a replacement by an equally strong individual, can diminish the team. This is as true in IT innovation as it is in sports. Political turbulence diminishes the ability to develop a healthy set of relationships among organizational players.

The Technology and the Technical Infrastructure Both Enable and Hinder

New technologies can provide new opportunities for organizations to embark on major transformations of their activities. We have seen this in retail and music distribution. This implies that the health care CIO must have not only superior business and clinical understanding but also superior understanding of the technology. This does not imply that CIOs must be able to rewrite operating systems as well as the best system programmers, but it does mean that they must have superior understanding of the maturity, capabilities, and possible evolution of various information technologies. Several innovations have occurred because an IT group was able to identify and adopt an emerging technology that could make a significant contribution to addressing a current organizational challenge. The studies also stress the importance of well-developed technical architecture. Great architecture matters. Possessing state-of-the-art technology can be far less important than having a well-architected infrastructure.

The Organization Must Encourage Innovation

The organization's (and the IT department's) culture and leadership must encourage innovation and experimentation. This encouragement needs to be practical and goal directed: a real business problem, crisis, or opportunity must exist, and the project must have budgets, political protection, and deliverables.

True Innovation Takes Time

Creating visionary applications, making major organizational changes, or establishing an exceptional IT asset takes time and a lot of work. In the organizations studied it often took five to seven years for the innovation to fully mature and for the organization to recast itself. Innovation will proceed through phases that are as normative as the passage from being a child to being an adult. Innovation, similar to the maturation of a human being, will see some variations in timing, depth, and success in moving through phases.

Evaluation of IT Opportunities Must Be Thoughtful

Visionary and even more pedestrian IT innovations should be analyzed and studied thoroughly. Nonetheless, organizations engaged in launching a major IT initiative should also understand that a large amount of vision, management instinct, and "feel" often guides the decision to initiate investment and continue investment. For example, what is the strategic and clinical value of an integrated EHR across the continuum? The organization that has had more experiences with IT, and more successful experiences, will be more effective in the evaluation (and execution) of IT initiatives.

Processes, Data, and Business Model Change Form the Basis of an IT Innovation

All the strategic initiatives studied were launched from management's fundamental understanding of current organizational limitations. Strategic initiatives should focus on the core elements to be discussed following in this chapter as the basis for achieving an IT-based advantage: significant leveraging of processes, expanding and capitalizing on the ability to gather critical data, and enabling new business models. Often an organization can pursue all three simultaneously.

Alignment Must Be Mature and Strong

The alignment between the IT activities and the business challenges or opportunities must be strong. It should also be mature in the sense that it depends on close working relationships rather than methodologies.

The IT Asset Is Critical

Strong IT staff members, well-crafted architecture, and a superb CIO are critical contributors to success. There is substantial overlap between the factors identified in these studies and the components of the IT asset.

An overall critical factor in organizations being effective in using IT is the skills and orientation of senior leadership. Earl and Feeney (2000) assessed the characteristics and behaviors of senior leaders (in this case CEOs) who were actively engaged and successful in the strategic use of IT. These leaders

---

PERSPECTIVE
Principles for Higher Performance

Robert Dvorak, Endre Holen, David Mark, and William Meehan have identified six principles at work in a high-performance IT function:

1. IT is a business-driven line activity and not a technology-driven IT staff function. Non-IT managers are responsible for selecting, implementing, and realizing the benefits of new applications. IT managers are responsible for providing cost-effective infrastructure to enable the applications.

2. IT funding decisions are made on the basis of value. Funding decisions require thorough business cases. IT decisions are based on business judgment and not technology judgment.

3. The IT environment emphasizes simplicity and flexibility. IT standards are centrally determined and enforced. Technology choices are conservative, and packaged applications are used wherever possible.

4. IT investments have to deliver near-term business results. The 80-20 rule is followed for applications, and projects are monitored relentlessly against milestones.

5. The IT operation engages in year-to-year operation productivity improvements.

6. A business-smart IT function and an IT-smart business organization are created. Senior leadership is involved in and conversant with IT decisions. IT managers spend time developing an understanding of the business.

Source: Dvorak, Holen, Mark, and Meehan (1997, p. 166).

were convinced that IT could and would change the organization. They placed the IT discussion high on the strategic agenda. They looked to IT to identify opportunities to make significant improvements in organizational performance, rather than viewing the IT agenda as secondary to strategy development. They devoted personal time to understanding how their industry and their organization would evolve as IT evolved. And they encouraged other members of the leadership team to do the same.

Earl and Feeney (2000) observed five management behaviors in these leaders:

1. They studied, rather than avoided, IT. They devoted time to learning about new technologies and, through discussion and introspection, developed an understanding of the ways in which new technologies might alter organizational strategies and operations.

2. They incorporated IT into their vision of the future of the organization and discussed the role of IT when communicating that vision.

3. They actively engaged in IT architecture discussions and high-level decisions. They took time to evaluate major new IT proposals and their implications. They were visibly supportive of architecture standards. They established funds for the exploration of promising new technologies.

4. They made sure that IT was closely linked to core management processes:
   o They integrated the IT discussion tightly into the overall strategy development process. This often involved setting up teams to examine aspects of the strategy and having both IT and business leaders at the table.
   o They made sure IT investments were evaluated as one component of the total investment needed by a strategy. The IT investments were not relegated to a separate discussion.
   o They ensured strong business sponsorship for all IT investments.
   o Business sponsors were accountable for managing the IT initiatives and ensuring the success of the undertaking.

5. They continuously pressured the IT department to improve its efficiency and effectiveness and to be visionary in its thinking.

CEOs and other members of the leadership team have an extraordinary impact on the tone, values, and direction of an organization. Hence, their beliefs and daily behaviors have a significant impact on how effectively and strategically information technology is applied within an organization.

THE COMPETITIVE VALUE OF IT

For many years organizations across many industries have attempted to use (and at times succeeded in using) IT to achieve a competitive advantage. Decades ago airlines used travel reservation systems as an advantage, listing their flights before those of a competitor. At one time banks used personal computer–based banking as an IT-based advantage, making it easier for customers to manage their assets from home and reducing the need to visit a branch bank. Amazon is a superb example of an organization that used IT to achieve an advantage over its retail rivals. Amazon was able to offer a very broad range of products without incurring the expense of setting up hundreds of retail stores.[4]

Sources of Advantage

These efforts have shown that IT can enable a significant improvement in organizational performance and assist in achieving an advantage, especially when it is used to leverage core organizational processes, support the collection of critical data, or enable the development of new business models.

Leverage of Organizational Processes

Information technology can be applied in an effort to improve organizational processes by making them faster, less error prone, less expensive, and more convenient. However, improved organizational competitive position through process gains is not an automatic result of IT implementation.

The right processes must be chosen. The leverage of processes is most effective when the processes being addressed are critical, core processes that customers use to judge the performance of the organization or to define the core business of the organization.

For example, patients are more likely to judge a provider organization on the basis of its ambulatory scheduling processes and billing processes than they are on its accounts payable and human resources processes. Making diagnostic and therapeutic decisions is a core provider organization process that is the backbone of its business.

Organizations must also examine and redesign processes. If underlying problems with processes are not remedied, the IT investment can be wasted or diluted. IT applications can result in existing processes continuing to perform poorly, only faster. Moreover, it can be harder to fix flawed processes after the application of IT because the new IT-supported process now has an additional source of complexity, cost, and ossification to address: the new computer system.

IT can be applied to significant competitive advantage if processes are chosen wisely and are reengineered skillfully.

Rapid and Accurate Provision of Critical Data

Organizations define critical elements of their plans, operations, and environment. These elements must be monitored to ensure the plan is working, service and care quality are high, the organization's fiscal situation is sound, and the environment is behaving as anticipated. Clearly data are required to perform such monitoring.

In addition to their utility in monitoring, data can be used to guide management actions. Internet-based retailers use purchase data to target their advertisements. Providers use data on care costs and quality to devise initiatives to improve outcomes. However, obtaining and reporting critical data is not easy.

Data quality may be limited and incomplete. For example, although physicians are using an EHR, they may not be recording all of a patient's problems, and many of their entries are unstructured free text. There may be confusion about which patients belong on specific physician panels. There can be significant disagreements about the definition of "a visit."

Using IT to improve performance through the capture of critical data requires addressing process problems that hinder data capture, developing user incentives to record good data, and engaging in difficult conversations about data meaning.

Developing New Business Models

A business model refers to an organization's plans about what it will do, how it will do it, and why that "what and how" will lead to revenue that will enable the organization to sustain itself. For example, a hospital will have a business model that looks something like this:

- We will cure you of your disease or repair you if you experience trauma (the what).
- We will do so by hiring clinicians, providing acute care beds, developing ancillary services such as the laboratory, and implementing clinical protocols (the how).
- You will pay us for doing so (primarily through health insurance).

When IT is used competitively to enable new business models, most of these efforts focus on the how. For example:

- Telehealth visits can be conducted virtually rather than face-to-face, which improves convenience.
- Uber uses information technology to replace taxi cab employees with renting of driver capacity by independent contractors and providing a very easy way to order a ride and pay for it (which lowers Uber's costs and improves rider convenience).
- The Internet of Things enables manufacturers of equipment to monitor equipment performance to detect potential issues and dispatch repair staff members before the equipment breaks, which improves the how of maintaining equipment.
- At times IT can enable capabilities that were previously impractical. Gathering real-time physiological data from a patient at home was not practical until the advent of mobile devices and the Internet. eBay enabled the development of a global auction using the Internet.

Observations on IT Use for Competitive Advantage

IT has been used competitively by hundreds of organizations across a range of industries over the course of multiple decades. These experiences have taught us several overall lessons.

Obtaining and Sustaining an Advantage

It is very difficult to obtain a competitive advantage based solely on the implementation of a particular application or technology. Competitors, noting the advantage, are quick to attempt to copy the application, lure away the original developers, or obtain a version of the application from the same or different vendor. Moreover, the advantage rarely results from the acquisition of a system but from skilled process changes that thoughtfully understand how to differentiate an organization from its competitors.

The advantage does not come from the application system. In an industry in which most applications can be purchased from a vendor, it is almost impossible for the application to provide an advantage. If you can buy an EHR from vendor x, so can your competitor, and any advantage is short-lived.

Any IT-enabled advantage results from using the technology to improve processes, gather critical data, and define new business models. Advantage lies in the application of the technology and not the possession of the technology.

Technology Is a Tool

Information technology can provide a competitive advantage. However, IT has no magic properties. In particular, technology cannot overcome poor strategies, inadequate management, inept execution, or major organizational limitations. IT implementation cannot overcome badly managed process change, insufficient political will to standardize data, or faulty business models.

The early experiences of Internet-based retailers have highlighted the problems created by sloppy inventory management, poor understanding of customer buying behaviors such as returning purchases, and insufficient knowledge of customer price tolerance.

Referring physicians will not find valuable and probably will not use a system that gives them access to hospital data if the consulting physicians at the hospital are remiss in getting their consult notes completed on time or at all.

McAfee and Brynjolfsson (2008) note a significant separation in the spread in the gross margin, over time, between those companies performing in the top 25 percent of their industry versus those performing in the bottom 25 percent as measured by variables such as return on capital (see Figure 13.2). Beginning in the late 1990s the gap between winners and losers was widening.

McAfee and Brynjolfsson (2008) made two major observations. First, IT had become sufficiently potent that its ability to advance organizational

Figure 13.2 Gross margin performance differences in high IT–use industries

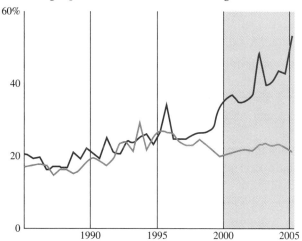

Source: McAfee and Brynjolfsson (2008). Reproduced with permission of Harvard Business School Publishing.

performance had become very significant. The personal computers of the 1980s were important but were not powerful enough to enable one organization to significantly outperform another. However, the Internet, which began to be used by business in the late 1990s, was powerful enough. Information technology had come of age. Second, although potent technologies had become available, they were available to all. So why did the separation in performance occur? Why didn't all organizations see improvement? The answer is simple—some organizations were very skilled at leveraging the technology to improve competitive performance and others were not.

As an analogy, a skilled carpenter and a novice will be similarly effective in constructing a house if both use crude tools. But if you give them sophisticated tools, the skilled carpenter will significantly outperform the novice.

When one looks back at organizations that have been effective in the strategic application of IT over a reasonably long time, one sees what looks like a series of singles punctuated by an occasional leap, a grand slam (McKenney, Copeland, & Mason, 1995). One doesn't see a progression of grand slams or, in the parlance of the industry, killer applications (Downes & Mui, 1998).

In the course of improving processes, changing business models, and gathering data, organizations carry out a series of initiatives that improve their performance. The vast majority of these initiatives do not by themselves fundamentally alter the competitive position of the organization, but in the aggregate they make a significant contribution, just as the difference between a great hotel and a mediocre hotel is not solely the presence of clean sheets or hot water but one thousand such things.

In addition, at various points in time, the organization may have an insight that leads to a major leap in its application of IT to its performance. For example, airlines, having developed their initial travel reservation systems, continued to improve them. At some point they realized that the data gathered by a reservation system had enormous potency and frequent flyer programs resulted. Google realized that it had a very large base of users that accessed the site often for searches. Google could capitalize on this base by introducing other, nonsearch offerings such as YouTube. No organization has ever delivered a series of killer, or grand slam, applications in rapid succession.

Organizations must develop their IT asset in such a way that they can affect the types of continuous improvement that managers and medical staff members will see as possible, day in and day out. For example, in an ideal world an organization would be able to capitalize on the improvements in ambulatory scheduling that a middle manager thinks up and also be able to capitalize on a thousand other good ideas and opportunities. The organization must also develop antennae that sense the possibility of a leap and the ability to focus that enables it to bring about the systems needed to make the leap. Ensuring that

Figure 13.3 Singles and grand slams

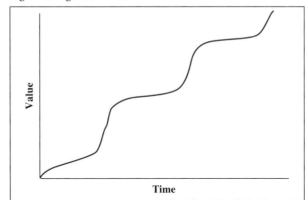

these antennae are working is one of the key functions of the CIO. The resulting pattern may look like the graph line in Figure 13.3—continuous improvement (singles) in performance using IT punctuated by periodic leaps or grand slams.

It is also clear that organizations have a limited ability to see more than one leap at a time. Hence, they should be cautious about visions that are too visionary or that have a very long time horizon. Organizations have great difficulty understanding a world that is significantly different from the one they inhabit now or that can be only vaguely understood in the context of the next leap. We might understand frequent flyer programs now, but they were not well understood, nor was their competitive value well understood, at the time they were conceived. Moreover, the organizational changes required to support and capitalize on a leap can take years—five to seven years at times (McKenney, Copeland, & Mason, 1995).

SUMMARY

The management and leadership of an organization play significant roles in determining the effectiveness of information technology. This chapter discussed the role of developing and maintaining IT governance mechanisms—the processes, procedures, and roles that the organization uses to make IT decisions. These decisions cover diverse terrain: budgets, roles, and responsibility distribution and the process for resolution of IT issues.

The processes and structure of developing the IT budget were reviewed. Budgets are critical. They turn strategy into reality by providing (or not) the resources needed to carry out the strategy.

Management is a major contributor to the success or failure of IT initiatives. The chapter discusses factors, under management's control, that often

PERPSECTIVE
How Great Companies Use IT

In his seminal book *Good to Great*, Jim Collins (2001) identified companies that made and sustained a transition from being a good company to being a great company. His research noted that these companies had several consistent orientations to IT:

- They avoided IT fads but were pioneers in the application of carefully selected technologies.
- They became pioneers when the technology showed great promise in leveraging that which they were already good at doing (their core competency) and that which they were passionate about doing well.
- They used IT to accelerate their momentum toward being a great company but did not use IT to create that momentum. In other words, IT came after the vision had been set and the organization had begun to move toward that vision. IT was not used to create the vision and start the movement.
- They responded to technology change with great thoughtfulness and creativity driven by a burning desire to turn unrealized potential into results. Mediocre companies often reacted to technology out of fear, adopting it because they were worried about being left behind.
- They achieved dramatically better results with IT than did rival companies using the exact same technology.
- They rarely mentioned IT as being critical to their success.
- They "crawled, walked, and then ran" with new IT even when they were undergoing radical change.

derail IT initiatives and suggested steps that can be taken to mitigate those factors. The chapter also reviewed attributes of organizations that have been highly effective in their use of IT for many years.

Finally, the chapter reviewed lessons learned from the use of IT to improve an organization's competitive position. Increased competiveness can occur when IT issues are applied to leverage critical organizational processes, address information needs, and enable new business models. However, we are reminded that IT is a tool and its use requires skill.

KEY TERMS

Effectiveness in IT
IT budget
IT governance
IT responsibilities

IT steering committee
Senior management responsibilities
User responsibilities

LEARNING ACTIVITIES

1. Interview a member of the senior leadership team of a health care organization on the subject of IT governance. Describe the organization's approach to IT governance and assess its effectiveness.

2. Interview a health care CIO and a member of the senior leadership team of the same health care organization separately. Ask each of them to describe the process of preparing the IT budget. Compare and discuss their responses.

3. Interview senior leaders of a health care organization and ask them to describe how they apply IT to improve their competitiveness.

4. Interview a health care CIO and a member of the senior leadership team of a health care organization separately. Ask each of them to describe the distribution of IT and user responsibilities. Compare and discuss their responses.

5. Assume that you are a consultant who has been asked to assess the effectiveness of an organization in applying IT. Construct a questionnaire (twenty questions) to guide the interviews of organizational leaders that you would conduct to determine effectiveness.

NOTES

1. List quoted from Applegate, Austin, & McFarlan, 2007, McGraw-Hill © 2007, is reproduced with permission of The McGraw-Hill Companies.

2. List quoted from Applegate, Austin, & McFarlan, 2007, McGraw-Hill © 2007, is reproduced with permission of The McGraw-Hill Companies.

3. List quoted from Applegate, Austin, & McFarlan, 2007, McGraw-Hill © 2007, is reproduced with permission of The McGraw-Hill Companies.

4. This section adapted with permission of Healthcare Financial Management Association from J. Glaser, "The Competitive Value of Healthcare IT," *Healthcare Financial Management,* July 2007, *61*(7), 36–40.

REFERENCES

Applegate, L., Austin, R., & McFarlan, W. (2007). *Corporate information strategy and management* (7th ed.). Boston, MA: McGraw-Hill.

Brown, C., & Sambamurthy, V. (1999). *Repositioning the IT organization to enable business transformation.* Chicago, IL: Society for Information Management.

Cash, J., McFarlan, W., & McKenney, J. (1992) *Corporate information systems management: The issues facing senior executives.* Chicago, IL: Irwin.

Collins, J. (2001). *Good to great.* New York, NY: HarperCollins.

Cook (2007, July 20). How to spot a failing project. *CIO.* Retrieved November 2008 from http://www.cio.com/article/124309/How_to_Spot_a_Failing_Project

Downes, L., & Mui, C. (1998). *Unleashing the killer app.* Boston, MA: Harvard Business School Press.

Drazen, E., & Straisor, D. (1995). *Information support in an integrated delivery system.* Paper presented at the annual Healthcare Information and Management Systems (HIMSS) conference, Chicago.

Dvorak, R., Holen, E., Mark, D., & Meehan, W., III. (1997). Six principles of high-performance IT. *McKinsey Quarterly, 3,* 164–177.

Earl, M., & Feeney, D. (2000). How to be a CEO for the information age. *MIT Sloan Management Review, 41*(2), 11–23.

Feld, C., & Stoddard, D. (2004). Getting IT right. *Harvard Business Review, 82*(2), 72–79.

McAfee, A., & Brynjolfsson, E. (2008). Investing in the IT that makes a competitive difference. *Harvard Business Review, 86*(7–8), 98–107.

McKenney, J., Copeland, D., & Mason, R. (1995). *Waves of change: Business evolution through information technology.* Boston, MA: Harvard Business School Press.

Ross, J., Beath, C., & Goodhue, D. (1996). Develop long-term competitiveness through IT assets. *MIT Sloan Management Review, 38*(1), 31–42.

Sambamurthy, V., & Zmud, R. (1996). *Information technology and innovation: Strategies for success.* Morristown, NJ: Financial Executives Research Foundation.

Weill, P., & Broadbent, M. (1998). *Leveraging the new infrastructure.* Boston, MA: Harvard Business School Press.

Weill, P., & Ross, J. (2004). *IT governance: How top performers manage IT decision rights for superior results.* Boston, MA: Harvard Business School Press.

CHAPTER 14

Health IT Leadership Case Studies

Faculty members and others who teach health administration students are often in search of case studies that can be used to help students apply theory and concepts to real-life IT management situations, encourage problem-solving and critical thinking, and foster discussion and collaboration among students. This chapter provides a compendium of case studies from a variety of health care organizations and settings. It is intended to serve as a supplement to the preceding chapters and as a resource to faculty members and students. Many of these case studies were originally written by working health care executives enrolled as students in the doctoral program in health administration offered at the Medical University of South Carolina. We wish to acknowledge and thank these students for allowing us to share their stories and experiences with you:

Penney Burlingame	Randall Jones
Barbara Chelton	Catrin Jones-Nazar
Stuart Fine	Ronald Kintz
David Freed	George Mikatarian
David Gehant	Michael Moran
Patricia Givens	Lorie Shoemaker
Shirley Harkey	Gary Wilde
Victoria Harkins	

Most of the cases begin with background information that includes a description of the setting, the current information system (IS) challenge facing the organization, and the factors that are felt to have contributed to the current situation. (All real names and identifying information have been changed from the original cases to protect the identity of the individuals and organizations involved.) Following each case is a set of recommended discussion questions. To the extent possible, the cases are organized by the corresponding chapter(s) to which they relate (see Table 14.1).

We hope you find the cases thought-provoking and useful in applying the concepts covered in this book to what is happening in health care organizations throughout our nation. We have also included at the end of the chapter a listing of other published cases and webinars that may be useful to you and your students.

CASE 1: POPULATION HEALTH MANAGEMENT IN ACTION

Although the integration of patient-centered medical homes and account-able care organizations into the health system is still emerging—as are best

Table 14.1 List of cases and corresponding chapters

Title of Case	Corresponding Chapter(s)
Case 1: Population Health Management in Action	Chapter 4
Case 2: Registries and Disease Management in the PCMH	Chapter 4
Case 3: Implementing a Capacity Management Information System	Chapter 5
Case 4: Implementing a Telemedicine Solution	Chapter 5
Case 5: Selecting an EHR for Dermatology Practice	Chapter 5
Case 6: Watson's Ambulatory EHR Transition	Chapter 5
Case 7: Concerns and Workarounds with a Clinical Documentation System	Chapter 6
Case 8: Conversion to an EHR Messaging System	Chapter 6
Case 9: Strategies for Implementing CPOE	Chapter 6
Case 10: Implementing a Syndromic Surveillance System	Chapters 6 and 12
Case 11: Planning an EHR Implementation	Chapters 6 and 12
Case 12: Replacing a Practice Management System	Chapters 6 and 13
Case 13: Implementing Tele-psychiatry in a Community Hospital Emergency Department	Chapters 6, 7, and 13
Case 14: Assessing the Value and Impact of CPOE	Chapter 7
Case 15: Assessing the Value of Health IT Investment	Chapter 7
Case 16: The Admitting System Crashes	Chapter 10
Case 17: Breaching the Security of an Internet Patient Portal	Chapter 10
Case 18: The Decision to Develop an IT Strategic Plan	Chapter 12
Case 19: Selection of a Patient Safety Strategy	Chapter 12
Case 20: Strategic IS Planning for the Hospital ED	Chapter 12
Case 21: Board Support for a Capital Project	Chapters 12 and 13

practices and key learnings from these early efforts—there have been myriad examples demonstrating encouraging returns and improvement in quality of care. The Patient-Centered Primary Care Collaborative recently profiled several organizations that have adopted patient health management (PHM) tools and strategies to address the preventive and chronic care needs of their patient populations.

Bon Secours Virginia Medical Group

Richmond, VA

Provider Type: Multispecialty group practice

Locations: 140

Patients: 25,000 (Virginia)

A pioneer in implementing medical home and accountable care initiatives, Bon Secours has dedicated itself to executing a sustainable care delivery model that is in alignment with health care reform across its providers and locations. Bon Secours's transformation into an organization that embraces PHM is the result of a systematic strategy to reengineer primary care practices, integrate new technologies into care team workflows, and engage patients in their care.

Bon Secours took a leap of faith in implementing these changes, acting on the belief that payers would come to them if they built a viable model. And payers did. The organization was selected as an early participant in the Medicare Shared Savings Program. It has also signed value-based contracts with two commercial payers—CIGNA and Anthem—and is in negotiations with several more. These contracts provide a financial mechanism to expand and scale the medical home initiative and support ACO models. This case study examines in more detail Bon Secours's approach to position itself to achieve quality outcomes and financial success in the changing health care environment.

Bon Secours's Care Team Model

The foundation of Bon Secours's strategy for value-based care is its medical home initiative—the Advanced Medical Home Project. The project began as a pilot five years ago. Since that time, eleven practices have earned NCQA recognition as patient-centered medical homes. One of the most significant objectives of the Advanced Medical Home Project is to improve capacity—making it possible for care teams to double the size of their patient panel without overburdening themselves or sacrificing quality of care.

At the heart of this medical home strategy is the effort to reengineer practices by creating high-performance physician-led care teams, which requires changes in workflow, new care coordination activities, and designed delegation of clinical responsibilities across the care team. To facilitate this process, Bon Secours has invested significantly in embedding care managers into the primary care team. These nurse navigators are registered nurses (RNs) who are either board-certified case managers or actively working toward certification.

Each nurse navigator is assigned a panel of approximately 150 high-risk patients. He or she cultivates a personal relationship with these patients, usually through repeated phone contacts. Although most outreach is telephonic, navigators have the skill to assess which patients require face-to-face intervention. And because they are embedded in the practice, they can spend time with these patients doing assessments, care planning, and education.

Bon Secours's eHealth Strategies

An important aspect of Bon Secours's strategy is implementing health information technology that empowers the care team to efficiently manage the health of their populations. They consider this technology—standardized across the medical group—as the key to enable them to scale their system for value-based care. As a first step, Bon Secours implemented an EHR and all its modules in every practice within the system. This gave them a strong foundation for documenting care and accessing health records across the enterprise.

Risk stratification. They were able to build a registry that could identify high-risk and high-utilization patients based on data such as number of medications or frequent visits to the emergency department. However, the organization recognized the need for a more robust, scalable registry that would drive efficient population health workflows in their practices and enable analytics and predictive modeling across multiple clinical conditions.

Integrating their EHR with a PHM platform, Bon Secours is able to aggregate all source data into a population-wide registry that enables the organization to implement multiple quality-improvement programs simultaneously. The registry stratifies the population by risk—providing a total population view while enabling each care team to drill down to the data they need about cohorts and individual patients. The system enables care teams within the practice to monitor their patients' health status and take action by delivering timely and appropriate care interventions. Because the system automates these interventions, care teams are able to communicate with many patients at once.

Automated outreach. A significant priority for Bon Secours has been preventing thirty-day readmissions. The medical group uses an automated outreach system to identify discharged patients, link them to a primary care provider (PCP), and pinpoint those who are at high risk for readmission. Flagged patients are then called within twenty-four to seventy-two hours to reinforce discharge instructions, make sure their medications are reconciled, and set up an appointment with the primary care team within five to ten days of discharge. Bon Secours will soon implement a readmissions solution to automate the process of calling discharged patients, asking them to complete a short assessment, and escalating cases as needed based on their feedback.

Personal health records. Another strategy for patient engagement is activating patients on an electronic personal health record (PHR), which allows patients to view clinical results and communicate conveniently with their caregivers via e-mail. Bon Secours works to gain physician consensus on policies that drive the use of PHR: physicians agreed to allow automatic release of normal results to the PHR, but abnormal results are held for 24 hours to enable the care team to contact the patient. The organization is relying on physicians and staff members to get patients active on the PHR to help them sign up on the spot in the exam room.

Challenges and Lessons Learned

Gaining physician buy-in for reengineering practice workflow. The concept of the care team can be difficult for some physicians because they see themselves as the clinician and the rest of the team as support staff members. To help physicians embrace the care team and delegate patient-care tasks, Bon Secours placed tremendous emphasis on physician education. The organization also allows physicians to adjust some of the standardized care team protocols to meet the needs of their practice, which fosters ownership of the process and assures physicians that they remain in control.

Paying for the transition to value-based care. As mentioned previously, Bon Secours implemented its medical home model with the hope that payers would come to them if they built a viable program. CIGNA currently gives the organization a per-member per-month (PMPM) adjustment for care coordination. Anthem, the group's biggest payer, pays a care coordination fee and will change to PMPM in the coming year. Several more commercial payers are lined up to sign contracts with the group. However, this payer involvement is a relatively new development. For the first few years of the project, Bon Secours shouldered the expense. The organization is now poised to reap the rewards of its investment.

Bon Secours is also demonstrating significant progress managing its CIGNA population. In the first six months of their value-based contract, they have achieved a 27 percent reduction in readmissions and are $1.8 million below their projected spend. They have hit many of their care quality metrics and need to improve their gap-in-care metrics only slightly to achieve the index necessary to qualify for gain sharing with CIGNA—a development that will bring a projected annual savings of $4 million.

Bon Secours's mantra for the future is "health care without walls." The organization is aggressively pursuing remote, noninvasive monitoring for highly acute case management. Their vision is to bring care outside the four walls of the hospital into the patient's home using technology. They are operationalizing a geriatric medical home that will enable patients to age in place with home visits for preventive and acute management. They are also expanding their implementation of the PHM platform to include performance measurement at the group, site, and provider levels; feedback to providers on variance in care; and quality reporting. This added functionality for analytics and insight on the clinical and administrative levels will help the organization ensure that it is meeting the triple aim (to improve the patient experience of care, including quality and satisfaction; to improve the health of populations; and to reduce the per capita cost of health care).

Innovation Impact

- Thirty-day readmission rate for medical home patients was < 2 percent for two years.

- Patient engagement scores were in the 97th percentile.

- Patient outreach efforts generated approximately forty thousand unique patient visits for preventive, follow-up, or acute care, leading to $7 million increased revenue.

Source: Shaljian, M., & Nielsen, M. (2013). *Managing populations, maximizing technology: Population health management in the medical neighborhood.* Patient-Centered Primary Care Collaborative. Retrieved from https://pcpcc.org/resource/managing-populations-maximizing-technology. Used with permission.

Discussion Questions

1. What do you think are the important take-home messages in this case?

2. What is your assessment of the approach Bon Secours has taken in embracing its commitment to population health management by investigating in different IT capabilities? How useful are capabilities such as risk stratification, automated outreach, and PHRs in improving quality while managing costs? Are there other tools that could have been useful? If so, what are they? How might they be used?

3. Bon Secours's mantra for the future is "health care without walls." What might success in achieving this vision look like? What challenges may they face? How might they overcome these challenges?

CASE 2: REGISTRIES AND DISEASE MANAGEMENT IN THE PCMH

Union Health Center (UHC)

New York, NY

Provider Type: Community Health Center

Medical Home NCQA Level 3

Patients: 11,000

Office Visits: 55,000

UHC's Care Team Model

Union Health Center (UHC) embraced the patient-centered care team model very early on, which helped ease the transition to new workflows, processes, and features that are critical to change management and quality improvement. UHC clinicians and staff members are assigned to clinical care teams, composed of physicians, nurse practitioners, physician assistants, nurses, medical assistants, and administrative staff members. The practice uses a full capitation model with standard fee-for-service and a fee-for-service plus care management payment model.

Ten years ago, UHC instituted the California Health Care Foundation's Ambulatory Intensive Caring Unit (AICU) model, which emphasizes intensive education and self-management strategies for chronic disease patients. The model relies heavily on the role of medical assistants (called *patient care assistants* or PCAs) and health coaches. Working closely with other members of the care team, PCAs and health coaches review and update patient information in the record, conducting personal outreach and self-management support, and providing certain clinical tasks. For instance, all PCAs have been trained to review measures (e.g., HgbA1C, blood pressure, and LDL cholesterol), provide disease education, and set and review patient health goals. A subset of higher-trained health coaches works more intensely with recently diagnosed diabetic patients or those patients whose condition is not well managed.

UHC's eHealth Strategies

Patient registries. UHC uses patient registries to identify patients with specific conditions to ensure that those patients receive the right care, in the right place, at the right time. In some instances, they use registries to target cases for chart reviews and assess disease management strategies. For example, patients with uncontrolled hypertension are reviewed to help identify treatment patterns, reveal any need for more provider engagement, and may indicate the need for care team workflow changes. In the future, UHC would like to construct queries that combine diagnosis groups with control groups and stratify patients by risk group. For example, care teams could pull a report of all patients over the age of sixty-five with multiple chronic conditions or recent emergency room admissions.

Maximizing time and expertise. UHC uses technology such as custom EHR templates to support PCAs and free up clinicians for more specialized tasks and complex patients. For example, a PCA or health coach taking the blood pressure of a high-risk diabetic patient has been trained to determine whether or not BP is controlled. If it is not controlled, the health coach checks the electronic chart for standard instructions on how to proceed and may carry out instructions noted in the record. Or, if no information is available he or she will consult with another provider to adjust and complete the note. Following all visits with PCAs or health coaches, the patient's record is electronically flagged for review and signed by the primary care physician.

Working with medical neighbors. The teams also collaborate with on-site specialists, pharmacists, social workers, physical therapists, psychologists, and nutritionists to enhance care coordination and whole-patient care. UHC has also adopted curbside consultations and e-consults to reduce specialty office visits. For example, if a hypertensive patient has uncontrolled blood pressure, the record is flagged by the PCA for further follow-up with a physician or nurse practitioner, who may opt for an e-consult with the nephrologist to discuss recommendations. UHC also has a specialty coordination team—composed of two primary care physicians, one registered nurse, one PCA, and one health coach—which functions as a liaison between primary and specialty providers.

Customized reporting. With their most recent upgrade to a Meaningful Use–certified version of their EHR, UHC will have the capacity to generate standardized Meaningful Use reports. UHC intends to construct queries that generate reports that group diagnosis groups with control groups and identify and manage subgroups of high-risk patients (or risk stratification). For example, care teams can run a report of all patients with diabetes that have an elevated LDL and have not been prescribed a statin.

Challenges and Lessons Learned

Recruiting staff members with IT and clinical informatics expertise. Over the years, UHC has faced challenges in identifying and recruiting staff members with the right mix of IT and clinical informatics skills. Although effective in troubleshooting routine issues and hardware maintenance, UHC felt there was a clinical data analysis gap. To resolve this, UHC works closely with an IT consultant and also recruited a clinical informatics professional to work with providers and performance improvement staff members.

Consistent data entry. UHC's lack of consistent data entry rules and structured data fields led to several challenges in producing reports and tracking patient subgroups. The problem stems from UHC's lack of internal data entry policies as well as the record's design. For instance, UHC cannot run reports on patients taking aspirin because this information may have been entered inconsistently across patient records. Moving forward, UHC will be implementing data entry rules and working closely with their vendor to maximize data capture.

Real-time data capture. UHC realized that by the time data reach the team, they may no longer be current. As a workaround they considered disseminating raw reports to clinical teams in real time, followed by tabulated, reformatted data. They are exploring the possibility of purchasing report writing software to streamline the process.

Managing multiple data sources. Similar to many practices, UHC pulls data from its billing system and clinical records, causing issues with data extraction. For example, pulling by billing codes does not provide the most accurate data when it comes to clinical conditions, health status, or population demographics. UHC recognized that to reduce errors in identifying patients and subgroups this will require custom reports.

Innovation Impact

- Forty-six percent reduction in overall annual health costs
- Eighteen percent reduction in total cost of care
- Significant decline in emergency room visits, hospitalizations, and diagnostic services
- Significant improvements in clinical indicators for diabetic patients

Source: Shaljian, M., & Nielsen, M. (2013). *Managing populations, maximizing technology: Population health management in the medical neighborhood.* Patient-Centered Primary Care Collaborative. Retrieved from https://pcpcc.org/resource/managing-populations-maximizing-technology. Used with permission.

Discussion Questions

1. Identify and discuss the various IT tools and staff resources UHC used to deploy its education and self-management strategies among patients with chronic disease. What are their strengths? Limitations?

2. UHC identified several challenges and lessons learned in this case. Discuss each of these including UHC's approach to overcoming the challenges. What other strategies or approaches might you have considered? Why? Explain your rationale.

3. UHC used curb-side consultations and e-visits to reduce specialty office visits. To what extent are these used by provider organizations in your community? Or others as evidenced by the literature? How effective have e-visits been? Are patients open to them?

4. How might other health care provider organizations learn from UHC's experiences? What are the critical take-home messages?

CASE 3: IMPLEMENTING A CAPACITY MANAGEMENT INFORMATION SYSTEM

Doctors' Hospital is a 162-bed, acute care facility located in a small city in the southeastern United States. The organization had a major financial upheaval six years ago that resulted in the establishment of a new governing structure. The new governing body consists of an eleven-member authority board. The senior management of Doctors' Hospital includes the CEO, three senior vice presidents, and one vice president. During the restructuring, the CIO was changed from a full-time staff position to a part-time contract position. The CIO spends two days every two weeks at Doctors' Hospital.

Doctors' Hospital is currently in Phase 1 of a three-phase construction project. In Phase 2 the hospital will build a new emergency department (ED) and surgical pavilion, which are scheduled to be completed in eleven months.

Information Systems Challenge

The current ED and outpatient surgery department have experienced tremendous growth in the past several years. ED visits have increased by 50 percent, and similar increases have been seen in outpatient surgery. Management has identified that inefficient patient flow processes, particularly patient transfers and discharges, have resulted in backlogs in the ED and outpatient areas. The new construction will only exacerbate the current problem.

Nearly a year ago Doctors' Hospital made a commitment to purchase a capacity management software suite to reduce the inefficiencies that have been identified in patient flow processes. The original timeline was to have the new system pilot-tested prior to the opening of the new ED and surgical pavilion. However, with the competing priorities its members face as they deal with major construction, the original project steering committee has stalled. At its last meeting nearly six months ago, the steering committee identified the vendor and product suite. Budgets and timelines for implementation were proposed but not finalized. No other steps have been taken.

Discussion Questions

1. Do you think the absence of a full-time CIO has had an impact on this acquisition project? Why or why not?

2. What steps should the CIO take to ensure that the capacity management system will be purchased and implemented? What do you see as the critical first step in this process? Why?

3. Discuss who you think should serve on the project steering committee. Who should serve as chair? Why?

4. At this point, what do you think is a realistic time frame for implementation of the capacity management system? What steps can be taken to ensure the new timeline is met despite competing priorities?

CASE 4: IMPLEMENTING A TELEMEDICINE SOLUTION

Grand Hospital is located in a somewhat rural area of a Midwestern state. It is a 209-bed, community, not-for-profit entity offering a broad range of inpatient and outpatient services. Employing approximately 1,600 individuals (1,250 full-time equivalent personnel) and having a medical staff of more than 225 practitioners, Grand has an annual operating budget that exceeds $130 million, possesses net assets of more than $150 million, and is one of only a small number of organizations in this market with an A credit rating from Moody's, Standard & Poor's, and Fitch Ratings. Operating in a remarkably competitive market (there are roughly one hundred hospitals within seventy-five minutes' driving time of Grand), the organization is one of the few in the region—proprietary or not-for-profit—that has consistently realized positive operating margins. Grand attends on an annual basis to the health care needs of more than 11,000 inpatients and 160,000 outpatients, addressing more than 36 percent of its primary service area's consumption of hospital services. In expansion mode and currently in the midst of $57 million in construction and renovation projects, the hospital is struggling to recruit physicians to meet the health care needs of the expanding population of the service area and to succeed retiring physicians.

Grand has been an early adopter of health care information systems and currently employs a proprietary health care information system that provides (among other components) these services:

- Patient registration and revenue management
- EHRs with computerized physician order entry
- Imaging via a PACS
- Laboratory management
- Pharmacy management

Information Systems Challenge

Since 1995, Grand Hospital has transitioned from being an institution that consistently received many more inquiries than could be accommodated concerning physician practice opportunities to a hospital at which the average age of the medical staff members has increased by eight years. There is a widespread perception among physicians that because of such factors as high malpractice insurance costs, an absence of substantive tort reform, and the comparatively unfavorable rates of reimbursement being paid physician specialists by the region's major health insurer, this region constitutes a "physician-unfriendly" venue in which to establish a practice. Consequently, a need exists for Grand to investigate and evaluate creative approaches to enhancing its physician coverage for certain specialty services. These potential approaches include the effective implementation of IT solutions.

The findings and conclusions of a medical staff development plan, which has been endorsed and accepted by Grand's medical executive committee and board of trustees, have indicated that because of needs and circumstances specific to the institution, the first areas of medical practice on which Grand should focus in approaching this challenge are radiology, behavioral health crisis intervention services, and intensivist physician services. In the area of radiology, Grand needs qualified and appropriately credentialed radiologists available to interpret studies twenty-four hours per day, seven days per week. Similarly, it needs qualified and appropriately credentialed psychiatrists available on a 24/7 basis to assess whether behavioral health patients who present in the hospital's emergency room are a danger to themselves or to others, as defined by state statute, and whether these patients should be released or committed against their will for further assessment on an inpatient basis. Finally, inasmuch as Grand is a community hospital that relies on its voluntary medical staff members to attend to the needs of patients admitted by staff members such as some ED personnel, it also needs to have intensivist physicians available around the clock to assist in assessing and treating patients during times when members of the voluntary attending staff members are not present within or immediately available to the intensive care unit.

The leadership at Grand Hospital is investigating the potential application of telemedicine technologies to address the organization's need for enhanced physician coverage in radiology, behavioral health, and critical care medicine.

Discussion Questions

1. What are the ways in which Grand's early adoption of other health care information system technologies might affect its adoption of telemedicine solutions?

2. What do you see as the most likely barriers to the success of telemedicine in the areas of radiology, behavioral health, and intensive care? Which of these areas do you think would be the easiest to transition into telemedicine? Which would be the hardest? Why?

3. If you were charged by Grand to bring telemedicine to the facility within eighteen months, what are the first steps you would take? Whom would you involve in the planning process? Defend your response.

CASE 5: SELECTING AN EHR FOR DERMATOLOGY PRACTICE

Suppose you've just been hired as the practice administrator of an eight-physician dermatology practice. After several years of contemplation and serious deliberations, the physicians have made the strategic decision to invest in the selection and implementation of a facility-wide EHR system. They also want to replace their practice management system (which includes patient scheduling and billing). It's an older system that is rather clunky. Ideally, they'd like to find an integrated practice management system that has an EHR component.

Dan Brown, the current CEO of the physician organization, has very little knowledge of information systems technology. He has been reluctant to move toward an EHR system for many years, primarily because he heard stories from a few his colleagues in other specialty areas who have implemented EHRs in their practices and have found the systems to be highly cumbersome and disruptive to the patient care process. One of his best friends claims he "spends an extra hour or two a night in the office because of the additional time demands of the EHR. He claims the system never seemed to work right."

Brown is convinced that there are not any great dermatology-related EHR products on the market, but with value-based payment looming, and the opportunity to improve quality of patient care, he's open to taking another look. In addition, one of their newest partners, Pam Martin, just finished her residency program where EHRs were an integral part of her training. She is a big champion of the effort to select and implement an EHR. She has offered to help lead the effort. One of the other partners, John Harris, came back from a conference impressed with the vendor presentation from Allscripts and convinced it's the way the practice ought to go. The other physicians are nearing retirement and a little nervous about the possible disruption to the office.

Information Systems Challenge

Even though the patient records at the dermatology practice are paper-based, the practice has been using computerized practice management systems for patient scheduling and billing for years. Six months ago, they started to have a nurse enter physician-dictated notes into the paper record while in the examination room with the patient. The physician then reviews the notes at the end of the visit or day and signs off on them. This is in an effort to decrease the dictation and transcription that the practice had historically done and to get the nurses and physicians ready for the EHR. The expectation is that nurses will do the bulk of the data entry in the exam room while the physicians are seeing the patients. However, the physicians will have to review the documentation and sign off on all entries.

The practice currently has approximately four thousand patient visits per month, including 40 percent Medicare and 10 percent Medicaid.

Discussion Questions

You are tasked with leading the team charged with the selection of the new practice management system, including EHR, for the practice.

1. You begin by convening a practice management–EHR selection team. Who would serve on the team? Who would serve as executive sponsor? Explain your rationale.

2. How might you conduct an EHR-readiness assessment for this practice? What factors will be important to consider? Why?

3. Develop a draft system selection plan for this practice. What do you envision will be the practice's greatest challenges in selecting a replacement practice management system and a new EHR? Explain your rationale.

CASE 6: WATSON'S AMBULATORY EHR TRANSITION

Primary care physicians play a key role in the US health care delivery system. These providers integrate internal and external information with their clinical knowledge to determine the patient's treatment options. An effective ambulatory EHR is critical to supply physicians with the information they need to provide quality care and maximize their efficiency. This case involves the decision-making process to replace an inadequate EHR system in a primary care network owned by a community hospital. The IT challenge reviewed in this case will be the decision-making process that optimizes provider support for the new EHR while addressing the strategic plan requirements of data integration, clinical application, and practice management functionality.

Watson Community Association is a private, not-for-profit corporation that operates Watson Community Hospital (WCH), a two hundred–bed acute care facility located in Arizona. WCH has pursued a strategy of employing primary care physicians in their primary service area to provide convenient points of access for patients and to secure a primary care base for the specialists who use the hospital. WCH employs thirty-six physicians and seven mid-level providers in eight clinics, specializing in internal medicine, family practice, infectious disease, and gynecology.

Several years ago, the WCH board of directors adopted a plan to implement a system-wide EHR to, among other things, improve patient safety, integrate information from ancillary systems, and provide access to patient information for all WCH caregivers. In addition, the plan calls for an evaluation of the effectiveness of the WCH physician clinic organization's EHR.

The WCH clinics currently use the XYZ Data Systems Integrated EHR and Practice Management System. This system has been operational for four years. The XYZ system was chosen because of its compatibility with the hospital's Meditech platform. Physician needs and application functionality were secondary considerations. As a result, physician system adoption and support has been poor. Under prior leadership, the hospital IT department provided limited support for the XYZ EHR. The clinic organization was left to develop its own internal IT capabilities to manage the XYZ system and, as a result, the system has not been routinely updated.

The hospital has decided to stay with the Meditech platform to address the IT strategic plan for an integrated EHR. The clinic organization must now evaluate whether it is in their best interest to stay with the XYZ system, with strong Meditech compatibility, or move to a different EHR platform. The path of least resistance from the IT perspective would be to upgrade the XYZ system. This option offers the greatest integration and could be implemented much sooner. A new platform would require an evaluation and selection process and a significant conversion. With either scenario, physician support will be critical to a successful transition.

EHR Project Plan

The following sections detail a description of the planning process developed by the leadership team to transition to a replacement EHR. Read and critique the plan by answering the questions that follow it.

Project Organization

The organizational phase of the project will involve establishing a project steering committee and identifying the leadership members who will ensure the project's success. WCH operates eight separate clinics, each with their unique teams and EHR experience. By necessity, the steering committee will need representation from each of these clinics. The project steering committee will likely have twenty to twenty-five members. In addition to provider representatives, the steering committee will also include nurses, medical assistants, and office managers from each clinic. IT representation is critical to the success of the project, and because the department provided poor IT support in the past, the CIO will play an active role on the steering committee. A representative from finance should also participate on the committee, given the importance of billing and collections and other practice management issues.

The leadership of the steering committee will ensure that the committee addresses key steps in the process and does so in a timely fashion. Ideally, the committee should be chaired by a provider who is respected within the group, is objective, and is a supporter of EHR technology. Although the clinic organization does not have a provider who meets all of these criteria, a physician with strong peer support and credibility will be selected to cochair the steering committee. To complement the clinical leadership, the CIO will serve as a cochair for the committee, providing technical expertise. This individual has implemented other EHR systems and will bring a structured process to the committee to ensure a thorough evaluation process.

Committee Development

Organizations often overlook the importance of understanding the emotional climate of a medical practice when implementing an EHR. Therefore, although the first task of the steering committee will be to define the project objectives, the existing concerns about an EHR transition require that a fair amount of time be devoted to addressing the emotional needs of the participants. Listening to practitioners and empathizing with their concerns will be critical to establish trust and overcome resistance during the EHR conversion.

To address this important issue, a series of discussion exercises will be used to encourage open dialogue and participant engagement. The first exercise will break the large group into teams of four to five members, and each team will discuss the lessons learned from the XYZ implementation that took place four years previously. Team leaders will be handpicked for their facilitation skills and ability to listen. The group discussions will address the "change readiness" and will surface the major issues associated with the implementation. It will also enable the group members to get to know each other in a less formal setting than the large group. The larger committee will reconvene to discuss their findings and prepare a master list of implementation lessons learned.

Although this exercise may raise a number of issues related to implementation, it is also important to openly discuss the current issues with the existing EHR. Once again, small groups will be asked to discuss these issues to ensure participation by all members of the steering committee. Small groups will report out to the large group, and a summary of issues will be developed. This list, as well as the list of implementation issues, will set the stage for a later discussion regarding the scope of the project.

Project Scope and Objectives

Once the group has had the opportunity to express personal concerns and key issues have been identified, the group can turn its attention to defining the project objectives. Anxious committee members are often tempted to begin discussing whether the steering committee should upgrade this system or consider alternatives. When this occurs, discussions and conclusions are usually based on the emotional attachment to or disappointment with the current system. A more systematic review process will help frame this discussion to ensure the conclusion is based on facts and the needs of the clinic organization.

The leadership must guide the committee in developing project objectives that are based on the needs of the organization, not individuals. Returning to the list of implementation and current issues, the group will be asked to prioritize the concerns that were raised. This prioritization will focus the committee on the most pressing issues that must be addressed. With this background work, the committee will be positioned to articulate the goals of the committee. It will also define the scope of the project by determining what the project is and isn't intended to address. Invariably, users will raise issues that may not be solved by an EHR application. It is important that the end users review all issues, even though some of those issues may not prove to be within the scope of the project. Users with unrealistic expectations can end up frustrated and disengaged as the process unfolds. Defining the scope and the objectives clarifies expectations before options are considered.

Communication

The steering committee will need to establish plans to communicate with the larger audience of clinic users and stakeholders. A plan will be developed that provides this audience with regular updates. The plan must also address how the committee can solicit feedback from stakeholders during the evaluation and selection process. Regular minutes establish the record of the committee's work and provide a means for communicating with stakeholders. Special meetings with individual clinic groups will also be necessary to address rumors or provide more detailed information regarding the process. The steering committee must communicate regularly to ensure information is flowing to individuals.

Plan of Work

Once project objectives are established, the committee will prepare a plan of work. This plan will outline the specific action steps required to achieve the project objectives and the timeline for their completion. The plan of work focuses on the decision to upgrade the existing XYZ application and remain with a Meditech platform or move to a different software solution. The plan of work provides the steering committee with the road map to achieve its goals.

The key steps in the plan of work are identifying possible vendors, establishing system requirements, and completing a request-for-proposal (RFP) process. Vendor identification can occur simultaneously with establishing the project goals. This is a reasonable assertion because it will save time and will engage the clinic representatives in the process. The steering committee will select individuals to attend trade shows to maximize exposure to EHR products. IT staff members will also participate in this review process to address technical requirements and issues.

Establishing system requirements is a critical step in the EHR decision-making process. The system requirements identify the needs of the organization and are the basis for the vendor evaluation process. The implementation and current issues lists developed by the committee will be used to develop the system requirements. Each clinic employee will receive a summary of these lists, and staff members will be asked to provide additional input to steering committee representatives. In addition, the IT department will conduct a thorough evaluation of new advancements in EHRs and regulatory requirements that may affect the EMR choice. The first draft of the system requirements will be preliminary. As the steering committee begins to interact with vendors and complete site visits, additional functionality may be added to the requirements. It would not be prudent to submit RFPs to all vendors who claim to have a functional EHR. The steering committee will need to determine the top five to seven vendors, judging by the initial survey of qualified vendors, trade shows, and market information.

Well-defined system requirements will need to be established and included in the RFPs. Packaging the system requirements in a format that provides structure for vendor responses and steering committee evaluations of vendor responses will be important, as will establishing a record of documentation throughout the acquisition process. The RFP document will provide the following:

- Instructions for vendors
- Organizational objectives
- Organization background information
- System goals and requirements

The vendors will be required to submit the following:

- Vendor qualifications
- Proposed solutions
- Criteria for evaluating proposals
- Contractual requirements
- Pricing and support

The vendor review process will also encompass technical calls, vendor fairs, reference checks, site visits, and vendor presentations. These elements of the review process are designed to ensure that sufficient information is gathered to augment the proposals submitted by the vendors. It will not be feasible for all steering committee members to participate in these activities; therefore, individuals will be appointed to participate on their behalf.

Prior to reviewing the vendor proposals, the steering committee will develop vendor criteria that can be used to evaluate the proposals. Each member of the steering committee will be asked to score the proposals based on the criteria, and a summary score report will be developed. The WCH

CEO will give the final approval to proceed with the conversion based on the report and recommendation from the steering committee. However, the final recommendation of the committee will not be based solely on the score report. Ideally, the final deliberations will involve a robust dialogue based on the mutual trust that has developed over time. Ultimately, the committee will balance its objective assessment of options with its intuition and considerable knowledge of the clinic organization.

Conclusion

The WCH clinic organization will undergo a significant EHR transition if they upgrade the XYZ system or purchase another product. The process that is outlined in this plan provides the organization the best opportunity to make the right decision for the organization and establish support with key stakeholders for an EHR conversion. A good IT decision-making process requires discipline and objectivity. The structural elements of the process involve leadership, committee structure, system requirements, and a thorough RFP and evaluation process.

Discussion Questions

1. What are the strengths of this plan? What aspects do you think are particularly important?

2. How could the plan be improved? What, if anything, might you do differently if you were leading the effort? Explain your rationale.

3. What factors should the leadership team consider when deciding whether to stay with a single vendor for supporting the hospital and primary care settings?

CASE 7: CONCERNS AND WORKAROUNDS WITH A CLINICAL DOCUMENTATION SYSTEM

Garrison Children's Hospital is a 225-bed hospital. Its seventy-seven-bed neonatal intensive care unit (NICU) provides care to the most fragile patients, premature and critically ill neonates. The twenty-eight-bed pediatric intensive care unit (PICU) cares for critically ill children from birth to eighteen years of age. Patients in this unit include those with life-threatening conditions that are acquired (trauma, child abuse, burns, surgical complications, and so forth) or congenital (congenital heart defects, craniofacial malformations, genetic disorders, inborn errors of metabolism, and so forth).

Garrison is part of Premier Health Care, an academic medical center complex located in the Southeast. Premier Health Care also includes an adult hospital, a psychiatric hospital, and a full spectrum of adult and pediatric outpatient clinics. Within the past six months or so, Premier has implemented an electronic clinical documentation system in its adult hospital. More recently the same clinical documentation system has been implemented at Garrison in pediatric medical and surgery units and intensive care units. Electronic scheduling is to be implemented next.

The adult hospital drives the decisions for the pediatric hospital, a circumstance that led to the adult hospital's CPOE vendor being chosen as the documentation vendor for both hospitals. A CPOE system was implemented at Garrison Children's Hospital several years prior to implementation of the electronic clinical documentation system.

Information Systems Challenge

A pressing challenge facing Garrison Children's Hospital is that nurses are very concerned and dissatisfied with the new clinical documentation system. They have voiced concerns formally to several nurse managers, and one nurse went directly to the chief nursing officer (CNO) stating that the flow sheets on the new system are grossly inadequate and she fears using them could lead to patient safety issues. Lunchroom conversations among nurses tend to center on their having no clear understanding of why the organization is automating clinical documentation or what it hopes to achieve. Nurses in the NICU and PICU seem to be most vocal about their concerns. They claim there is inconsistency in what is being documented and a lack of standardization of content. The computer workstations are located outside the patients' rooms, so nurses generally document their notes on paper and then enter the data at the end of the shift or when they have time.

The system support team, consisting of nurses as well as technology specialists, began the workflow analysis, system installation, staff training, and go-live first with a small number of units in the adult hospital and the children's hospital beginning in January. The NICU and PICU did not implement the system until May and June of that year. System support personnel moved rapidly through each unit, working to train and manage questions. The timeline for each unit implementation was based on the number of beds in the unit and the number of staff members to be trained. No consideration was given to staff members' prior experience with computers and keyboarding skills or to complexity of documentation and existing work processes.

Although there are similarities between the adult and pediatric settings, there are also many differences in terms of unit design, computer resources (hardware), level of computer literacy, information documented, and work processes, not to mention patient populations. Little time was spent evaluating or planning for these differences and completing a thorough workflow analysis. After the initial units went live, less and less time was spent on training and addressing unit-specific needs because of the demands placed on training staff members to stay on the timeline in preparation for the next system implementation involving electronic scheduling.

The clinical documentation system was implemented to the great consternation and dissatisfaction of the end users (physicians, nurses, social workers, and so forth) at Garrison, yet the Premier clinicians are happy with it. Many Garrison physicians and nurses initially refused to use the system, stating it was "unsafe," "added to workload," and was not intuitive. A decision to stop using the system and return to the paper documentation process was not then and is not now an option. Physician "champions" were encouraged to work with those who were recalcitrant, and nursing staff members were encouraged to "stick it out" with the hope that system use would "get easier."

As a result, with their concerns and complaints essentially forced underground, Garrison clinical staff members developed workarounds, morale was negatively affected, and the expectation that everyone would eventually "get it" and adapt has not become a reality. Instead, staff members are writing on a self-created paper system and then translating those notes to the computer system; physicians are unable to retrieve important, timely patient information; and the time team members spend trying to retrieve pertinent patient information has increased. There have been clear instances when patient safety has been affected because of the problems with the appropriate use of this system.

Discussion Questions

1. What is the major problem in this case? What factors seem to have contributed to the current situation?

2. The nurses at Garrison argue that pediatric hospitals and intensive care units, in particular, are different from adult hospitals and that these differences should be clearly addressed in the implementation of a new clinical documentation system. Do you agree with this argument? Why or why not? Give examples from the literature to support your views.

3. How might the workflow issues and concerns mentioned in this case have been detected earlier?

4. Assume you are part of the leadership team at Garrison. How would you assess the current situation? What would you do first? Next? Explain the steps you would take and why you feel your approach is necessary.

5. What lessons can be learned from this case and applied to other settings?

CASE 8: CONVERSION TO AN EHR MESSAGING SYSTEM

Goodwill Health Care Clinic is the clinical arm of Jefferson Health Sciences Center in a large Southern city. The clinic was founded in the early 1950s as a place for faculty physicians to engage in clinical practice. Over the years the clinic has grown to nine hundred faculty physicians and two thousand employees, with over one million patient visits per year. Clinic services are spread across eleven primary care and specialty care units. Each unit operates somewhat independently but shares a common medical record numbering system that enables consolidation of all documentation across units. Paper charts were used until two years ago, when the clinic adopted an EHR system.

Goodwill Health Care Clinic uses a centralized call center to receive all patient calls. Patients call a central switchboard to schedule appointments, request medication refills, or speak to anyone in any of the eleven units. Call center staff members are responsible for tracking all calls to ensure that each is dealt with appropriately. Currently the call center uses a customized Lotus Notes system that can be accessed by anyone in the system who needs to process messages. Messages can be tracked and then closed when the appropriate action has been taken. Notes created from closed messages are printed and filed in the appropriate patients' paper records. These notes cannot be accessed via the EHR.

Clinic staff members are very comfortable with the current Lotus Notes system, and it is used routinely by all units.

Information Systems Challenge

Goodwill Health Care Clinic requires all medication lists and refill information to be kept up-to-date in the EHR. Therefore, the existence of the current Lotus Notes system means that the same information must be documented in two locations—first in the call center note and then in the EHR. This leads to duplication of effort and documentation errors. The potential for serious error is present. Physicians and other health care providers look in the EHR for the most up-to-date medication information.

Although the adoption of the EHR has been fairly successful, not all units use all of the available components of the EHR. A companion paper record is needed for miscellaneous notes, messages, and so forth. All units are recording office visits into the EHR, but not all have activated the lab results or the prescription writing features. Several units have been experiencing physician resistance to adding more EHR functions.

The EHR system has a messaging component that works similar to a closed e-mail system. Messages can be sent, received, and stored by EHR-authenticated users. Pertinent patient care messages are automatically stored in the correct patient record. In addition, the EHR messaging system works seamlessly with the prescription writing module, which includes patient safety checks such as allergy checks and drug interactions.

The challenge for Goodwill Health Care Clinic is to implement the messaging feature and prescription writing component (where it is not currently being used) of their current EHR in the call center and the clinical units, replacing the existing Lotus Notes system and improving the quality of the documentation, not only of medication refills but also of all patient-related calls. The long-term goal is to add a patient portal feature where patients can schedule appointments, send messages to their providers, and refill prescriptions electronically.

Discussion Questions

1. Outline the steps that you would take to ensure a successful conversion from the existing call center system to the new EHR-compatible system. Defend your response.

2. Who should be involved in the conversion planning and implementation? Discuss the roles of the people on your list and your reasons for selecting them.

3. What are some strategies that you would employ to minimize physicians' and other users' resistance to the conversion?

4. Do you think that making sure all units are running the same EHR functions is a necessary precursor to the conversion to the messaging and prescription writing components? What information would be helpful in making this determination?

5. How might the implementation of the patient portal feature address some of the current issues? What workflow considerations will need to be made?

CASE 9: STRATEGIES FOR IMPLEMENTING CPOE

Health Matters is a newly formed nonprofit health system comprising two community hospitals (Cooper Memorial Hospital and Ashley Valley Hospital), nine ambulatory care clinics, and three imaging centers. Since its inception two years ago, the information services (IS) department has merged and consolidated all computer systems under one umbrella. Each of the facilities within the health system is connected electronically with the others through a fiber optic network. The organizational structure of the two hospitals is such that each has its own executive leadership team and board.

Seven years ago, the leadership team at Cooper Memorial Hospital made the strategic decision to choose Meditech as the vendor of choice for its clinical and financial applications. The philosophy of the leadership team was to solicit a single-vendor solution so that the hospital could minimize the number of disparate systems and interfaces. Since then, Meditech has been deployed throughout the health system and applications have been kept current with the latest releases. Most nursing and clinical ancillary documentation is electronic, as is the medication administration record. Health Matters does have several ancillary systems that interface with Meditech; these include a picture archiving and communication system (PACS), a fully automated laboratory system, an emergency department tracking board, and an electronic bed board system. The leadership team at Ashley Valley Hospital chose to select non-Meditech products, because at the time Meditech did not offer these applications or its products were considered inadequate by clinicians. However, the current sentiment among the leadership team is to continue to go with one predominant vendor, in this case, Meditech, for any upgrades, new functionality, or new products.

The IS group at Health Matters consists of a director of information systems (who reports to the chief financial officer) and fifteen staff members. The IS staff members are highly skilled in networking and computer operations but have only moderate skills as program analysts and project managers. The CEO, Steve Forthright, plans to hire a CIO to provide senior-level leadership in developing and implementing a strategic IS plan that is congruent with the strategic goals of Health Matters.

Currently, the senior leadership team at Health Matters has identified the following as the organization's top three IS challenges. The current director of IS has been somewhat involved in discussions related to the establishment of these priorities.

- To implement successfully computerized provider order entry (CPOE)
- To increase the variety and availability of computing devices (workstations or handheld devices) at each nursing station
- To implement successfully medication administration using bar-coding technology

Information Systems Challenge

The most pressing IS challenge is to move forward with the implementation of CPOE. The decision has already been made to implement the Meditech CPOE application. Several internal and external driving forces are at play. Internally, the physician leaders believe that CPOE will further reduce medication errors and promote patient safety. The board has established patient safety as a strategic goal for the organization. Externally groups such as Leapfrog and the Pacific Business Group on Health have strongly encouraged CPOE implementation. CEO Steve Forthright has concerns, however, because Health Matters does not yet have a CIO on board and he feels the CIO should play a pivotal role. Much of Steve's concern stems from his experience with CPOE implementation at another institution, with a different vendor and product. Steve had organized a project implementation committee, established an appropriate governance structure, and the senior leadership team thought it had "covered the bases." However, according to Steve, "The surgeons embraced the new CPOE system, largely because they felt the postoperative order sets were easy to use, but the internists and hospitalists rebelled. The CPOE project stalled and the system was never fully implemented." Steve is not the only person reeling from a failed implementation. The clinical information committee at Health Matters is chaired by Mary White, who was involved in a failed CPOE rollout at another hospital several years ago. She was a strong supporter of the system at the time, but she now speaks of the risks and challenges associated with getting physician buy-in and support throughout the health system.

Members of the medical staff at Cooper Memorial Hospital have access to laboratory and radiology results electronically. They have access through workstations in the hospital; most physicians also access clinical results remotely through smartphones. An estimated 35 percent of the physicians take full advantage of the system's capabilities. Almost all active physicians use the PACS to view images, and most use a computer to look up lab values. Fewer than half of the physicians use electronic signatures to sign transcribed reports.

Discussion Questions

1. Assume you are part of a team charged with leading the implementation of CPOE within Health Matters. How would you approach the task? What would you do first? Next? Who should be involved in the team? Lead the team?

2. The CIO hasn't been hired yet. Do you see that as a problem? Why or why not? What role, if any, might the CIO have in the CPOE implementation project?

3. To what extent does the fact that Health Matters is a relatively new health system simplify or complicate the CPOE implementation project? How do other health systems typically implement CPOE or other clinical information system projects of this magnitude?

4. How might you solicit the wisdom and expertise of others who may have undergone CPOE projects similar to this one? Or who have used Meditech's CPOE application? How might Steve Forthright's and Mary White's prior experiences with partially and fully failed implementations affect their views in this case?

5. Develop a high-level implementation plan of key tasks and activities that will need to be done. How will you estimate the time frame? The resources needed? What role does the vendor have in establishing this plan?

CASE 10: IMPLEMENTING A SYNDROMIC SURVEILLANCE SYSTEM

Syndromic surveillance systems collect and analyze pre-diagnostic and non-clinical disease indicators, drawing on preexisting electronic data that can be found in systems such as EHRs, school absenteeism records, and pharmacy systems. These surveillance systems are intended to identify specific symptoms within a population that may indicate a public health event or emergency. For example, the data being collected by a surveillance system might reveal a sharp increase in diarrhea in a community and that could signal an outbreak of an infectious disease.

The infectious disease epidemiology section of a state's public health agency has been given the task of implementing the Early Aberration Reporting System of the Centers for Disease Control and Prevention. The agency views this system as significantly improving its ability to monitor and respond to potentially problematic bioterrorism, food poisoning, and infectious disease outbreaks.

The implementation of the system is also seen as a vehicle for improving collaboration among the agency, health care providers, IT vendors, researchers, and the business community.

Information Systems Challenge

The agency and its infectious disease epidemiology section face several major challenges.

First, the necessary data must be collected largely from hospitals and in particular emergency rooms. Developing and supporting necessary interfaces to the applications in a large number of hospitals is very challenging. These hospitals have different application vendors, diverse data standards, and uneven willingness to divert IT staff members and budget to the implementation of these interfaces.

To help address this challenge, the section will acquire a commercial package or build the needed software to ease the integration challenge. In addition, the section will provide each hospital with information it can use to assess its own mix of patients and their presenting problems. The agency is also contemplating the development of regulations that would require the hospitals to report the necessary data.

Second, the system must be designed so that patient privacy is protected and the system is secure.

Third, the implementation and support of the system will be funded initially through federal grants. The agency will need to develop strategies for ensuring the financial sustainability of the application and related analysis capabilities, should federal funding end.

Fourth, the agency needs to ensure that the section has the staff members and tools necessary to appropriately analyze the data. Distinguishing true problems from the noise of a normal increase in colds during the winter, for example, can be very difficult. The agency could damage the public's confidence in the system if it overreacts or underreacts to the data it collects.

Discussion Questions

1. If you were the head of the agency's epidemiology section, how would you address the four challenges described here?

2. Which of the challenges is the most important to address? Why?

3. If you were a hospital CEO being asked to redirect IT resources for this project, what would you want in return from the agency to ensure that this system provided value to your organization and clinicians?

4. A strong privacy advocacy group has expressed alarm about the potential problems that the system could create. How would you respond to those concerns?

CASE 11: PLANNING AN EHR IMPLEMENTATION

The Leonard Williams Medical Center (LWMC) is a 240-bed, community acute care hospital operating in a small urban area in upstate New York. The medical center offers tertiary services and has a captive professional corporation, Williams Medical Services (WMS). WMS is a multispecialty group employing approximately fifty primary care and specialty physicians.

WMS has its own board, made up of representatives of the employed physicians. The WMS board nominations for members and officers are subject to the approval of the medical center board. The capital and operating budgets of WMS are reviewed and approved during the LWMC budget process. The WMS board is responsible for governing the day-to-day operations of the group. LWMC serves a population of approximately 215,000. There are five other hospitals in the region. One of these, aligned with a large clinic, is viewed as the primary competitor.

In its most recent fiscal year, LWMC had an operating margin of 0.4 percent. LWMC has $40 million in investments and has a long-term debt-to-equity ratio of 25 percent.

Information Systems Challenge

LWMC has been very effective in its IT efforts. It was the first hospital in its region to have a clinical information system. Bedside computing has been available on the inpatient units since the 1990s. The CIO and IT department are highly regarded. LWMC has received several industry recognitions for its efforts.

The LWMC information systems steering committee recently approved the acquisition and implementation of a CPOE system. This decision followed a thorough analysis of organizational strategies, the efforts of other hospitals, and the vendor offerings. LWMC is poised to begin this major initiative.

During a recent steering committee meeting, it was learned that the WMS physicians were anxious to acquire an EHR system. Two years ago a rival physician group had purchased an EHR system. WMS, concerned about a competitive threat, obtained approval of $300,000 to acquire its own EHR. The rival group has since encountered serious difficulties with implementation and has de-installed the system. This troubled path caused WMS to slow down its efforts.

Now WMS has decided to return to its plans to implement a certified EHR. The physicians have begun to look at vendor offerings but have not involved the LWMC CIO and IT staff members. The physicians have ignored the CIO's technical and integration advice and requirements during their EHR search.

The CEO is concerned about the EHR process and its disconnect from the medical center's IT plans.

Discussion Questions

1. What is your assessment of this situation? What are the physician group's possible reasons for deciding to proceed on an independent path?

2. If you were the CEO, what steps would you take to bring the hospital and physician group IT plans back into alignment? Should the EHR effort proceed or wait until the CPOE initiative is complete? Should you require that both systems come from the same vendor? Explain your rationale.

3. The LWMC board is concerned that the physicians are being naive about the challenges of EHR implementation, have established no measurable goals for the system, and have only weak incentives to make the implementation successful. How would you address these concerns?

CASE 12: REPLACING A PRACTICE MANAGEMENT SYSTEM

University Physician Group (UPG) is a multispecialty group practice plan associated with the College of Osteopathic Medicine (COM). UPG employs 90 physicians and 340 clinical and business support personnel.

UPG has recently been profitable (with revenue from operations this fiscal year of $32 million and a retained profit of $500,000 from operations). However, prior year losses make UPG a break-even organization.

Management and the physicians are focusing on strengthening the fiscal position of the organization. This focus has led to plans to restructure physician compensation, establish a self-insurance trust for professional liability, and improve the financial budgeting and reporting processes.

UPG has entered into a preliminary agreement to merge with Northern Affiliated Medical Group (NAMG). NAMG is a 150-physician multispecialty group located in the same city as UPG. NAMG holds a contract with the local county hospital to provide indigent care and serve as the faculty for the graduate medical education programs in family medicine.

Both organizations believe that the merged organization would be able to reduce expenses through the elimination of redundant functions and, because of greater geographical coverage and size, would improve their ability to obtain more favorable payer contracts.

Information Systems Challenge

For many years UPG has obtained practice management systems from Gleason Solutions (GS). The applications are hosted in a GS data center, reducing UPG's need for IT staff members.

Prior to the merger, UPG was in the process of examining replacements for GS. UPG had become displeased because of the GS application failure to incorporate new technologies and application features, limited ability to generate reports, and inflexible integration approaches to other applications.

Despite its displeasure, UPG now appears to be on the path to renewing the GS contract. GS executives have effectively lobbied several important physicians and administrators, and UPG's limited cash position makes the GS low-cost financial proposal attractive.

NAMG uses the GS applications and has also been examining replacing the system. NAMG has a strong IT department and will be providing IT support to the newly merged organization. After examining the market, NAMG has identified four potential vendors, including GS.

Discussion Questions

1. Would you suspend both organizations' pursuit of a new system until an IT strategic plan for the merged organization has been developed? Why?

2. What steps would you take to integrate the system selection processes of the two organizations?

3. Implementing a practice management system is always challenging. What additional implementation risks are introduced by the merger?

4. Both organizations expect the result of the merger to be lower costs, improved patient service, and increased market power. What steps would you take to make sure that the new practice management system furthers these objectives?

CASE 13: IMPLEMENTING TELE-PSYCHIATRY IN A COMMUNITY HOSPITAL EMERGENCY DEPARTMENT

Westend Hospital is a midsize, not-for-profit, community hospital in the Southeast. Each year, the hospital provides care to more than twelve thousand inpatients and sixty thousand emergency department (ED) patients. Over the past decade, the hospital has seen increasing numbers of patients with mental illness in the ED, largely because of the implementation of the state's mental health reform act, which shifted care for patients with mental illness from state psychiatric hospitals to community hospitals and outpatient facilities. Westend ED has in essence become a safety net for many individuals living in the community who need mental health services.

Largely considered a farming community, Westend County has a population of 120,000. Westend Hospital is the third largest employer in the county. However, Westend is not the only hospital in the county. The state still operates one of three psychiatric facilities in the county. Within a five-mile radius of Westend Hospital is a 270-bed inpatient psychiatric hospital, Morton Hospital. Morton Hospital serves the citizens of thirty-eight counties in the eastern part of the state.

Westend Hospital is fiscally strong with a stable management team. Anika Lewis has served as president-CEO for the past fifteen years. The remainder of the senior management team has been employed with Westend for eight to thirteen years. There are more than 150 active or affiliate members of the organized hospital medical staff and approximately 1,600 employees. The hospital has partnered with six outside management companies for services when the expertise is not easily found locally, including HighTech for assistance with IT services.

In terms of its information systems, Westend Hospital has used Meditech since the 1990s, including for nursing documentation, order entry, and diagnostic results. The nursing staff members use bar-coding technology for medication administration and have done so for years. CPOE was implemented in the ED four years ago and hospital-wide two years ago along with a certified EHR system.

The Challenge

Westend Hospital has seen increasing numbers of mental health patients in the ED over the past decade. For the past three years, the ED has averaged one hundred mental health patients per month. Depending on the level of patient acuity and availability of state- or community-operated behavioral health beds, the patient may be held in the ED from two hours to eight days before a safe disposition plan can be implemented.

The ED mental health caseload is also rapidly growing in acuity. Between 20 percent and 25 percent of the behavioral health patients are arriving under court order (involuntary commitment). The involuntary commitment patients are the most difficult in terms of developing a safe plan for disposition from the ED. The Westend Hospital's inpatient behavioral health unit is currently an adult, voluntary admission unit and does not admit involuntary commitment patients. The length of stay for involuntary commitment patients in the ED can be quite long. In some cases, it may take three to four days to stabilize the patient on medication (while in the ED) before the patient meets criteria for discharge to outpatient care. Approximately 40 percent of the mental health patients in the ED, both involuntary commitment and voluntary, are discharged either to home or outpatient treatment.

The psychiatrists and the emergency medicine physicians have met multiple times during the past six years to develop plans to improve the care of the mental health patients in the ED. Defining the criteria for an appropriate Westend psychiatrist consultation remains a challenge. The daily care needs of the mental health patients boarding in the ED are complex. The physicians have not been able to reach an agreement on this topic. Senior leaders have suggested that tele-psychiatry may be a partial solution to address this challenge.

Tele-psychiatry as a Strategy

Westend Hospital has chosen to consider contracting with a tele-psychiatry hospital network to provide tele-psychiatry services in the ED. The network has demonstrated good patient outcomes and is considered financially feasible at a rate of $4,500 per month. This fee includes the equipment, management fees, and physician fees. The director of tele-psychiatry in the hospital network has verbally committed to work very closely with the Westend Hospital team to ensure a smooth implementation.

Technology to support tele-psychiatry uses two-way, real-time, interactive audio and video through a secure encrypted wireless network. The patient and the psychiatric provider interact in the same manner as if the provider were physically present. The provider performing the patient consultation uses a desktop video conferencing system in the psychiatric office.

Tele-psychiatry as a solution to the mental health crisis in the ED was not immediately embraced by the medical staff members. They did agree to the implementation of tele-radiology four years previously. However, the most recent revision of the medical staff bylaws to support telemedicine explicitly states that the medical executive committee must approve, by a two-thirds vote, any additional telemedicine programs that may be introduced at the hospital. The medical staff leaders wanted to preserve their ability to maintain a financially viable medical practice in the community as well as protect the quality of care.

The idea of tele-psychiatry was introduced to portions of the medical staff. The psychiatrists realized that tele-psychiatry could relieve them of the burden of daily rounds in the ED for boarding patients. They were also concerned about their workload when tele-psychiatry was not available.

The emergency medicine physicians immediately verbalized their disapproval on several levels. First, they were concerned about the reliability of the technology based on their experiences over the past several years with video remote interpreting. Then, the emergency medicine physicians were skeptical about the continued support from the psychiatrists when an in-person consultation might be clinically necessary.

Physicians outside of the ED and psychiatry could not understand why the current psychiatrists could not meet the needs of the ED. The barriers to adoption of tele-psychiatry crossed three arenas: financial, behavioral, and technical. Subsequently, many conversations were conducted. Eventually, the medical executive committee approved tele-psychiatry as a new patient care service on June 25 of this year.

Implementation Plan

The CEO appointed the vice president of patient services as the executive sponsor. The implementation team includes the IT hardware and networking specialist, IT interface specialists, nursing informatics analyst, ED nurse director, behavioral health nurse director, assistant vice president patient services, physician clinical systems analyst, and the medical staff services coordinator. These individuals represent the major activities for implementation: provider credentialing, physician documentation, equipment and technical support, and patient care activities. Because of competing projects and psychiatry subject matter expertise, the executive sponsor will also serve as the project manager.

The mental health crisis affecting the ED is the focal driver for change. Patient safety is at risk. Barriers to implement tele-psychiatry have been well documented. The strategies to overcome the barriers include defining the new role for the Westend psychiatrists, developing a process for ease of access and reliability of equipment for the ED physicians, and development of a plan when the tele-psychiatry program is not available.

An unexpected barrier has been recently identified. On initiation of the tele-psychiatry provider credentialing process, the medical staff services coordinator discovered that the bylaws do not have a provision for credentialing of physician extenders in the telemedicine category. The tele-psychiatry providers include six board-certified psychiatrists and twelve mental health–trained nurse practitioners. The medical executive committee has agreed to ask the medical staff bylaws committee to convene and revise the bylaws accordingly. The original go-live date of September has been changed to December.

The executive sponsor along with the implementation team will be responsible for managing the organizational changes necessary to support the introduction of technology and new patient care flow processes. Managing organizational change will be essential to the success of this project. Some items in the project will be viewed as incremental change and other items will be viewed as step-shift change. Communication strategies will be developed to support the change.

Discussion Questions

1. What are the benefits associated with using tele-psychiatry services in the ED? To the patient? To the hospital? To the medical staff members? What are the potential barriers or challenges?

2. Based on the information provided in this case, how equipped is Westend Hospital to implement tele-psychiatry services? What resources do they have in place? What other resources might they consider?

3. How might the Westend Hospital evaluate or measure the success of its tele-psychiatry services? What metrics might they use?

CASE 14: ASSESSING THE VALUE AND IMPACT OF CPOE

The University Health Care System is an academic medical center with more than 1,200 licensed beds and more than 9,000 employees. The system comprises the University Hospital, Winston Geriatric Hospital, Jefferson Rehabilitation Hospital, and two outpatient centers in the metropolitan area. The system has a history of being a patriarchal, physician-driven organization. When University Health Care first started taking patients, it was viewed as a mecca to which community physicians throughout the South referred difficult-to-treat patients. That referral mentality persisted for decades, so physicians within the system had a difficult time making the transition to an organization that had to compete for patients with other health care entities in the region.

In recent years, University Health Care System has evolved and has given physicians proportionately more clout in decision making, in part because the health care leadership team has not stepped forward. Creating a balance between clinician providers and administrative leadership is a real issue. In the midst of the difficulty, both groups have agreed to embark on the EHR journey. Currently about 55 percent of the system's patient record is electronic; the remainder is on paper. The physicians as a whole, however, have embraced technology and view the EHR as the right road to take in achieving the organization's goal of providing high-quality, safe, cost-effective patient care.

Information Systems Challenge

Currently, the University Health Care System is in the midst of rolling out the CPOE portion of the EHR project. A multidisciplinary decision-making project was established before beginning the initiative, and leaders and clinicians tried to educate themselves on what the CPOE project would entail. They were familiar with cases such as one at Cedars-Sinai in which CPOE was halted after physician uproar over the time it took to use it and patient safety concerns. To help ensure this did not happen at the University Health Care System, the leadership team decided to take a slower, phased-in approach. Team members visited similar organizations that had implemented CPOE, attended vendor user-group conferences, consulted with colleagues from across the nation, and articulated the following project goals:

- Optimize patient safety.
- Improve quality outcomes and reduce variation in practice through the use of evidence-based practice guidelines.
- Reduce risk for errors.
- Accommodate regulatory standards expectations.
- Enhance patient satisfaction.
- Standardize processes.
- Improve efficiency.

The board has made it very clear that it wants regular updates on the progress of the project and expects to see what the return on the investment has been.

Discussion Questions

1. How might you evaluate the CPOE implementation process at University Health Care System? Give examples of different methods or strategies you might employ.
2. How would you respond to the board's desire for a "return on investment" from this initiative? Is it a reasonable request? Why or why not?

3. Assume you are to lead the evaluation component of this project. You have reviewed the goals for the project. What process would you use to develop a plan for assessing the value of CPOE? Who would be involved? What roles would they play? How would you decide on the best metrics to use? What baseline data would you want to collect or review?

CASE 15: ASSESSING THE VALUE OF HEALTH IT INVESTMENT

Five years ago, senior leadership at the Southeast Medical Center made the decision to embark on the implementation of a host of new clinical applications in the inpatient units enterprise-wide. The four hospitals that comprise Southeast Medical Center include the Main Adult Hospital, the Children's Hospital, McKinsey Hospital, and the Institute of Psychiatry. They contracted with McKesson to implement the following applications:

- ED tracking system
- Replacement pharmacy information system
- Clinical documentation system (for all nurses and ancillary personnel; does not include physician notes)
- Medication administration using bar-coding technology
- Computerized provider order entry (CPOE)

In addition, several administrative applications were implemented, including a new operative scheduling system and materials management system. They also upgraded their clinical data repository viewer (referred to as Oacis). All applications are now operational.

Most recently, the board of trustees has approved replacement of Southeast's ambulatory care EHR. A system known as EasyDoc (a McKesson product) has been in use for years. However, the system was viewed by clinicians and IT staff members as antiquated and cumbersome to navigate. It is also very difficult to retrieve aggregate data from the system. Much of this is apparently because of its underlying database architecture and structure. EasyDoc also did not interface with the hospital clinical applications, and leaders were concerned that the system was not going to enable Southeast to achieve meaningful use criteria.

Clinicians have also been frustrated that Southeast has been using two different EHR systems, one for inpatient and another for outpatient, and the two don't interface or give a complete picture of the patient's health record. With payment reform and the need to be able to more effectively manage patient care quality and outcomes, senior leaders recommended, and the board approved, replacement of the EasyDoc EHR with Epic ambulatory care

EHR. The patient registration and billing system used in ambulatory care will also be replaced with Epic's practice management application. Long-term plans are to eventually replace the McKesson clinical applications with Epic in the inpatient sector as well.

The total cost of ownership for the replacement ambulatory EHR and practice management system is approximately $30 million. Included in this estimate are not only the software and hardware upgrades but also the staff members needed to implement and support the new applications. Replacing the McKesson clinical products with Epic inpatient EHR will cost an additional $90 million. Again, this is an estimated total cost of ownership.

The primary purpose of the Epic EHR project is to provide clinicians with access to a single, complete EHR that spans the patient's continuum of care and improves collaboration and coordination of care. Community providers and patients will have access to the system. Community partners (such as primary care providers) will be able to retrieve important patient information. Currently a local HIE exists that provides ED visit information to all local hospitals. This is to be expanded to include continuity of care documents (CCDs) and other relevant health information. Patients will be given access to their health information such as lab tests, X-ray results, and medications. They will also be able to schedule appointments and pay their bills online through a patient portal known as MyChart. Southeast physician leaders view patients as partners in their own care and are pleased to provide them access to information electronically.

Southeast providers treat a large population of patients with multiple chronic conditions. Managing chronic diseases using evidence-based, real-time support is considered essential. In addition, Southeast Medical Center has available a secure data warehouse of patient data that researchers and clinicians will be using more fully in the future to ensure that clinical research drives best care.

Discussion Questions

Assume you've been tasked with developing a plan to assess the value of Southeast's investment in the Epic outpatient and inpatient systems and expansion of its use of the data warehouse. The board is interested in knowing how these new and replacement systems have affected or will affect Southeast's ability to offer coordinated, collaborative care in a cost-effective manner. The facility fully intends to meet Meaningful Use criteria and report on quality outcomes. They realize that the traditional fee-for-service system in which providers are paid on volume will be a thing of the past.

1. How would you determine which metrics to use? Who would be involved in the process?

2. How would you know that a change is attributable to the EHR or data warehouse system and not something else?

3. Do you think traditional return-on-investment methods are useful in this case? Why or why not?

CASE 16: THE ADMITTING SYSTEM CRASHES

Jones Regional Medical Center is a large academic health center. With nine hundred beds, Jones had forty-seven thousand admissions last year. Jones frequently has occupancy in excess of 100 percent, requiring diversion of ambulances. In addition, Jones had 1,300,000 ambulatory and emergency room visits in the past three years.

Jones is internationally renowned for its research and teaching programs. The IT staff members at Jones are highly regarded. They support more than three hundred applications and twelve thousand workstations.

The admitting system at Jones is provided by the vendor Technology Med (TechMed). The TechMed system supports the master patient index; registration; inpatient charge and payment entry; medical records abstracting and coding; hospital billing and patient accounting; reporting; and admission, discharge, and transfer capabilities.

The TechMed system was implemented twelve years ago and uses now-obsolete technology, including a rudimentary database management system. The organization is concerned about the fragility of the application and has begun plans to replace the TechMed system two years from now.

Information Systems Challenge

On December 20, the link between the main data center (where the TechMed servers were housed) and the disaster recovery center was taken down to conduct performance testing.

On December 21, power was lost to the disaster recovery center, but emergency power was instantly put in place. However, as a precaution, a backup of the TechMed database was performed.

During the afternoon of December 21, the TechMed system became sluggish and then unresponsive. Database corruption was discovered. The backup performed earlier in the day was also corrupt. The link to the disaster recovery data center had not been restored following the performance testing.

Because there was no viable backup copy of the database, the Jones IT and hospital staff members began the arduous process of a full database recovery from journaled transactions. This process was completed the evening of December 22.

The loss of the TechMed system for more than thirty-six hours and the failure during that time of registration transactions to update patient care and ancillary department systems resulted in a wide variety of operational problems. The patient census had to be maintained manually. Reports of results were delayed. Paper orders were needed for patients who were admitted on December 21 and 22. Charge collection lagged.

Once the TechMed system was restored, additional hospital staff members were brought in to enter, into multiple systems, the data that had been manually captured during the outage. By December 25, normal hospital operations were restored. No patient care incidents are believed to have resulted.

Discussion Questions

1. If you were the CIO of Jones Regional Medical Center during this system failure, what steps would you take during the outage? What steps would you take after the outage to reduce the likelihood of a reoccurrence of this problem?

2. The root cause analysis of the outage showed that process, technology, and staffing factors all contributed to the problem. What are some of the likely factors? Which of these factors do you believe are likely to have been the most important?

3. If you were a member of the audit committee of the Jones board of trustees, what questions would you ask the CIO?

4. What issues and problems should a disaster recovery plan prepare for? How does an organization determine how much to spend to reduce the occurrence and severity of such episodes?

CASE 17: BREACHING THE SECURITY OF AN INTERNET PATIENT PORTAL

Kaiser Permanente is an integrated health delivery system that serves more than eight million members in nine states and the District of Columbia. In the late 1990s, Kaiser Permanente introduced an Internet patient portal, Kaiser Permanente Online (also known as KP Online). Members can use KP Online to

Note: Information for this case was taken from Collmann, J. C., & Cooper, T. (2007). Breaching the security of the Kaiser Permanente Internet patient portal: The organizational foundations of information security. *Journal of the American Medical Informatics Association, 14*(2), 239–243.

request appointments, request prescription refills, obtain health care service information, seek clinical advice, and participate in patient forums.

Information Systems Challenge

In August, there was a serious breach in the security of the KP Online pharmacy refill application. Programmers wrote a flawed script that actually concatenated over eight hundred individual e-mail messages containing individually identifiable patient information, instead of separating them as intended. As a result, nineteen members received e-mail messages with private information about multiple other members. Kaiser became aware of the problem when two members notified the organization that they had received the concatenated e-mail messages. Kaiser leadership considered this incident a significant breach of confidentiality and security. The organization immediately took steps to investigate and to offer apologies to those affected.

On the same day the first member notified Kaiser about receiving the problem e-mail, a crisis team was formed. The crisis team began a root cause analysis and a mitigation assessment process. Three days later Kaiser began notifying its members and issued a press release.

The investigation of the cause of the breach uncovered issues at the technical, individual, group, and organizational levels. At the technical level, Kaiser was using new web-based tools, applications, and processes. The pharmacy module had been evaluated in a test environment that was not equivalent to the production environment. At the individual level, two programmers, one from the e-mail group and one from the development group, working together for the first time in a new environment and working under intense pressure to quickly fix a serious problem, failed to adequately test code they produced as a patch for the pharmacy application. Three groups within Kaiser had responsibilities for KP Online: operations, e-mail, and development. Traditionally these groups worked independently and had distinct missions and organizational cultures. The breach revealed the differences in the way groups approached priorities. For example, the development group often let meeting deadlines dictate priorities. At the organizational level, Kaiser IT had a very complex organizational structure, leading to what Collmann and Cooper (2007, p. 239) call "compartmentalized sensemaking." Each IT group "developed highly localized definitions of a situation, which created the possibility for failure when integrated in a common infrastructure."

Discussion Questions

1. How serious was this e-mail security breach? Why did the Kaiser Permanente leadership react so quickly to mitigate the possible damage done by the breach?

2. Assume that you were appointed as the administrative member of the crisis team created the day the breach was uncovered. After the initial apologies, what recommendations would you make for investigating the root cause(s) of the breach? Outline your suggested investigative steps.

3. How likely do you think future security breaches would be if Kaiser Permanente did not take steps to resolve underlying group and organizational issues? Why?

4. What role should the administrative leadership of Kaiser Permanente take in ensuring that KP Online is secure? Apart from security and HIPAA training for all personnel, what steps can be taken at the organizational level to improve the security of KP Online?

CASE 18: THE DECISION TO DEVELOP AN IT STRATEGIC PLAN

Meadow Hills Hospital is a 211-bed acute care hospital with four hundred members on its medical staff. Meadow serves a population of three hundred thousand. There are three other similarly sized hospitals in the region. As an organization, Meadow Hills is very well run. It has a good reputation in the community and is considered to be technically advanced based on its investments in imaging technology. The organization is also in a strong financial position, with $238 million in reserves. Meadow Hills has never had an IT strategic plan.

Information Systems Challenge

The IT function reports to the Meadow Hills chief financial officer (CFO). The CEO and other members of the senior leadership team have largely left IT decisions up to the CFO. As a result, the organization's financial systems are very well developed. Computerized provider order entry (CPOE), an EHR system, and a PACS have not been implemented. IT support for departments such as nursing, pharmacy, laboratory, imaging, and risk management is limited.

The Meadow Hills IT team is well regarded and the limited IT support for clinical processes has not drawn complaints from the nursing or medical staff. The organization does not currently have a CIO.

The CEO has never felt the need to pay attention to IT. However, he is worried that reimbursement based on care quality will arrive at Meadow Hills soon. He also believes that the Meadow Hills Clinical Laboratory and Imaging Center would be more competitive if it had stronger IT support; rival labs and imaging centers are able to offer electronic access to test results. And he suspects that the lack of IT support may eventually lead to nurses and physicians choosing to practice elsewhere.

Discussion Questions

1. What steps should the CEO take to develop an IT strategy for the organization?
2. Are there unique risks to the ability of Meadow Hills Hospital to develop and implement an IT strategy?
3. Meadow Hills appears to have been successful despite years without an IT strategy. Why is this?

CASE 19: SELECTION OF A PATIENT SAFETY STRATEGY

Langley Mason Health (LMH) is located in North Reno County, the largest public health care district in the state of Nevada, serving an 850-square-mile area encompassing seven distinctly different communities. The health district was founded in 1937 by a registered nurse and dietician who opened a small medical facility on a former poultry farm. Today the health system comprises Langley Medical Center, a 317-bed tertiary medical center and level II trauma center; Mason Hospital, a 107-bed community hospital; and Mason Continuing Care Center and Villa Langley, two part-skilled nursing facilities (SNFs); a home care division; an ambulatory surgery center; and an outpatient behavioral medicine center.

In anticipation of expected population growth in North Reno County and to meet the state-mandated seismic requirements, LMH developed an aggressive facilities master plan (FMP) that includes plans to build a state-of-the-art 453-bed replacement hospital for its Langley Medical Center campus, double the size of its Mason Hospital, and build satellite clinics in four of its outlying communities. The cost associated with actualizing this FMP is estimated to be $1 billion. Several years ago, LMH undertook and successfully passed the largest health care bond measure in the state's history and in so doing secured $496 million in general obligation bonds to help fund its massive facilities expansion project. The remaining funds must come from revenue bonds, growth strategies, philanthropic efforts, and strong operational performance over the next ten years. Additionally, $5 million of routine capital funds will be diverted every fiscal year for the next five years to help offset the huge capital outlay that will be necessary to equip the new facilities. That leaves LMH with only $10 million per year to spend on routine maintenance, equipment, and technology for all its facilities. LMH is committed to patient safety and is building what the leadership team hopes will be one of the safest hospital-of-the-future facilities. The challenge is to provide for patient safety and safe medication practices given the minimal capital dollars available to spend today.

LMH developed an IT strategic plan and identified the following ten goals:

- Empower health consumers and physicians.
- Transform data into information.
- Support the expansion of clinical services.
- Expand e-business opportunities.
- Realize the benefits of innovation.
- Maximize the value of IT.
- Improve project outcomes.
- Prepare for the unexpected.
- Deploy a robust and agile technical architecture.
- Digitally enable new facilities, including the new hospital.

Information Systems Challenge

LMH has implemented Phase 1—an enterprise-wide EHR system developed by Cerner Corporation at a cost of $20 million. Phase 2 of the project is to implement CPOE with decision-support capabilities. This phase was to have been completed previously, but has been delayed because of the many challenges associated with Phase 1, which still must be stabilized and optimized. LMH does have a fully automated pharmacy information system, albeit older technology, and Pyxis medication-dispensing systems on all units in the acute care hospitals. Computerized discharge prescriptions and instructions are available only for patients seen and discharged from the LMH emergency departments.

Currently, the pharmacy and nursing staff members at LMH have been working closely on the selection of a smart IV pump to replace all of the health system's aging pumps and have put forth a proposal to spend $4.9 million in the next fiscal year. Smart pumps have been shown to significantly reduce medication administration errors, thus reducing patient harm. This expenditure would consume roughly half of all of the available capital dollars for that fiscal year.

The CIO, Marilyn Chen, understands the pharmacists' and nurses' desire to purchase smart IV pumps but believes the implementation of this technology should not be considered in isolation. She sees the smart pumps as one facet of an overall medication management capital purchase and patient safety strategic plan. Marilyn Chen suggests that the pharmacy and nursing leadership team lead a medication management strategic planning process and evaluate a suite of available technologies that taken together could optimize medication safety (for example, CPOE, electronic medication administration records [e-mar], robots, automated pharmacy systems, bar coding, computerized discharge prescriptions and instructions, and smart IV pumps), the costs associated with implementing these technologies, and the organization's readiness to embrace these technologies. Paul Robinson, the director of pharmacy, appreciates Marilyn Chen's suggestion but feels that smart IV pumps are critical to patient safety and that LMH doesn't have time to go through a long, drawn-out planning process that could take years to implement and the process of gaining board support. Others argue that all new proposals should be placed on hold until CPOE is up and running. They argue there are too many other pressing issues at hand to invest in yet another new technology.

Discussion Questions

1. Describe the current situation as you see it. What are the major issues in this case?

2. Marilyn Chen, CIO, and Paul Robinson, director of pharmacy, have different views of how LMH should proceed. What are the pros and cons of their respective approaches? Which approach, if either, seems like an appropriate course of action to you? Explain your rationale.

3. Assume you are to mediate a discussion on this issue and that participants are to come to consensus on how best to proceed. What would you do?

CASE 20: STRATEGIC IS PLANNING FOR THE HOSPITAL ED

Founded in 1900, Newcastle Hospital today is a 375-bed, not-for-profit community hospital that serves more than two hundred thousand residents of Newcastle County, New York. The hospital is approximately thirty miles from midtown Manhattan. It provides a full range of primary and secondary medical and surgical services and is an affiliate of one of the large New York City hospital systems for tertiary referrals and select residency programs. Newcastle Hospital has an independent governing body with 25 trustees, 604 active physicians, and 1,121 full-time equivalent (FTE) staff members. Revenues of approximately $130 million per year come from 15,600 inpatient admissions, 71,000 outpatient visits, and 65,000 home care visits. Newcastle Hospital operates in a difficult environment characterized by relatively poor reimbursement and severe competition. There is one other acute care hospital in the county and a total of thirty-five others within a twenty-mile radius.

The sentinel event in the hospital's recent history occurred four years ago—a six-month nursing strike that alienated the workforce, decimated public confidence, and directly cost at least $19.5 million, effectively eradicating the hospital's capital reserves. Most of the senior management was replaced after the strike. When hired, the new CEO and CFO uncovered extensive inaccuracies that resulted in a reduction of reported net assets by almost $30 million and the near-bankruptcy of the hospital. The new management restated financial statements, began resolving extensive litigation, and set out to reestablish immediate operations, future finances, and a long-term strategy. The new CEO states that "years of board and management neglect, plus the ravages of the strike complicated recovery, because standards, systems, and middle managers were universally absent or ineffective."

Among its many issues, the challenges within the hospital's emergency department (ED) are particularly important to the overall recovery effort. The ED is described by the hospital CEO as the organization's "financial, clinical, and public relations backbone." The ED sees 34,000 patients per year and admits 24 percent of them, constituting 51 percent of all inpatient admissions. In addition, the ED is a clinically distinguished Level II trauma center, with a long legacy of outcomes that compare favorably against regional, state, and national benchmarks. Finally, most community members have experience with the ED and consider it a proxy for the hospital as a whole, whether or not they have experienced an inpatient stay.

Currently, Newcastle ED patient satisfaction compared to patient satisfaction among peer organizations ranks at the 14th percentile in the Press Ganey New York State survey and the 5th percentile in national surveys. Since the start of the new millennium, three organized initiatives to improve these results (especially regarding walkouts and waiting times) have failed, even though two involved prestigious consultants. After the management change, the new CEO diagnosed two core barriers to overcoming the ED problems: first, inflexibility and unwillingness to change among the ED physician management group that had been in place for ten years, and, second, an almost complete absence of the data required to define, measure, and improve the

ED's service performance. The first barrier was addressed via an RFP process that resulted in engaging a new physician management group two years ago.

Information Systems Challenge

The present IS challenge follows directly from Newcastle Hospital's overarching strategic objectives: "satisfying patients and staff," "supporting ourselves," and "getting better every day" (that is, improving performance). The ED as presently structured has ill-defined manual processes and no information system. The challenge is selecting an ED information system with an emphasis on informing, not just automating, key ED processes in order to support the overall strategic initiatives of the organization.

Several organizational and IT system factors that affect this IT challenge have been identified by the hospital CEO.

Organizational Factors

Undefined strategy. Newcastle Hospital operated without a formal strategic action plan and corresponding tactics until two years ago. As a result, systematic prioritization and measurement of institutional imperatives such as improving the ED did not occur.

Data integrity. Data throughout the hospital were undefined and unreliable. For example, two irreconcilable daily census reports made timely bed placement from the ED impossible.

Culture. "Looking good," that is, escaping accountability, was valued more highly than "doing good," that is, substantively improving performance. Serious problems in the ED were often masked or dismissed as anecdotes, even in the face of regulatory citations and six- to eight-hour waiting times. The previous ED contract had contained no quality standards, and the ED physicians claimed to be busy "saving lives" whenever their poor service performance was questioned.

IT System Factors

IT strategy. Paralleling the hospital, the IS department had no defined strategies, objectives, or processes. Alignment with hospital strategy and IT performance measurements were not considered. Although some progress has been made, this remains an area needing attention.

IT governance. There is no IT steering committee at either the board or management level. IT policies, service-level agreements, decision criteria, and user roles and responsibilities do not exist.

Functionality. The IT applications portfolio is missing critical elements (for example, order entry, case management, nursing documentation, radiology) that would greatly benefit the ED, even without a dedicated ED system. The hospital's core information system is three versions out-of-date and certain functions have been bypassed by users altogether.

IT infrastructure and architecture. The data center and most IT staff members are located twelve miles away from the hospital, isolating IT physically and culturally from users and patients. Software and networks have been arbitrarily and extensively customized over the years, without documentation, and inadequate hardware capacity has often been given as an excuse for not pursuing an ED system.

IT organization and resources. IT spending has been, on average, less than 1 percent of the hospital's budget and IT staff members have lacked essential training in critical applications and tools. Newcastle Hospital has been dependent on multiple IT vendors for a variety of implementation and operations support activities.

Discussion Questions

1. Outline the steps you would take to initiate a strategic planning process for improving the ED information system. How will you ensure that this plan is in alignment with the hospital's and department's overall strategic plans?

2. Multiple factors have contributed to the current state of the ED at Newcastle Hospital and are listed in the case. Which of these do you think will be the most difficult to overcome? Why?

3. The new CEO has good insight into the ED issues. Assuming that his assessment of the situation is accurate, discuss how his continued support could affect the outcome of any ED IS strategic plan.

4. Assume the CEO has appointed you to spearhead the ED IS strategic planning effort. What are the first steps you will take? Outline a general plan of action for the next three months. Indicate, by title, whom you would involve in the process. Explain your choices.

CASE 21: BOARD SUPPORT FOR A CAPITAL PROJECT

Lakeland Medical Center is a 210-bed public hospital located in the Southeast. It is governed by a politically appointed nine-member board and serves a market of approximately one hundred thousand people. The hospital has been financially successful, but in recent years several capital investments have not brought high returns. As a result, project investment decisions became more conservative and oriented toward financial returns. Competitive forces have continued to grow in the market, and significant internal expense items (such as the organization's pension program, paid leave bank, and health insurance program) have put strains on Lakeland's financial resources.

Revenue continues to grow at an average rate of about 10 percent each year, but controlling expenses remains a challenge. Bad debt has grown from $5 million last year to a budgeted amount of $14 million this year. The hospital continues to accomplish high patient and employee satisfaction scores, high quality scores, and an A+ credit rating. Debt is approximately $55 million, and cash reserves are approximately $95 million. Total operating revenues are approximately $130 million. The hospital employs 940 staff members. The average length of stay is 4.3 days. Annual capital expenditure is $4 million.

Information Systems Challenge

Three years ago, the installation of computed radiography (CR) components to build a picture archiving and communication system (PACS) began, at an estimated total cost of $1 million. The following year, $400,000 was spent for additional CR components. Most recently the board of directors (with three new members) did not approve the request of $1.9 million for completion of the PACS, saying that it represented far too large a percentage of the organization's annual capital budget. Lakeland is still in need of completing the PACS program, with a board that is unlikely to approve the expenditure.

A number of factors are contributing to the board's decision not to authorize the additional $1.9 million for completion of the PACS:

- Leadership's inability to guarantee to the board's satisfaction a financial return on the proposed investment
- The board's perception that the radiologists are not committed to the hospital and to the community because none of the radiologists live in the community
- The board's perception that the cardiologists are not committed to the hospital or to the community; the five cardiologists on staff are considered to be uncooperative among themselves and not supportive of the hospital's goals
- Poor leadership within the IT department for providing the proper guidance on acquisition and implementation

- The board's philosophy that Lakeland Medical Center should be more high-touch and less high-tech, and thus there is a philosophical difference over the need for a PACS

- Jealousy among the medical staff members that the diagnostic imaging department continues to obtain capital approvals for large items representing a major percentage of the annual capital budget; thus, many influential members of the medical staff, such as surgeons, are not supportive of the expenditure

- A few vocal employees speaking directly to board members expressing their concern that the PACS implementation will result in job loss for them

- Leadership's inability to make a connection between this capital project and the strategic goals of the organization

The chief of staff, Iesha Brown, firmly believes that a PACS will increase patient and physician satisfaction because waiting times for results will decrease, enhance patient education, improve staff member and physician productivity, improve clinical outcomes, improve patient safety, eliminate lost films, reduce medical liability, assist in reducing patient length of stay, and increase revenue potential. She believes it is management's challenge to understand the key issues of the board and to present the necessary supportive information for ultimate approval of the PACS program.

Discussion Questions

1. Conduct a role-play. Divide into four teams—the Lakeland Medical Center administrative team, the board, the medical staff members, and the hospital and community at large. Assume the role of your constituent group and answer these questions: What are your views on this proposal? What are your major concerns? What questions do you have? And for whom? Do you think this is a case of someone failing to do his or her homework in putting together a sound business plan for the PACS project, or do you think there are bigger issues at play here? Explain your answers as necessary.

2. Assume that the CEO believes that the PACS project is well aligned with Lakeland's strategic goals but that this case hasn't been made clear to the board. How might Lakeland build this case? Who should lead that effort? What work needs to be done that has not occurred yet?

3. Are the board's concerns about medical staff commitment relevant in this case? Why or why not?

4. Develop a strategy for addressing the board's concerns and winning their buy-in and approval for the PACS project. Include in your description the who, what, where, when, and how.

SUPPLEMENTAL LISTING OF RELATED CASE STUDIES AND WEBINARS

Enabling Change in Health Care

by Martha Hostetter, Sarah Klein, and Douglas McCarthy

Source: The Commonwealth Fund. Retrieved July 27, 2016, from https://medium.com/@CommonwealthFund/penn-medicine-center-for-health-care-innovation-enabling-change-612703a8f53b#.9ssb2vzab

Publication date: August 2015

The University of Pennsylvania Health System founded the Center for Health Care Innovation in 2012 to test new models of care and build evidence of their effectiveness. The center is also designed to help Penn Medicine—a $4.9 billion system based in Philadelphia—prepare for payment models that reward clinicians for the value of the care they deliver.

Penn Medicine's working premise is that innovation relies not on inspiration but on having a ready infrastructure to develop, test, and implement new strategies for delivering health care. The health system also sees innovation as a discipline that can be learned. This case describes the methods used by the Center for Health Care Innovation to test new models of care and lessons learned. Analytics is an integral part.

The Road to Accountable Care: Building Systems for Population Health Management

by Douglas McCarthy, Sarah Klein, and Alexander Cohen

Source: The Commonwealth Fund. Retrieved July 27, 2016, from http://www.commonwealthfund.org/publications/case-studies/2014/oct/road-to-accountable-care-synthesis

Publication date: October 2014

This case study series describes how three diverse organizations are developing accountable care systems to improve the quality, reduce the costs of care, and ultimately improve the health of populations of patients insured by Medicare, Medicaid, and commercial health plans. They employ a constellation of strategies to identify and address unmet medical needs, improve care transitions, and reduce inefficiencies and unnecessary variation in care. Care managers, outreach workers, and virtual care teams help improve outcomes for patients with complex needs that are costly to treat. Data integration and analytics are key to their efforts, although the sophistication of these capabilities varies. Two study sites have established a record of savings, and the third is still proving the potential of its approach. Their progress to date suggests that payment reforms can foster the will and accountability necessary to transform care.

Webinar: Engaging Physicians in the Health Care Revolution

by Thomas Lee

Source: *Harvard Business Review*. Retrieved July 25, 2016, from https://hbr.org/webinar/2016/03/engaging-physicians-in-the-health-care-revolution

This webinar discusses how today's health care marketplace is driven by competition based on value. Health care providers must focus on meeting patients' needs, delivering and measuring outcomes that matter to patients, and doing so as efficiently as possible.

In this new competitive market, value will be created by teams and collaboration will be the strategic differentiator. Social capital will be as important as financial capital, and social network science will be an essential tool for driving the spread of values throughout a provider organization. The webinar may be helpful background information in discussions on strategy and IT implications in health care.

Uber: Changing the Way the World Moves

by Youngme Moo

Source: *Harvard Business Review*. Prod. No.: 316101-PDF-ENG

Publication date: November 1, 2015

In 2015, Uber is building what may be the largest point-to-point transportation network of its kind; it is literally changing the way the world moves. But unlike traditional transportation logistics companies such as FedEx, Uber has an incredibly lightweight infrastructure: It owns no vehicles, employs no drivers, and pays no vehicle maintenance costs. Instead, its network relies on peer-to-peer coordination between drivers and passengers, enabled by sophisticated software and a clever reputation system. But despite its remarkable early success, Uber is an extremely polarizing company. Its business model is highly disruptive, and although disruptive innovation can be a good thing, it is also true that disruptive companies tend to break things. This is certainly true for Uber, and it is one of the key tensions in the case: Uber's innovative business model is outpacing many of the laws regulating its industry, and although it is going to take the regulatory system some time to catch up, Uber doesn't appear to be willing to wait.

Inciting a Computer Revolution in Health Care: Implementing the Health Information Technology Act

by Pamela Varley

Source: Harvard Business Review. Prod. No.: HKS874-PDF-ENG

Publication date: April 4, 2011

This case poses this question: given the ambitious goals of the 2009 Health Information Technology for Economic and Clinical Health (HITECH) Act and the hurdles to its successful implementation, how should incoming national coordinator for health information technology David Blumenthal proceed? It is ideal for a class on strategic leadership. The case describes Blumenthal's resources, most notably the following:

- $27 billion in Medicare and Medicaid incentives to hospitals, physicians, and other eligible providers who invested in "certified" electronic health systems and made "Meaningful Use" of them
- $2 billion in other funds to address specific obstacles to widespread acquisition of health IT systems
- Broad regulatory authority to define "Meaningful Use" and set certification criteria

It also describes Blumenthal's major challenge: to persuade thousands of hospitals and hundreds of thousands of doctors—many of them skeptical— that health IT systems were worth the time and trouble it would take to buy them and integrate them into daily clinical practice. Small, cash-strapped community hospitals and individual practitioners constituted a particular concern. Finally, it describes the nature of Blumenthal's regulatory task: to define Meaningful Use quickly and to strike the right balance. Define Meaningful Use too strictly, and large numbers of health care providers might turn down the proffered incentives. Define it too loosely, and the expensive federal initiative would deliver little more than the market would have produced anyway. The case may be used on its own. It may also be used as the second part of a two-case unit with HKS Case 1937.0, "A. Inciting a Computer Revolution in Health Care: Weighing the Merits of the Health Information Technology Act." HKS Case Number 1938.0.

Information Technology and Clinical Operations at Beth Israel Deaconess Medical Center

by Richard Bohmer and F. Warren McFarlan

Source: Harvard Business School. 24 pages. Prod. No.: 607150-PDF-ENG

　Publication date: June 4, 2007

Describes the history of clinical computing at Boston's Beth Israel Hospital and the development, since the 1996 merger to form the Beth Israel Deaconess Medical Center, of an information system designed to support the delivery of patient care. The hospitals' CIO, John Halamka, has overseen the development of an information system that places physicians at its center. Describes the design and function of five major components of the system: the online medical record, e-prescribing, physician order entry, the emergency department dashboard, and the performance manager. Provides students with an opportunity to identify key design principles for health care information systems and to discuss the unique implementation challenges that the health care delivery setting raises for CIOs and CEOs.

Partners Healthcare System: Transforming Health Care Services Delivery through Information Management

by Richard M. Kesner

Source: Richard Ivey School of Business Foundation. 15 pages. Prod. No.: 909E23-PDF-ENG

　Publication date: February 26, 2010

This case considers the process of organizational transformation undertaken by Partners Healthcare System (PHS) since the 1990s as their hospital and affiliated ambulatory medical practices have adopted EHR and CPOE systems. Encompassing a strategic investment in information technologies, widespread process change, and the pervasive use of institutional clinical decision-support and knowledge management systems, this story has been fifteen years in the making, culminating in 2009 with the network-wide use of EHR and CPOE by all PHS doctors. These developments in turn opened the door to the redefinition of services delivery and to the replacement of established therapies through the leveraging of the knowledge residing in 4.6 million now-digitized PHS patient records. As such, the PHS experience serves as a window into how one organization strove to address the daunting challenges of twenty-first-century health care services information management, as a template for success in the implementation of large-scale information systems among research-based hospitals across the United States and more broadly as a learning platform for industry executives in their efforts to transform health care delivery through data and knowledge management.

Mount Auburn Hospital: Physician Order Entry

by Andrew McAfee, Sarah MacGregor, and Michael Benari

Source: Harvard Business School. 18 pages. Prod. No.: 603060 PDF-ENG

Publication date: December 17, 2002

Mount Auburn Hospital is preparing to introduce a physician order entry (POE) system throughout the hospital, starting with the labor and delivery ward. POE systems replace paper-based and oral medication ordering processes with an information system; the physician uses the system to enter medication orders, which are then transferred to the hospital's pharmacy. This is Mount Auburn's first experience with POE systems, and the implementation team must determine how best to introduce the technology to the physicians and other personnel who will use it.

Moore Medical Corporation

by Andrew McAfee and Gregory Bounds

Source: Harvard Business School. 21 pages. Prod. No.: 601142-PDF-ENG

Publication date: April 23, 2001

Moore Medical is a medium-sized distributor of medical supplies to practitioners such as podiatrists and emergency medical technicians. At the time of the case, it has relied on traditional customer channels such as catalogues, phones, and faxes to communicate product offerings, promotions, and availability, and to take orders. It is now attempting to shift to a "bricks and clicks" distributor with a strong Internet presence. It has already made substantial investments in an e-commerce website and in "back office" enterprise resource planning (ERP) software to improve the fulfillment performance of its four distribution centers. The ERP software has not lived up to expectations in all areas, and the company must decide whether to invest in more modules for this system that might address its shortcomings. It must also decide whether to make a significant additional investment in customer relationship management software.

CareGroup

by F. Warren McFarlan and Robert D. Austin

Source: HBS Premier Case Collection. 22 pages. Prod. No.: 303097-PDF ENG

Publication date: January 29, 2003

Describes the circumstances leading to the three-and-a-half-day collapse of a major hospital group's IS capabilities. Identifies the technical reasons for the failure, management steps in dealing with the problem short term, and the long-term lessons they believe they learned from the incident. This case is accompanied by a short video for educators to show in class.

University Health Network: The MOE-MAR Initiative

by Darren Meister and Ken Mark

Source: Richard Ivey School of Business Foundation. 22 pages. Prod. No.: 906E13-PDF-ENG

Publication date: February 9, 2010

The director of acute care information management at University Health Network is thinking about how to form a steering committee and several working groups to manage the implementation and ongoing operation of the medication order entry and medication administration record module. This initiative would be the most challenging and complex the IT department had ever undertaken. The director would need to address the concerns of administration, physicians, and nurses.

STARS Air Ambulance: An Information Systems Challenge

by Malcolm Munro and Sid L. Huff

Source: Richard Ivey School of Business Foundation. 12 pages. Prod. No.: 908E04-PDF-ENG

Publication date: February 26, 2008

Shock Trauma Air Rescue Society (STARS) in Calgary, Canada, provides a safe, rapid, highly specialized, emergency medical transport system for the critically ill and injured by dispatching helicopters and air medical crew at any time. STARS operates a sophisticated communication system that links together hospitals, ground ambulance services, police, firefighters, search and rescue organizations, and park wardens. The recently appointed CIO expected to inherit a sound IS operation but soon discovered a number of problems that seriously impeded his ability to manage progress. These included a poorly organized department, excessive and undisciplined use of consultants, inadequate project management, independent IS operations, IS staff members in other departments, other managers possibly resistant to change, and an IS department with no clearly organized role or mission. The basic issue in this case concerns what action the new CIO must undertake to ensure that the IS department can fully support the organization's mission.

Secrets of HIE Success Revealed: Lessons from the Leaders

by National eHealth Collaborative

Source: Retrieved from http://www.nationalehealth.org/ckfinder/ userfiles/files/REPORT%20SecretsofHIESuccessRevealed.pdf

Publication Date: July 2011

This report features twelve case studies of health information exchange (HIE) organizations that are leaders in achieving sustainable enterprises built on the value created by efficiently exchanging health information and mobilizing its effective use at the point of care. These organizations have focused on building a successful HIE through innovation, continuous learning, and business discipline with the end goal of improving quality, care coordination, and cost-effectiveness of health care. Although each organization's business model and strategy is unique, reflecting the local, community-based nature of health care, each profile offers a rich source of ideas and guidance to help HIE organizations that are at earlier stages of their life cycle succeed.

Overview of the Health Care IT Industry

The health care information technology (IT) industry is composed of companies that provide hardware, software, and a wide range of services, including consulting, implementation, and outsourcing to health care organizations. The industry also includes associations that support the professional advancement of the health care IT professions and organizations that put on industry conferences and put out publications that cover current topics and issues in the industry.

It is not possible to develop an IT strategy and implement that strategy without engaging this industry.

This appendix provides an overview of this industry:

- The size, structure, composition, and evolution of the health care IT industry
- Sources of industry information
- Health care IT associations

THE HEALTH CARE IT INDUSTRY

Health care is the largest sector of the US economy, $3.0 trillion in 2014 (CMS, 2015). It is not surprising that a large, diverse, and robust industry has developed to provide IT products and services to that sector.

Table A.1 IT interests of different health care organizations

Type of Organization	Example Care Provision Interests	Example Relevant Information Technology Applications
Providers, such as hospitals and physician practices	Making diagnoses Providing treatment	Electronic health records Revenue cycle Analytics of care costs and quality
Health plans (including self-insured employers and government payers)	Managing care costs and quality Keeping patients healthy	Patient engagement technologies Analytics of care costs and quality
Pharmaceutical companies	Ensuring medication compliance	Patient engagement technologies
Public health departments	Monitoring disease patterns Ensuring preventive care measures are occurring	Health information exchanges

The industry focuses on organizations that play a role in providing care to patients. These organizations are diverse and address different aspects of care provision (see Table A.1). Within that diversity the industry centers on health care providers.

Table A.1 does not represent a complete overview of the interests of the organizations or a complete overview of the IT that is acquired by these organizations. Nonetheless the table does illustrate the different types of organizations that are served by the health IT industry and the substantial overlap in interests and relevant technologies.

This book and this appendix focus on health care providers because the provider IT market is the most well developed and the largest portion of the overall health care IT market.

The provider portion of the market is also very diverse. Table A.2 displays the taxonomy of the health care provider industry as defined by the North American Industry Classification System (NAICS). Some IT companies focus on the federal health care system, others on nursing homes, and yet others on physician offices. Some focus even more narrowly. Within the hospital sector (NAICS code 6222), for example, some IT companies focus

Table A.2 Health care provider market: NAICS taxonomy

Health care providers	Ambulatory services	Physician offices Dentist offices Other health Outpatient centers Laboratories Home health
	Hospitals	General medical and surgical Psychiatric and substance abuse Specialty hospitals
	Nursing and residential care	Nursing care Mental care Elderly care
Insurance	Health	Accident and health insurance Hospital and medical Service plans
Government health		Federal hospitals Local hospitals Government psychiatric and long-term care

Source: Gartner (2008).

on large academic medical centers and others focus on small community hospitals.

Transition of the Health Care IT Market

The significant changes in the business model of health care that were discussed in the Preface are resulting in a transition in the health care IT market. This transition is occurring across several dimensions.

First, these changes have resulted in the development of new types of applications and accelerated development of existing applications; some of these are summarized in Table A.3.

Second, Table A.1 depicted several areas of overlapping application interests by different types of health care organizations. The overlap centers on technologies that improve patient engagement, analytics to assess care quality and costs, health information exchanges, and population health management applications. The overlap is growing stronger and becoming more extensive as payment reform gains steam; all of these organizations have

Table A.3 Changes in application focus resulting from changes in the health care business model

Business Model–Driven Change	Impact on Application Focus
Consolidation of providers and the formation of health systems	Health information exchanges
	Implementation of a common electronic health record across the continuum
Payment based on managing the health of populations	Population health applications
	Patient engagement technologies
	Analytics to assess care quality and costs
Pressures to improve operational efficiency	Applications that improve efficiency, streamline processes, and measure productivity, such as referral management

strong commercial interests in keeping patients healthy and managing their utilization of care services.

Providers will be held accountable for the care of patients but so will be employers, Medicaid, and health plans. These organizations will seek many of the applications and services that are sought by providers. The provider health care IT market is expanding into adjacent types of health care organizations.

Third, from 2010 through 2016, the provider market focused on the adoption of EHRs and the implementation of health information exchanges. This focus was driven by the Meaningful Use incentive program discussed in Chapter One. Over the next two decades we should anticipate that this focus will shift.

The high levels of EHR adoption that have resulted from Meaningful Use will mean a de-emphasis on adoption and a shift to an emphasis on leveraging the EHR to achieve gains in care quality, efficiency, and safety. Having made the substantial implementation investment, providers will focus on achieving the value discussed in Chapter Seven. This will lead to additional demand for services such as process optimization as well as investing in the applications shown in Table A.3.

Fourth, with the tremendous changes being seen, health care entrepreneurs and venture capital and private equity firms see opportunity. In 2010 $194 million was invested in emerging companies in 150 deals. In 2015 those numbers had reached $1.1 billion in 490 deals. An extraordinary increase in industry innovation has been unleashed (Startup Health, 2016).

Major Suppliers of Health Care IT Products and Services

There are many different types of companies that serve the health care market.

- Some companies strive to have a product and service line that covers the full spectrum of health care settings. Hence, these companies will offer hospital information systems, physician office systems, nursing home applications, and applications for ancillary departments, such as radiology.
- Several companies focus on a specific setting, for example, hospitals or the physician's office, but not both.
- Some companies offer products that support an application needed by multiple sectors, for example, pharmacy systems, health information exchanges, or analytics.
- Some companies offer infrastructure, for example, mobile devices, networks, and servers that are used by all sectors. These companies usually do not offer applications.
- Several companies offer services used by multiple sectors, for example, IT strategic planning, application implementation, and consulting services.
- Some companies focus their service offerings on a specific type of organization, for example, improving the operations of physician practices—or a specific type of service—for example, improving collections of overdue payments for a provider billing office.

There are literally thousands of companies that support the IT needs of the health care industry. In any given year, hundreds of companies may go out of business and hundreds of new companies may emerge. You can gain an appreciation of the diversity of health care IT companies by attending a large health care IT conference, such as the annual conference of the Healthcare Information and Management Systems Society (HIMSS), and visiting the exhibit hall. In 2016 there were 1,300 companies exhibiting.

Table A.4 provides a summary of the top vendors in the industry. These data, collected by the publication *Healthcare Informatics* (2016), rank companies according to their health information technology (HIT) revenue. Use such lists with caution, of course. In any given year, some companies will be acquired, and others will experience dramatic upturns and downturns in financial performance. Companies will disappear from the list, and companies will arrive on the list over the course of time. The products and services listed in Table A.4 are illustrative but do not make up a comprehensive list. Moreover, the fact that a company is large does not mean that it has the best solution for a particular need of a particular organization.

Nonetheless, the data in Table A.4 are interesting for several reasons:

- Health care leadership should know the names and have a reasonable understanding of the major IT vendors that serve their type of organization; sooner or later the organization will be doing business with some of these vendors.
- The size of some of these companies is apparent, with the listed companies taking in over $1 billion in revenue.
- The diversity of products and services is also apparent. Some companies focus on applications, whereas others focus on consulting, outsourcing, imaging, and analytics.
- The companies have diverse parentage. Cerner and Epic have traditional EHR roots. Phillips and GE have a medical imaging and device core. Optum is a subsidiary of a health plan (United). Dell, Cognizant, and Xerox provide IT services and products across a

Table A.4 Major health care IT vendors, ranked by revenue

Company	HIT Revenue	Types of Products and Services
Optum	$6.2 B	Applications, analytics, consulting services
Cerner	$4.4 B	Applications, analytics, consulting services and infrastructure services
Cognizant	$3.7 B	Application services
McKesson	$3.1 B	Applications, analytics, consulting services
Dell	$2.9 B	Infrastructure, consulting services
Phillips	$2.4 B	Imaging and point of care applications
Xerox	$2.1 B	Implementation and outsourcing services
Epic	$2.0B	Applications, analytics
EMC	$1.5B	Hardware, systems software
GE	$1.5B	Applications, imaging

Source: Company and revenue data from *Healthcare Informatics* (2016).

wide range of industries. McKesson is a distributor of supplies and medications to health care providers.

When an organization needs to turn to the market for applications, infrastructure, or services, its leadership would be well served by reviewing several of the sources of information described in this appendix, talking to colleagues who may have recently pursued similar IT products and services, and engaging the services of consultants who keep close tabs on the health care IT industry.

Size of the Industry

The global health care IT market is expected to grow from $115 billion in 2015 to $220 billion in 2020, a compound annual rate of 13 percent (Markets and Markets, 2015). Approximately 40 percent of that market is in the United States with Europe accounting for 33 percent of the market.

In general, growth in IT spending among health care providers is attributed to providers' pursuing IT "answers" to a range of challenges and issues facing them:

- Concerns over patient safety can lead to investments in computerized provider order entry (CPOE) and medication administration record systems.
- Cost pressures can lead to the use of IT to improve organizational efficiency.
- Problems with shortages of health care professionals and cost pressures can result in efforts to use IT to improve operational efficiency and reduce staff workloads.
- Compliance with new health care regulations, such as rules designed to improve the security of information systems or reduce fraudulent billing, often requires an IT response.
- Desires to improve patient service can lead to new systems designed to improve the process of obtaining an appointment or to reduce test result turnaround time.
- Initiatives designed to prepare the organization for payment reform will lead to needs for population health applications and advanced analytics to assess care performance.

Such answers are identified during the IT strategy and alignment process that was discussed in Chapter Twelve.

SOURCES OF INDUSTRY INFORMATION

It is essential for the health care professional to identify sources that he or she can trust for current information on health care IT. This textbook cannot examine all the terrain covered by this industry. Moreover, the face of the industry can change quickly. New companies arrive as others disappear. New technologies emerge, and people's understanding of current technologies improves. Federal legislation that affects what health care IT is expected to do can surface rapidly.

These sources of information should be diverse: colleagues, consultants, vendors, conferences, and trade press. It takes time and some effort to identify your best sources. You will find some consultants helpful and others not so helpful. You will note that some publications are insightful and others are not.

The following sections provide a brief overview of publications you may find useful.

Periodicals

These are among the high-quality health care information technology periodicals (journals and magazines):

- *Health Data Management*
- *Health Management Technology*
- *Healthcare Informatics*
- *Healthcare IT News*

All the following associations discussed in this appendix also publish journals, magazines, or newsletters.

These publications can be supplemented with periodicals that cover the overall IT industry:

- *CIO*
- *CIO Insight*
- *Computerworld*
- *Information Week*

Several periodicals focus on vertical segments of technology; *Network World* and *eWeek* are examples.

Several periodicals address cross-industry management issues, including IT:

- *BusinessWeek*
- *The Economist*
- *The Harvard Business Review*
- *MIT Sloan Management Review*

In addition, there are magazines and journals that cover health care broadly. They often publish articles and stories on IT issues:

- *Health Affairs*
- *Hospitals & Health Networks*
- *Modern Healthcare*

You can obtain subscription information for these publications by visiting their websites. An afternoon at a university library, medical library, or large public library spent perusing these publications is worthwhile.

Books

In any given year, several books that cover various aspects of health care IT are published. Following are the publishers that routinely produce such books and publish conference proceedings:

- Elsevier
- Healthcare Information and Management Systems Society
- John Wiley & Sons
- Jossey-Bass
- Springer-Verlag

Industry Research Firms

Finally, there are industry research firms that routinely cover IT generally and health care specifically. Such firms include KLAS, Gartner, the Advisory Board, and HIMSS Analytics. These firms, and others, do a nice job of analyzing industry trends, critiquing the products and services of major vendors, and assessing emerging technologies and technology issues. They provide written analyses, conferences, and access to their analysts.

HEALTH CARE IT ASSOCIATIONS

All health care professionals should join associations that are dedicated to advancing and educating their profession. Health care chief financial officers (CFOs) often join the Healthcare Financial Management Association, and health care executives routinely join the American College of Healthcare Executives. These associations serve several useful purposes for the person who joins:

- Publications on topics of interest to the profession
- Conferences, symposiums, and other educational programs
- Information on careers and career development opportunities
- Data that can be used to compare performance across organizations
- Opportunities to meet colleagues who share similar jobs and hence have similar challenges and interests
- Staff members who work with legislators and regulators on issues that affect the profession

These association products and services can be invaluable sources of information and experience for any organization or individual.

The health care IT industry has several associations that serve the needs of the health care IT professional. People who are not health care IT professionals will find that their own profession's association also routinely provides periodical articles and conference sessions that cover IT issues. For example, the Healthcare Financial Management Association may present conference sessions on IT advances in analyzing the costs of care or in streamlining patient accounting processes.

The health care IT industry associations are discussed in the following sections. Additional information on these associations can be obtained through each association's website.

American Health Information Management Association (AHIMA)

AHIMA is an association of health information management professionals. AHIMA serves largely what has been known historically as the medical records professional. AHIMA's members confront a diverse range of issues associated with paper and electronic medical records, including privacy, data standards and coding, management of the record, appropriate uses of medical record information, and state and federal regulations that govern the medical record.

AHIMA sponsors an annual conference, produces publications, makes a series of knowledge resources available (news, practice guidelines, and competency tests), posts job opportunities, supports distance learning opportunities, and engages in federal and state policy lobbying. AHIMA also offers local and state chapters, which have their own conferences and resources.

The health information management profession has a process for certifying the skill levels of its professionals. AHIMA manages that certification process.

American Medical Informatics Association (AMIA)

AMIA is an association of individuals and organizations "dedicated to developing and using information technologies to improve health care." AMIA focuses on clinical information systems, and a large portion of its membership has an interest and training in the academic discipline of medical informatics. AMIA brings together an interesting mix of practitioners and academics.

AMIA offers an annual symposium, a spring congress, a journal, a series of working groups and special interest groups, and a resource center with job opportunities, publications, and news. AMIA carries out initiatives designed to influence federal policy on health care IT issues.

College of Healthcare Information Management Executives (CHIME)

CHIME is an association dedicated to advancing the health care chief information officer (CIO) profession and improving the strategic use of IT in health care (CIOs were discussed in Chapter Twelve). CHIME provides two annual forums, a newsletter, employment information, a data warehouse of information contributed by its members and vendors, distance learning sessions, and classroom-style training. CHIME is partially supported by the CHIME Foundation, established as a nonprofit organization by a group of vendors and consultants committed to advancing the CIO profession.

Healthcare Information and Management Systems Society (HIMSS)

HIMSS is an association dedicated to "providing leadership for the optimal use of health care information technology and management systems for the betterment of human health." HIMSS members are diverse, covering all segments and professions in the health care IT industry.

HIMSS sponsors an annual conference and series of symposiums and smaller conferences. It publishes books, a journal, and newsletters. HIMSS member services include employment information, industry and vendor information, certification programs, distance learning, and white papers. The association has special interest groups and local chapters, and it is actively working with the federal government to develop policy.

Other Industry Groups and Associations

Within the health care IT industry, organizations also exist that serve the needs of health care organizations (in contrast to the individual professional). This section will not attempt to list and describe them. However, examples include the University Health System Consortium, which serves academic health centers and the Scottsdale Institute, whose members are large integrated delivery systems. These and other similar organizations have a partial or dedicated focus on health care IT.

All the associations and groups mentioned in this discussion provide publications and conferences. In addition, companies whose business is putting on conferences sometimes offer health care IT events. Quality publications in addition to those listed previously are available. The reader who is interested in developing a deeper appreciation of the wealth of conference and publication opportunities can type "health care IT publications" and "health care IT conferences" into a web search engine to locate many online sources of information.

SUMMARY

The health care IT industry is large and growing. The many pressures on health care organizations to perform and comply are leading them to invest in IT. The industry is served by a multitude of companies that provide products and services. These companies are diverse in revenue and in their choice of focus within the submarkets that compose the health care industry.

Professionals in the health care IT industry have formed associations that serve their information and development needs. These associations and industry publications are terrific sources of information on industry issues, emerging technologies, and the strengths and weaknesses of companies serving the industry.

LEARNING ACTIVITIES

1. Identify two companies that serve the health care IT market. Write a summary that lists each company's products, services, market focus, and size. Compare the two companies.

2. Pick one of the health care IT associations listed in this appendix. Develop a summary that describes the association's membership, activities, products, and services.

3. Select two periodicals that serve the health care IT industry and review an issue of each one. Comment on the types of topics and issues that these publications address.

REFERENCES

CMS. (2015). *National health care expenditures 2014 highlights.* Retrieved April 2016 from https://www.cms.gov/Research-Statistics-Data-and-Systems/Statistics-Trends-and-Reports/NationalHealthExpendData/Downloads/highlights.pdf

Gartner, Inc. (2008). *Forecast: Healthcare IT spending worldwide, 2006–2011.* Stamford, CT: Author.

Healthcare Informatics. (2016). *2015 Healthcare Informatics 100 list.* Retrieved June 2016 from http://www.healthcare-informatics.com/HCI100?sort_by=field_hci100_rank_value&sort_order=ASC

Markets and Markets. (2015). *Healthcare IT Market by product (EHR, RIS, PACS, VNA, CPOE, mHealth, Telehealth, healthcare analytics, supply chain management, revenue cycle management, CRM, claims management, fraud management) by end user (provider, payer)—Global forecast to 2020.* Retrieved April 2016 from http://www.marketsandmarkets.com/Market-Reports/healthcare-it-252.html

Startup Health. (2016). *Digital health fund rankings Q1 2016.* Retrieved April 2016 from http://www.startuphealth.com/content/insights-2016q1

Sample Project Charter, Sample Job Descriptions, and Sample User Satisfaction Survey

SAMPLE PROJECT CHARTER

Information Systems

Mobile Mammography Van

Project Charter

Version 1.0

Created: 08/01/2017

Printed:

Prepared by: Sam Smith

Presented to: Karen Zimmerman

Project Charter Table of Contents

REVISION HISTORY

FOREWORD

The purpose of a Project Charter is to document what the Project Team is committed to deliver. It specifies the project timeline, resources, and implementation standards. The Project Charter is the cornerstone of the project and is used for managing the expectations of all project stakeholders. (See Table B.1.)

Table B.1 Revision history

Name	Date	Reason for Changes	Ver./Rev.

A Project Charter represents a formal commitment among Business Sponsors, Business Owners, Steering Committees, the Project Manager, and the Project Team. Therefore, it is the professional responsibility of all project members to treat this agreement seriously and make every effort to meet the commitment it represents.

BUSINESS REQUIREMENTS

Background

Sponsored by the Ogilvey Cancer Institute in partnership with the Boston Public Health Commission, neighborhood health centers, and community groups, Boston's Mammography Van provides mammography screening and breast health education throughout the City of Boston to all women, regardless of ability to pay, with a priority on serving uninsured and underserved women right in their neighborhoods. The Mammography Van program began in April of 2017, using GE software for registration, scheduling, and billing. All clinical documentation of the mammography screening has been performed manually since April 2017. Statistical reports generated to maintain state and federal guidelines are all done manually.

Project Overview

The project has two major objectives:

- Implementation of Mammography Patient Manager software to allow for online documentation of the clinical encounter with the patient.
- Implementation of a wireless solution on the van at the time of the new software implementation. This will allow real-time updating of the patient appointment information as well as registering walk-on patients on the spot. Online documentation will allow ease of reporting to the state and federal agencies.

The products evaluated for implementation are specific to the needs of a mobile program and will meet most, if not all, of the needs of the program.

Project Objectives

Boston's Mobile Mammography Van program will benefit monetarily with a software system because of the reporting capabilities available with online documentation. Grant money, as well as state and federal money, is available to the program if evidence is produced to support the needs of the grant and/ or the state and federal guidelines of mammography programs. The program will be more easily able to report on the information required by grants and governments to receive funding. There is also the current possibility that we are losing funding as a result of our current manual reporting practice.

The current program's resources spend valuable time manually calculating statistics. A software system will automate these processes, thus freeing the resources to perform more valuable functions. The van's mammography technician spends a lot of time manually updating and calculating which clients require additional follow-up. A software system will allow real-time reporting of which clients require which type of follow-up. This will decrease the amount of time the technician will spend manually determining which patient requires which follow-up letter. The program will be secure in its adherence to state and federal reporting guidelines for the van program as well as for the technicians working in the program.

Value Provided to Customers

- Improved productivity and reduced rework
- Streamlined business processes
- Automation of previously manual tasks
- Ability to perform entirely new tasks or functions
- Conformance to current standards or regulations
- Improved access to patient clinical and demographic information via remote access
- Reduced frustration level compared to current process

Business Risks

The major risk associated with the implementation is the selection of an incompatible vendor. There is always the concern that with a program that is new to the institution, the understanding needed to fully anticipate the needs of the program is incomplete. In addition, there is the risk that the software solution will increase workload as it offers more functions than are currently available to the user in a manual system.

Risk mitigation action items include this charter, which should clearly state the "in scope" objectives of the implementation. This should address both risks identified here.

VISION OF THE SOLUTION
Vision Statement

The Mobile Mammography Van program will be a more efficient and safe environment. The current lack of a software system introduces risks due to potential regulatory issues, patient safety issues due to potential missed follow-up, as well as program risks due to potential loss of funding. The proposed implementation of a software system alleviates these risks as well as introduces the prospect of future expansion of the program that is not easily achieved in the current environment.

The program should be able to handle more patients with the new software. The registration and scheduling process will stay the same, but the introduction of remote access will increase efficiency. Changes to appointments or patient demographic data can now occur on the van. An interface with the GE scheduling and registration software to the mobile mammography software will ensure no duplicate entry of patient data. The ability to document patient history online on the van will decrease the amount of paperwork filled out at the end of the day by the technician. There will also be the opportunity to track patients better by entering data during the day rather than at the end of the day.

The current transcription process is not expected to change. Films will still be read in the current manner, but reports will be saved to a common database. This will allow the technician or program staff to access the reports online. Entry of the BIRAD result (mammography result) will occur much more quickly and efficiently. Patient follow-up based on the BIRAD will be done more quickly as well. Letters can be automatically generated based on the results and printed in batches. All patient follow-up, including phone calls, letters, and certified letters can be captured in the system with a complete audit trail. This ensures the program's compliance with regulations concerning patient follow-up.

The film-tracking functions will also allow more accurate tracking of the patient's films. Accurate film tracking will increase the turnaround time for film comparisons and patient follow-up.

The ability to customize the software will increase the grant funding possibilities for the program. The program can introduce new variables or queries to the clients in order to produce statistical reports based on the gathered information. Increases in funding can lead to increases in the program's expansion. The increased expansion will increase the availability of free mammography to underprivileged women.

Major Features

- Interface can be implemented from GE system to OmniCare system (OmniCare supports clinical documentation) for registration information.
- Mammography history questionnaires can be preprinted and brought on the van for the patient to fill out.
- OmniCare will allow entry of BIRAD results.
- Transcribed reports can be uploaded or cut and pasted into OmniCare from the common database.
- Patient letters are generated from and maintained in OmniCare.
- Follow-up, including pathology results, will be maintained in OmniCare.
- Communication management functions will be maintained with full audit trail.
- Film tracking will be done in OmniCare.
- Statistical reporting will be facilitated.

Assumptions and Dependencies

The assumptions and dependencies for this project are few, but all are crucial to the success of the implementation. The software and hardware to be purchased for this implementation are key aspects of the project. The project is dependent on the remote access satellite hardware working as expected. The software vendor chosen during the vendor selection project is assumed to be the best fit for this program. The GE interface is a crucial assumption in this project. This working interface is key to the efficiencies this program is looking to achieve with the implementation. Resources are an assumption inherent in the budget. Appropriate resources to effectively implement the solution are important to the success of the implementation.

Related Projects

There are no related projects for this project. All needed work is included in this implementation project.

SCOPE AND LIMITATIONS

Scope of Initial Release

- GE interface for patient demographic and registration information
- Film tracking (possible bar coding for film tracking)
- Mammography history questionnaires
- BIRAD result entry
- Patient follow-up management
- Communications management
- Statistical reporting
- Custom fields management
- Remote access satellite installation

Interface Scope

- GE registration data

Organizational Scope

The OmniCare implementation will focus on the implementation of the software with the Ogilvey Cancer Institute program of the Boston Mobile Mammography Van. No other partner institutions are involved for the rollout. The film reads done at Metro Hospital are not included in this scope.

Conversion Scope

No data conversion is planned for this project.

Scope of Subsequent Releases

Future releases may try to include the Metro Hospital radiologists. Currently, as Metro reads the film, the radiologist dictates and the text is transcribed. It would be more efficient in future if the readings were automatically part of OmniCare.

Out of Scope

- Billing functions are not within the scope of this implementation. Billing is currently done via the GE system and will continue this way.

- A results interface is not within the scope of this implementation. The results of the mammograms will be available only on paper in the medical record or within the OmniCare solution. There will be no integration with the results application.

- Scheduling and registration functions are not in scope for this implementation. These functions are currently done via the GE system. An interface from GE to provide this information in the OmniCare solution is planned.

- Entry of radiologists' data is not in scope for this implementation. It is listed as a possible scope of subsequent releases.

PROJECT SUCCESS FACTORS

- Increased turnaround time for patient follow-up
- Decreased turnaround time with films by film tracking
- Decreased time creating and managing reports
- Increased numbers of mammographies taken
- Decreased time spent by staff on administrative tasks

BUDGET HIGHLIGHTS

Capital budget	$52,550
Hardware	$10,000
Software	$30,000
Remote access	$6,200
First year remote service	$1,350
Contingency	$5,000

Project Staff Resources

IS analyst = .50 FTE for 6 months

Network services = .25 for 3–6 months

Karen = 40 hr./wk. for 4 months

Program asst. (Sarah) = 40 hr./wk. for 4 months

New person to be hired

Temp to do data entry conversion

TIMELINE

Project will commence on November 1, 2017, and be completed July 1, 2018. Approximate date of completion of major phases:

Analysis	January 1, 2018
Satellite installation	February 1, 2018
Registration interface	March 1, 2018
Film tracking	March 1, 2018
History questionnaires	May 1, 2018
Result entry	June 1, 2018
Communications management	June 1, 2018
Patient follow-up	June 1, 2018
Reporting	June 15, 2018

PROJECT ORGANIZATION

Business Sponsor(s)	Anne Jones, VP of External Affairs
Business Owner(s)	Karen Ruderman, Program Director
Steering Committee	Karen Zimmerman, Program Director
	Anne Johnson, Director of Planning
	Jerry Melini, Technical Director of Radiology
Project Manager	Charles Leoman
Project Team	IS analysts TBD
	Network Services IS staff TBD
	Karen Zimmerman, Program Director
	Sarah Smithson, Program Assistant
	Data Entry temporary staff

PROJECT MANAGEMENT STRATEGIES

Project Meetings

In order to maintain effective communication with Project Team members and the Mobile Mammography Van community, a series of standing meetings will be conducted. Meeting minutes will be documented and stored on the shared core team directory. The following meetings and facilitated sessions will be held.

Issue Management

Issue identification, management, and resolution are important project management activities. The Project Manager is responsible for the issue management process and works with the Project Team and Steering Committee (if needed) to agree on the resolution of issues.

Effective issue management enables

- A visible decision-making process
- A means for resolving questions concerning the project
- A project issue audit trail

The standard IS project issue management process and forms will be used and attached to this charter as needed. (See Table B.2.)

Scope Change Management

Scope change management is essential to ensure that the project is managed to the original scope, as defined in this charter. The purpose of a scope management process is to constructively manage the pressure to expand scope.

Scope expansion is acceptable as long as

- Users agree that the new requirements are justified
- Impact to the project is analyzed and understood
- Resulting changes to project (cost, timing, resources, quality) are approved and properly implemented

Any member of the Project Team or other member of the Mobile Mammography Van community may propose a change to the scope of the project. The requester will initiate the process by completing a Change Request Definition Form. When necessary, the Project Manager will review and seek advice from the Steering Committee on scope changes that affect the project schedule or budget, or both.

The standard IS project scope management process and forms will be used and attached as appendixes to this charter, as needed.

Training Strategy

Training Scope

The program personnel consist of a program administrator, one mammography technician, one assistant to the administrator, and one patient educator

Table B.2 Issue management

Decision-Making Level	Steering Committee	Project Team
Role	Resolves show-stopper issues and changes in scope. Acts as a sounding board for decisions and actions that affect user acceptance of the project. This includes anything that affects project milestones and outcomes. Reviews decisions, recommendations, and requests that are high in integration and complexity and that are not resolved at the Project Team level. Scope management and planning. Chaired by Business Sponsor.	Governs the actual work and the progress of the project. Reviews project work and status: —Resource issues —Vendor issues —Project risks Serves as working or focus group to report daily progress. Responsible for implementation decisions that have integration impact and that are of medium or high complexity. Cochaired by IS Project Manager and Business Owner.
Participants	Key stakeholders on business and IS sides.	All resources assigned to the project.
Meeting frequency	Meets regularly to ensure steady project progress.	Meets, as needed, weekly to monthly, for project status and updates.

and administration person. All of the employees will receive training for their specific role related to the process. The program administrator will learn all of the roles in order to fill in when needed. Additional training will be given to the other employees for backup purposes.

Training Approach

The vendor will provide the training during the initial implementation. The employees of the program will then train new employees.

Training Material Development

The vendor will provide training materials.

Documentation Development Strategy

The team will develop the following documentation:

- Technical operations procedure manual
- Policies and procedures related to the use and management of the system
- Application manuals, if needed
- OmniCare technical and application maintenance and support manuals, if needed

Project Work Paper Organization and Coordination

In order to keep the project documentation, meeting minutes, and deliverables organized and accessible to the core team, a project folder on the shared network will be established and maintained.

SAMPLE JOB DESCRIPTIONS

Sample CIO Job Description

«XX» Health Care System, Inc.

<u>**JOB DESCRIPTION**</u>

POSITION TITLE: Chief Information Officer (CIO)

DEPARTMENT: Information Systems & Telecommunications

POSITION REPORTS TO: Chief Financial Officer (CFO)

POSITION SUPERVISES: Information Systems Department, Telecommunications Department

POSITION REQUIREMENTS:

Master of Science Degree in Information Systems or other related field. Five to ten years' progressive management experience in Information Systems required. Experience with a multi-uni/integrated health care system preferred. Demonstrated successful leadership in planning, developing, and implementing management information processes, mechanisms, and systems is required. Excellent communication skills, leadership skills, negotiation skills, and motivational abilities are a must.

POSITION SUMMARY:

Responsible for «XX» Health Care System's Information Systems Division. This division includes Information Management, Health Information Management, and Telecommunications for our multilocation/integrated health care system operating 24 hours a day, 365 days a year. This job description is congruent with the human and community development philosophy of the «XX». The philosophy emphasizes responsibility for human life and the dignity and worth of every person. It also promotes the creation of caring communities in which the needs of those serving and being served are met. It is expected employees will perform their jobs in accordance with the philosophy.

<u>**ESSENTIAL FUNCTIONS:**</u>

1. Knows, understands, incorporates, and demonstrates the «XX» Health Care System Mission, Visions, Values, and Management Philosophy in leadership behaviors, practices, and decisions.
2. Montiors the health care delivery environment in order to anticipate any impact on information systems and communications networks to ensure appropriate utilization of information technology.
3. Examines new systems and develops strategies directed toward increased productivity by improving the work environment through systems and people consistent with the Mission, Vision, Values, and Management Philosophy of the «XX» system.
4. Establishes systemwide information management/technology standards and strategies for achieving integration and interoperability of information systems, technology architecture, and selection of software applications.

5. Maintains responsibility for the information system operations including the development and management of operating and capital budgets, policies, human resource utilization, mission effectiveness, and the overall performance of information technology within «XX» Health Care System.

6. Develops long-range plans and associated capital and expense budgets and monitors the achievement of these plans in order to ensure the successful performance of the organization.

7. Develops information system plans and programs to improve organization effectiveness and efficiency, ensuring that the information needs of «XX» Health Care System information technology staff are met.

8. Creates a seamless process to gather information regarding operational, human resources, financial, and clinical outcomes.

9. Maintains internal and external relationships with all system users and vendors.

10. Is responsible for the installation of all new information systems and telecommunication systems for «XX» Health Care System.

11. Is a member of the Executive Team providing leadership to «XX» Health Care System.

12. Maintains the integrity and security of «XX» Health Care System's information systems, complying wtih all regulatory agencies and statutes.

13. Provides for professional growth and career opportunities for the Information System division staff.

OTHER FUNCTIONS:
All other duties as assigned.

_____

APPROVED BY:

      _____

      DEPARTMENT HEAD   **DATE**

      _____

      PRESIDENT'S COUNCIL MEMBER   **DATE**

      _____

      HUMAN RESOURCES DEPARTMENT   **DATE**

REVISION DATES:

FOR HUMAN RESOURCES DEPT. USE ONLY: ___EXEMPT ___NONEXEMPT

JOB DESCRIPTION FOR CHIEF MEDICAL INFORMATION OFFICER

BACKGROUND

The position of Chief Medical Information Officer is a newly created position and reports to the Senior Vice President Information Services, CIO. This individual will lead the development and implementation of automated support for clinicians and clinical analysts through researching, recommending, and facilitating major and advanced clinical information system initiatives for the health care system.

In this role, the incumbent will provide reviews of medical informatics experiences and approaches, develop technical and application implementation strategies, manage implementation of advanced clinical information systems, assist in the development of strategic plans for clinical information systems, and provide project management for codevelopment relationships with the vendor community.

Information technology at THE HOSPITAL is becoming highly user driven. Governed by the Quality Council, a Clinical Informatics Steering Committee and subcommittees reporting to the Clinical Informatics Steering Committee will be formed to provide a user forum for input, coordination, and integration of information technology with THE HOSPITAL. The Director of Medical Informatics will chair, lead, and support the Clinical Informatics Steering Committee.

The following are ongoing responsibilities of the CHIEF MEDICAL INFORMATION OFFICER:

Lead the implementation of a computerized patient record (CPR) system for the health care system (hospitals, clinics, physicians offices, ancillary, and therapy units). This system should embody an information model focused on the diagnosis, treatment, and process data that will be required in future treatment and preventive care.

Engage providers with varying roles including independent and employed physicians and clinicians, medical records professionals, and clinical analysts to contribute to the development and use of the CPR and analysis tools.

Lead and support the Clinical Informatics Steering Committee which serves as the principal user governance forum to determine organizational priorities in this area.

Stay attuned to the national effort to develop comprehensive, functional, and uniform medical records, and take an active role in areas where the national effort and health care system can mutually benefit.

Be highly responsive to users' needs, including training, to ensure widespread acceptance and provider use of the clinical systems.

The following are expected accomplishments of the Chief Medical Information Officer for the first 12 to 24 months.

Gain a thorough understanding of the personality and culture of the organization and community; evaluate and refine the strategic information plan as it relates to clinical informatics.

Develop empathy and understanding of physician needs; build relationships with physicians to gain the support of physician leadership.

Together with a team leader, evaluate the skills of the current clinical informatics team, identify needs and build a strong team by enhancing team members' skill base, motivating them and fostering a collaborative approach that values their contribution.

Design a model of the clinical database(s) to support the enterprise-wide CPR. The database(s) should support individual patient care and clinical studies across the full continuum of care.

Guided by the Quality Council, determine an approach and plan for the development and implementation of clinical systems that are components of a computerized patient record. The CPR will be designed to support clinicians in the care of patients throughout the network.

Select the products and vendors for the components of the initial phase of CPR implementation. Be on schedule, according to plan, with the implementations.

Implement physician network services, the transfer of clinical information between network sites, and the presentation of that information on a physician workstation.

The following are the desired credentials, skills, and personality characteristics of the ideal candidate (not listed in priority order):

A licensed physician with recent medical practice experience, graduate degree in medical informatics, and one year of work experience in medical informatics. In lieu of graduate training in medical informatics, a minimum of three years' work experience in medical informatics systems will be required.

A personable individual with excellent interpersonal and communication skills who can handle a diversity of personalities and interact effectively with people at all levels of the organization.

A strong leader with a mature sense of priorities and solid practical experience to implement the vision for the organization.

An individual who is politically savvy, has a high tolerance for ambiguity, and can work successfully in a matrix management model.

A systems thinker with strong organizational skills who can pull all the pieces together and understand how to deliver ideals.

A strong manager who is adaptable and has a strong collaborative management style.

A creative thinker with high energy and enthusiasm.

A team player and consensus builder who promotes the concept of people working together versus individual performance.

A contemporary clinician who understands major trends in health care and managed care and has extensive knowledge of currently available point-of-care products and medical informatics development.

SAMPLE USER SATISFACTION SURVEY

Office of the Chief Information Officer (OCIO)

1. Personnel from the OCIO have positive attitudes and are willing to work with me to determine my specific needs and/or resolve my information technology problems.
   - Strongly Agree
   - Agree
   - Disagree
   - Strongly Disagree

2. Personnel from the OCIO understand my department's information technology requirements.
   - Strongly Agree
   - Agree
   - Disagree
   - Strongly Disagree

3. Personnel from the OCIO participate actively during meetings to help ensure that my information technology needs are met.
   - Strongly Agree
   - Agree
   - Disagree
   - Strongly Disagree

4. The OCIO personnel effectively communicate.
   - Strongly Agree
   - Agree
   - Disagree
   - Strongly Disagree

5. The OCIO personnel provide effective results.
   - Strongly Agree
   - Agree
   - Disagree
   - Strongly Disagree

6. Please select a category to leave us detailed feedback or comments.
   - Customer Service
   - Communication
   - Timeliness/Follow-Up
   - Training and Education
   - System Issues
   - Strategic Planning
   - Staffing
   - Leadership
   - Equipment Needs
   - Diversity
   - Project Management
   - Workflow

   Comments:

7. Please provide us any additional suggestions on how we can improve the services that we provide to you.

Source: Adapted from the Medical University of South Carolina (2016).

Index

Page references followed by *fig* indicate an illustrated figure; followed by *t* indicate a table.

Rehabilitation service documentation systems, 69t

Reimbursement: DRG (diagnosis related group) used for, 37; patient record purpose in, 26. *See also* Patient billing

Research–patient record relationship, 27

Revenue cycle management systems, 69t, 115

RFI (request for information): development and distribution of, 156–157; evaluating systems vendor, 160–162

RFP (request for proposal): development and distribution of the, 155–157; evaluating systems vendor, 160–162; overdoing or underdoing the, 168

The Road to Accountable Care: Building Systems for Population Health Management (McCarthy, Klein, and Cohen), 518–519

Rules engines, 115–116

Rutledge Retirement Community case study, 184

RxNorm, 365, 374–375

S

St. Luke's Medical Center case study, 184

SCAD (spontaneous coronary artery dissection) registry, 125

Scheduling systems, 68t

Scorecards (population health management), 118–119

SCRIPT Standard for e-Prescribing, 364

Secrets of HIE Success Revealed: Lessons from the Leaders (National eHealth Collaboration), 524

Security: description of, 288–289; HIPAA Security Rule on, 291, 295–300; as important health information privacy issue, 288; Kaiser Permanente case study on breaching patient portal, 507–509; multiple and everyday threats to, 288; viruses, Trojans, spyware, worms, ransomware threats to, 305–306; vulnerabilities of, 296, 309–311t. *See also* Cybersecurity

Security program development: step 1: lead your culture, select your team, and learn, 307–308; step 2: document your process, findings, and actions, 308; step 3: review existing security of ePHI, 308–309; step 4: develop an action plan, 309–311t; step 5: manage and mitigate risks, 311; step 6: attest for Meaningful Use security related objective, 311; step 7: monitor, audit, and update security on an ongoing basis, 311

Security programs: issues to consider when developing, 306–307; ONC's *Guide to Privacy and Security of Electronic Health Information* on a, 307; ONC's seven-step approach for implementing, 307–311t; resources for conducting a comprehensive risk analysis, 309t

Senior leadership organization forum, 437–438

Senior leadership. *See* IT senior leadership roles

Senior management responsibilities, 433–436

Sequoia Project, 15

Slope of enlightenment phase (hype cycle), 422fig, 423

Small data: big data versus, 43–44; disease and procedure indexes examples of, 44

SNOMED CT (Systematized Nomenclature of Medicine—Clinical Terms), 365, 370, 371, 372–373

SOAP format of progress notes, 30

Social media: ALS Ice Bucket Challenge example of power of, 125; health care benefits of patient and consumer use of, 124–127; as patient engagement tool, 120–121; PatientsLikeMe website, 124–125

Software as a services (SaaS), 158

Software bugs, 278

South Carolina Standards for Licensing Hospitals and Institutional General Infirmaries, 326e–327e

Southeast Medical Center case study: assessing the value of health IT investment focus of, 504–506; four hospitals comprising Southeast Medical Center, 504

SPECIALIST Lexicon and Lexical Tools, 376

Spyware, 305

Staff scheduling systems, 68t

Staff time and attendance systems, 69t

Staff training: project plan on, 190–191, 194–196; provide adequate, 207–208; train the trainer approach to, 195

Standards developing organizations (SDOs): description and functions of, 360, 361t, 362; list of ANSI-accredited and non-ANSI accredited, 362–363

Standards development process: description of, 360; European Committee for Standardization (CEN) and international, 363; four categories of the, 360–361; major developers of HIT standards in the United States, 362–363; profiling bodies of the, 363; relationships among standards-setting organizations during, 361t–362